ARKANA

THE HEALING PATH

Marc Ian Barasch is an editor at *Psychology Today* and *Natural Health* magazines and the former editor-in-chief of *New Age Journal*. He is also an award-winning writer-producer for television and film.

THE
HEALING
PATH

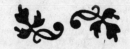

A SOUL APPROACH TO ILLNESS

Marc Ian Barasch

Foreword by Bernie S. Siegel, M.D.

PENGUIN

ARKANA

ARKANA
Published by the Penguin Group
Penguin Books USA Inc., 375 Hudson Street, New York, New York 10014, U.S.A.
Penguin Books Ltd, 27 Wrights Lane, London W8 5TZ, England
Penguin Books Australia Ltd, Ringwood, Victoria, Australia
Penguin Books Canada Ltd, 10 Alcorn Avenue, Toronto, Ontario, Canada M4V 3B2
Penguin Books (N.Z.) Ltd, 182–190 Wairau Road, Auckland 10, New Zealand

Penguin Books Ltd, Registered Offices: Harmondsworth, Middlesex, England

First published in the United States of America by G. P. Putnam's Sons 1994
Published in Arkana 1995

3   5   7   9   10   8   6   4   2

Some of the ideas presented in this book are speculative. The author does not recommend against consultation, diagnosis, and treatment by licensed medical practitioners.

THE LIBRARY OF CONGRESS HAS CATALOGUED THE HARDCOVER AS FOLLOWS:
Barasch, Marc.
The healing path: a soul approach to illness/Marc Ian Barasch.
p.   cm.
Includes bibliographical references and index.
ISBN 0-87477-743-7 (hc.)
ISBN 0 14 019.486 X (pbk.)
1. Mental healing.   2. Alternative medicine.   3. Mind and body.   I. Title.
RZ400B186   1994
615.8´51—dc20   93–704

Printed in the United States of America
Set in New Baskerville

To Leah, whose bravery,
love, and wisdom gave me
every reason to live

Vocatus atque non vocatus deus aderit.
Invoked or not invoked, the god is present.

—Motto chiseled into stone over the front door
of Carl Jung's house in Küsnacht, Switzerland

CONTENTS

FOREWORD

CARL JUNG REMARKED that a clinical diagnosis may be indispensable to the doctor, but only rarely helps the patient. "The crucial thing," the great physician observed, "is the story. For it alone shows the human background and the human suffering. Only at that point can the doctor's therapy begin to operate."

This book is a wonderful example of that essential truth, for it weaves together some powerful stories. One of them is a lyrical account of the author's own struggle with illness. His moving tale, which crossed my own path years ago, provides luminous insight into the inner dimensions of healing. Then there are the often startling journeys of patients, presented here with a compassion born of the rigors of fellow traveling. But most important, this book is the story of anyone who has ever had to walk the narrow path of suffering toward a more spiritual life—a story as old as the Bible.

Disease can teach us to live by confronting us with our own mortality, with the uncertainty embedded in every life. If we have the courage to follow where our fate leads us, a great rebirth can occur. Unfortunately, doctors do not always help the patient on this course. We physicians are still not educated to honor the inner life of a person in crisis. The medical perspective often depersonalizes the patient even as it treats the disease. The medical profession, with its various specialties and subsocieties, is only slowly awakening to the deeper needs of those who are ill. My life as a physician was changed when one of my patients told me, "What I need to know is how to live *between* office visits."

What help do patients need? Just as the title states: *The Healing Path.* They need—we *all* need—to learn how to let go of the reins and find the intuitive, authentic way to our home and our healing. This path, which the author aptly names "the soul approach," is totally distinct from curing every disease. But it is inseparable from healing any sickness, for it is no less than the way of life itself. As long as we are *in* life, *in* our bodies, we will inevitably experience pain. But if we can approach illness consciously, it becomes the labor pain of rebirthing ourselves, so we can start living *now*. Then whatever medical treatment we choose becomes part of the process of transforming our lives.

This book sheds a unique, even brilliant light on the patient's transformative struggle. Here a highly accomplished journalist encountered firsthand a painful aspect of the human condition, then insisted on pursuing its profoundest meaning. Marc left his career to spend seven years passionately seeking an underlying pattern, so that his experience and that of others could benefit us all. He reveals, with clarity and heartfelt eloquence, something I deeply believe: Healing is not something that comes only after you are free from the prison of disease and pain. It can come even while you are still *in* prison, and it can transform that prison into a place of love and wholeness.

As much as any work on such a paradoxical subject *could* be, *The Healing Path* is a marvelous guidebook, one made by and for explorers. But even more, it is a helpful, honest companion along the way.

—BERNIE S. SIEGEL, M.D.

ACKNOWLEDGMENTS

THE READER will indulge me as I thank those who gave me gifts and tools, words and deeds for my own healing path:

My parents, for indomitable love. Susan Noel, for literary conscience and all-purpose relentlessness. Rick Fields, for aid, comfort, and a contagious knack for living in the present.

Connie Zweig, for getting this off the ground, keeping it in the air, and seeing that it finally landed. Jeremy Tarcher, who waited patiently for me to resolve Xeno's Paradox. Adam Moss, for insisting I had a story. Maggie Tibbetts, for devoted running around.

Art Hermann of the Institute of Human Development, David Kay, Wiley T. Buchanan III, Ella Alford, the Authors Guild, the A.S.J.A., and PEN, for shepherding through timely grants and loans.

Richard Ratliff, for nonjudgmental caring.

Jeanne Achterberg, Larry Dossey, Michael Lerner, Dan Goleman, and Bernie Siegel for critical encouragement.

Those who are gone: Ronnie Laing, for teaching me there is laughter in Hell; Nancy Wilson Ross, keeper of the Mellon Elixir, whose sanity is sorely missed; Norman Cousins, for pivotal eggings-on; Peter Livingston, who conned me into books; and Chogyam Trungpa, for helping me remember who I was (or wasn't).

And those whose unpremeditated kindness meant more than they could suspect: Ken Ausubel, John Bailes, Doug Barasch, Latha Barasch, Christine Brotherson, Henrik Drescher, Mark and Shelley Gerzon, Annie Gottlieb, Bruce Green, Richard Grossinger, Sarah Harman, Joan Hyman, Helen Jensen, Doris Kuller, Richard Levy, Angelika Lizius, Barbara Meier, Alan Menken, Ignis Molasses, Alison Moore, Neva Newman, Kathleen Priest, John Steiner, John and Jillian Stevenson, Suzanne Taylor, Ellin Todd, Peter Wagg, Eve Wallace, Merle Worth, and Donna Zerner.

And most especially, all my fellow journeyers along the path of healing.

PREFACE

THIS BOOK BEGINS with an event that changed my life as violently as an earthquake wrenches a river from its course. Its medical label, "cancer," means little. Like other words that try to describe deep human experience—love, hatred, joy, grief—it only hides the enormity it signifies. Our most personal moments remain immune to language. If anything, disease is so ineffably *ours,* so much a part of our own irreproducible tale, that we are almost obliged to call it by our own name.

But to personalize disease is anathema. Like most people, when I became ill I felt as if I had been invaded by some alien Thing with little relation to the "real me." I was shocked when sickness reached into me and summoned up every unresolved emotional issue, every still-fertile hope and smoldering fear, every power of the body or mind to hurt and to heal. Cancer seemed to plunge me into an altered state, a separate reality that, despite years of inner exploring, was as unfamiliar to me as the dark side of the moon.

At the time, I had thought myself quite knowledgeable about the realms of healing. As the editor of *New Age Journal* I could recite the holistic canon chapter and verse. I understood—or thought I did—that mind and body were a seamless unity, that brain, glands, and organs engaged in mysterious commerce, that thoughts and feelings ricocheted off cell walls. But such formulations—now grouped under headings like "psychoneuroimmunology" and bristling with the terms and tools of molecular biology—were of little help. They failed utterly to explain how a condition of the flesh could become an inescapable dilemma of the spirit.

In part, my problem was cultural: Western science and religion have so long policed the border between consciousness and material existence that even our subjective experience seems circumscribed, cut-off. But there is also an instinctive response to the body's betrayal: repulsion. Sickness is an outrageous, Kafkaesque metamorphosis. I peered in the mirror one morning to see a face that refused to resolve itself into my familiar features. I blinked, but what blinked back was an image of one of the unfortunate ill. At such times, we

can only stand transfixed by the reflected stare of our own unsuspected fragility. It is scarcely surprising that we would want to avert
our gaze, to declare this image to be an Other, separate from the
substance of our lives.

"First take care of the physical problem," I remember my doctor
counseling me, "and then you can go back to worrying about your
inner life." At the time, my hesitation to rush into treatment seemed
to him like settling down with a good book when the house was
afire. A disease was a mandate for total war. Any departure from
a soldierly lockstep could prove deadly. All domestic resources were
to be diverted to the front, all inquiry subjected to provisional military censorship. By such reckoning, when we are faced with a threat
to our physical survival, psychological development is an afford-
able luxury.

From my present vantage point—closer now to that of those tribal
cultures which see illness as a disharmony in the larger web of our
lives—I would argue the precise opposite: It is in moments of crisis
that we most need inward centering. It is only then that we may
crucially distinguish between those aspects of ourselves that sabotage
well-being, and those that support it; only then that we may understand the roots of health and sickness. It is even possible that
doing "inner work" sometimes unleashes the hidden powers of the
bodymind: In 1989, Dr. David Spiegel of Stanford University Medical School, an avowed skeptic, pronounced himself "stunned" when
his own ten-year study revealed that women with metastatic breast
cancer survived twice as long when group therapy and self-hypnosis
were added to their treatment.

The women in that now-classic study were not magically cured.
Their lives were extended; but only two of the original eighty-six
have survived. The dark labyrinth of illness does not have a simple
escape route. Still, each juncture of our journey presents a choice,
a turning point: whether to split ourselves off from our own experience, or make what is happening, horrific though it may be,
part of our larger process of Becoming. For if we can fully inhabit
our life when it is both most painfully constricted and paradoxically
fraught with potential—if, even as our feet carry us into the maze,
we can proceed with our eyes open rather than squeezed shut—we
will inevitably discern a path of creative response.

I do not wish to romanticize illness as some True Path to Enlight-
ment. There are other ways to unearth our inner treasure than to
excavate it from the flesh with a backhoe. Nor will the most earnest

self-discovery necessarily heal our bodies. Still, I and others have learned that sickness may thrust upon us an unexpected requirement: to attend to what is generally called the soul.

By "soul" I do not mean some diaphanous eternal Essence, an astral double that will one day abandon this mortal shell like a butterfly flitting from a chrysalis. Rather, "soul" here describes a quality of subjective experience, an *approach* to life that embraces the often partitioned elements of our being: emotion and reason, thought and sensation, our social and private selves. For disease confronts us with a paradox: To reclaim what we have lost, we have to use what we may not know we already possess. We have visibly fallen apart, yet to become whole again, we must bring our whole self—heart, mind, body, and spirit—to the task of recovery. Healing, as shamans have long maintained, is the business of soul-retrieval.

For the past five years, through research, interviews with other patients, and painstaking self-inquiry, I have attempted to broaden my understanding of the role that the soul, or psyche, plays in disease and healing. This has not been an academic pursuit, but a survival exercise: I was urgently seeking a coming-to-terms, a way to ride out the aftershocks of my own catastrophe, to fit back the pieces of a life unexpectedly scattered. Almost incidentally, I began to see that a map was emerging, crude but unmistakable, of what might be called the Healing Path.

The map is not the territory, nor even a guide to it. Rather, it is an *interpretation*. Some maps reveal topography, others geography and geology, and still others populations or patterns of vegetation. Each chart is a reformulation of the truth, a fresh perception of the same terrain. Each journey, by necessity, is a new cartography.

What you hold in your hand, then, are field notes—the speculations, meditations, and sketches of fellow travelers. It is not a how-to, nor could it ever be: The route that heals one person may ravage his neighbor; what destroys one life may deliver another from death. But certain common features seem to dot the landscape of healing. What was particularly striking to me was how many disease survivors I spoke with had found, in the midst of their terrible ordeal, an unexpected unfolding of the authentic self.

In the course of my own quest, I have visited what, before the world shrank, used to be called "faraway lands"; crisscrossed the country to talk with some forty people who experienced unusual recoveries; been driven, a very amateur researcher, into medical libraries and sometimes out of doctors' offices. I heard answers that moved and amazed me, some prosaic, and others giddily dislocating. But strangest of all were the forays—by turns comforting and agonizing, illuminating and baffling—into my own still dark and unknown interior. To speak of this, I will have to tell you my dreams.

PROLOGUE:
WHERE LADDERS BEGIN

Now that my ladder's gone
I must lie down where all the ladders start:
In the foul rag and bone shop of the heart.

—WILLIAM BUTLER YEATS,
"The Circus Animals' Escape"

I T IS THE DAWN of my daughter's ninth birthday, and I am having a nightmare.

The top of my head has been drilled with three neat, bloody holes. An iron pot filled with red-hot coals has been hung under my chin. My arms are tied with lengths of clear plastic tubing. "We're going to boil your brains out," one of my invisible torturers announces. His voice is flat, matter-of-fact; he is a technician, not a sadist. I feel the heat sear my throat and I scream, the sound becoming hoarser, a raw, animal desperation, as the coals gnaw my larynx. "Please God"—though I can't now believe in God—"Please . . ." I feel an emotion I have never known in my waking life—complete hopelessness; a black, no-exit despair. As I wake up, slathered in fear-sweat, my heart beating hooves on my ribcage, I become aware that I am yelling aloud.

I'm still trying to shake free of it when the phone rings. It's my girlfriend, Susan, calling from back home in Colorado. I glance at the clock: five A.M. her time, seven here in Boston. What is she doing up at this hour? "Honey, are you all right?" she asks. Her voice sounds uneven, fluttery.

"I have cancer," I blurt out before I can think about it. "I have cancer growing in my throat." She laughs nervously. Months later, when my life—and hers—came churning down around us, furious as an avalanche, I would wonder how I had been so sure.

I had had a number of strange dreams that year—not passing strange, but the kind Robert Louis Stevenson once called "raw-head-and-bloody-bones nightmares." Certain themes—neck wounds, decapitations, sacrifice—kept recurring, in such crystalline Technicolor I was unable to forget them. In one, I had shot myself in the throat and a middle-aged Chinese surgeon removed a bullet tipped with a large hypodermic needle. In another, I was frantically trying to unscrew the head from a murderous robot that was about to kill me. In yet another, I found myself crawling through the dusty, bone-filled corridors of an ancient Maya "necropolis" in the shape of a truncated—headless—pyramid. (The *real* city of the dead, I was told, was "down the road.") "Neck-cropolis?" I remember musing, but I was too busy—and too unsettled by the morbidity of these night wanderings—to try to decipher it all.

I'd been living in Boston for a little over a year, the result of a phone call from a friend at *New Age Journal,* then a small health-food magazine that had in a decade slid from leading edge to near bankruptcy. A young Boston PR man with family money—"a socially conscious aristo," as my friend called him—was proposing to bail it out with half a million dollars, but they were stuck for an editor. "Why don't you throw your hat into the ring?" my friend asked. "You could use the work."

I was intrigued. The magazine, long before the term "new age" had turned into a marketeer's bonanza, had been a keeper of the then-countercultural flames of environmentalism, holistic health, and human potential. The few times I picked it up I had seen an earnest blend of social action and self-discovery, though sometimes obscured by transcendental pixie-dust.

I'd been an Ivy League activist in the late sixties, until politics grew so superheated that even my Yale classmate Garry Trudeau's fledgling "Doonesbury" strip was labeled "reactionary swill" by the campus left. After a few years on the demonstration circuit (I have a clear, diorama-like memory of being teargassed on the steps of the Justice Department), I landed in Colorado to study with a Tibetan Buddhist lama.

Like other former radicals, when marriage and children suddenly came into view, I began clambering up the career ladder as fast as I could get my hands on the rungs. I quickly went from overeducated menial laborer and monk *manqué* to up-and-coming editor. Though I kept up with my Buddhist studies, I had little outlet for the nagging idealism that some cohorts, in the Yuppie salad days of the early Reagan era, were uncomfortably edging away from.

When the magazine's publishers had asked for a résumé, I sat down and wrote a rambling, fevered manifesto describing how I thought the magazine could bring the "new paradigm" to the mainstream. To my surprise, they responded with enthusiasm, offering me the job over the phone. On the spur of the moment, I decided to take it. It meant leaving behind, with only a few weeks' notice, my entire life: my daughter, Leah, who regularly shuttled the few blocks separating me and my ex-wife, and a relationship with Susan that had arrived at a vertiginous overlook—to move in or not to move in—from which we seemed unable either to backpedal or to jump. Perhaps things would somehow sort themselves out if I took the plunge into what I only half-jokingly called "national life."

I arrived in the office just outside Boston hefting three falling-apart alligator-skin suitcases filled with Rolodexes and files—"The Exorcist!" one wit yelled as I stood silhouetted in the doorway. When I discovered over the next few days what a mess I was inheriting, my first impulse was to turn around and go home. *New Age Journal* was little more than a nameplate and some fresh-painted loft space in a dingy suburban shopping center. Not one story had been assigned for the launch issue only a month away; the editorial staff was skeletal; and, worse, the good writers had long since left ("Whale-shit," one snorted contemptuously when I called to beg him for a story, any story). The saccharine cheer around the office made me feel a piercing of despair.

In no time, I found myself performing a grueling one-man show, eating dinners at my desk, assigning, editing, and when necessary rewriting every story, every column, every headline, sleeping some nights on the stuffing-sprung office couch. "You must really love your work," the publisher would remark flippantly as he left, at five P.M. sharp, to play squash at his health club. But as the 100-hour workweeks stretched into months, love became an increasingly minor part of the equation: I was more like the proverbial man holding a live electrical cable, his muscles rigid with shock, incapable of loosening his grip.

Susan and I fell into a commuter romance, sustained, like my relationship with my daughter, by occasional weekend flights and forty-dollar phone calls. I had initially promised I wouldn't stay in Boston beyond a few months of consultant work. But it was as if a lifetime of pent-up energies, of hunger for recognition, were erupting. On the job, I was wired, effusive, light-emitting, a 78-rpm version of myself.

Susan, even at a distance, was becoming alarmed: "You can't do, or feel, or want, or accomplish anything at all if you die of a heart attack," she wrote after a flurry of phone calls during a particularly panic-stricken deadline. "The mind and body have many defenses, and will not allow you to go on much longer this way. If it isn't a stroke, or cancer, it will be a car wreck. It's odd that someone I think is so smart, sweet, and intuitive can treat himself so cruelly."

But I thought she was just being fainthearted: the girl back home, fretting over rumors from the front. After all, the hard work was paying off. Subscriptions had doubled. The magazine began winning awards. My phone calls were at last being returned. "The caricature of the Yuppie is going to change," I enthused a bit mindlessly to an *Adweek* reporter, who went on to characterize that change in print as "how to live with your money and some values."

When Susan next came out to visit, I found myself ranting to her one night that she didn't understand, that I was building a new national institution, that I now belonged—like Walter Mondale, for God's sake—to the public arena; I couldn't just walk away in the middle of the campaign. It took me a few minutes to notice her helpless laughter. "Walter Mondale?" she choked out, ludicrously elongating the name of the doomed presidential hopeful whose handlers had, with obtuse bravado, dubbed "Fightin' Fritz." "You want to be like Wal-ter *Mon*-dale?" It took me a minute to see it, and then we howled till we couldn't breathe.

But it wasn't really funny. Egged on by visions of glory, uncertain if I was publishing's boy wonder or a jerkwater in way over his small-time head, I had managed to ignore the disappearance of anything resembling normal human life. The magazine was the perfect trap for an idealist who—though I didn't yet know it—had never quite learned to love.

When I was offered a hefty ownership percentage of the company if I agreed to stay on, I started to talk to my ex-wife about moving east with my daughter, Leah. Susan decided to come, too; the last straw, she said, was the day a stray cat appeared at her back porch holding a scrap of newspaper in its mouth listing special fares to Boston. I began to look forward to life becoming real again after the awful haze of deadlines and loneliness that had stretched out to a year.

I had been looking forward to celebrating my daughter's birthday, her first in her new home, but the harrowing dream of my throat burning shadowed the occasion. My preoccupied glumness was contagious. A few weeks afterward, I suddenly began finding myself too exhausted to lift myself out of bed in the morning. I felt as if, I told a friend, my bones were filled with lead shot. My kidneys began to ache unmercifully; I began putting on weight. Susan, when she arrived a few weeks later, worriedly insisted I get a checkup.

When I told the doctor, a bearded man who looked only a few years out of internship, that I thought I had cancer, he looked at me quizzically. "You don't even have swollen glands," he said as he palpated my throat. "Your blood tests are all within normal range. It's probably the flu." Not caring how unhinged I might sound, I told him of the increasingly weird dreams I had been having almost nightly, including the one of a ritual circle of black and Indian "medicine men" who had stuck hypodermic needles into something called "the neck-brain." I could almost see the thought balloon—*hypochondriac*—rise over the doctor's head like a small cumulus cloud, but at my insistence he scheduled a full checkup.

It was then that he found the lump. "Nothing to worry about," he said, patting me when he was done kneading my neck. "But we'd better schedule a scan."

"Of what?" I demanded. I felt, oddly, not fear, but the kind of exhilaration you get when a rollercoaster car crests the first hump and begins its stomach-dropping swoosh to the ground. "Your thyroid gland," he said, then smiled grudgingly. "Your neck-brain."

The scan, which required swallowing several radioactive pellets—they slid down cold and heavy as ball bearings—revealed the presence of a plump nodule in the left thyroid lobe. My doctor, looking grave but sounding chipper, motioned me to sit down on the padded examination table. "It's most likely benign," he said comfortingly. "Ninety percent of them are."

But I was certain he was wrong. Nearly every night, I had been waking bolt upright, tangled in sopping sheets. I was usually being chased: by Nazis; by blond children with knives; by a monster billed as "the greatest mass murderer in the history of mankind"; by an ax-wielding executioner dragging me into a freight elevator to lop off my head; by a black jeep roaring toward me from a Brazilian jungle, a mask of the Hindu death god Yama mounted on its hood.

While my dreams relentlessly pursued me each night, my days filled up with medical talk. My doctor already had begun talking about removing the thyroid gland entirely, even if it turned out that it wasn't malignant. It was, he said, the safest route. Its function was easily replaced, he claimed, by "a little one-a-day tablet" of synthetic hormone.

But the sample hormone pills my doctors prescribed made me feel jangled and irritable, like the diet pills I had once taken during college finals. I threw them away after a week. I started reading all I could about the thyroid, "a juicy, bloody little gland," as my doctor put it, perched on either side of the voicebox. "The thyroid secretion is the great controller of the speed of living," said one book. Too much of it, and you zipped through life nervous as a whippet. Low levels of it could cause people to become "stupid and slow and abnormally deliberate." Congenital deprivation of the hormone created what one medical writer called "the 'human plant' type . . . apathetic, indifferent, dirty, awkward, apparently idiotic . . . a condition in which the burning taper we call life flickers and smolders and smokes." Complete absence of the hormone would lead to coma and death.

The idea of removing such a vital organ, leaving a daily pill standing between me and a state in which, according to the book, "there can be no complexity of thought, no learning, no responsive energy" seemed horrific. It in no way allayed my anxiety that my doctors classed what seemed a major alteration of the body as "just routine surgery." I decided to delay a diagnostic biopsy, sensing that the minute I had it, the momentum would quickly build, and the pressure to go along with doctors' "protocols"—to submit to the impressive and well-oiled machinery of medicine—could become irresistible.

I remembered how fast things had moved when, ten years before, my sister had been diagnosed with acute leukemia. A college student and budding concert flutist, she endured a series of caustic rounds of chemotherapy that had won her a precious, shaky year-long respite. When her remission collapsed, she had been rushed to the hospital for experimental treatment. After being given radiation to kill off her cancerous bone marrow and a transfusion of fresh cells from my brother to replace it, she had been sequestered in a sterile environment modeled after the germ-free rooms used in the U.S. space program. We were permitted occasional visits; masked and gowned, we stood behind a white line, shouting to her over the hum of the filtration fan or clumsily gesticulating our love. I remember my father making shoveling motions from his chest, a desperate grin pushing at the corners of his mask.

Until she went into a coma, my sister's doctors insisted that she still had a chance. I was there that afternoon; saw it happen through the thick rectangular window above her food slot: her head flopping back, her eyes rolling loose as two white marbles as she tried to curl her mouth into a lopsided smile—sweet and self-deprecating, as if to say, "Excuse me, I'm sorry, I'm dying now." And then she was gone.

But not entirely. Her body, pale as alabaster, its purple and green needle bruises fading, its blond hair splayed back, remained behind, its chest still gently soughing. When they finally moved her out of isolation, we were allowed to touch her all we wanted. But she never woke up. She was the hospital's twelfth failure in twelve attempts.

Once my father and I had watched in the hospital lobby as a man in what looked like an oversized Halloween mask made his way toward us. When he finally shuffled past, pushing a wheeled pole hung with intravenous fluids, we realized that the loose, rubbery thing on the lower half of his face was what remained after the surgical removal of his lower jaw.

"If I ever had to have that kind of thing done to me," my father whispered fiercely as the sideshow apparition—the no-mandible man—silently receded, "I'd kill myself." I argued with him about that, about the sanctity of life at all costs.

But now, ten years later, searching for my own alternative to surgery, I found myself arguing with him from a pay phone in New York and an antipode away.

"You're not seriously thinking of *not* getting surgery, are you?" he spat out angrily. "If you are, I want to tell you right now you're crazy."

I was taken aback by his vehemence. "Look," I said, almost pleading, suddenly discomforted by the perforated plastic against my ear, "what I most need you to do right now is love me. Have a little faith. I need your support." There was a silence on the line.

"If you are telling me that you are seriously talking about not having a routine operation," my father finally adjudicated, "then, no, I can't do that."

Nearly three years would pass before we spoke again. Looking back, I suppose my father was scared. Even my most adventurous friends were echoing the doctors. "Don't play rebel on this, man," said one, a journalist and ex–Vietnam grunt. "This could be for all the chips."

I went to consult a head-and-neck surgeon at a leading New York hospital for a second opinion. An eminence in his field, he had a packed schedule. Patients were seeded into four small examining rooms, their charts dropped into plastic slots on the door. I would catch glimpses of him as he sallied from one to the other, snatching up a folder and booming the same jocular greeting: "Good morning! How's the throat?" I was amazed at this display of virtuosity. I idly timed him as I waited; his consultations, as he wheeled in and out like a figure in a Swiss clock, averaged two-and-a-half minutes.

"A tiny scar and you're out in a week," he told me as he threw away the gauze he had used to pull on my tongue and set his instrument tray aside with an emphatic clack. "You'll never notice it's gone." When I hesitatingly asked him if he had ever seen tumors reverse their course of growth, he gave me a thin, perfunctory smile. "Never," he said.

"One of those holistic types," I heard him remark to his nurse as he asked her about his next patient. Leaving his waiting room, I was startled to hear a strange, grating electronic voice behind me. I turned to see a patient holding a device like a child's Speak & Spell pressed tightly against her throat, an artificial replacement for her surgically removed larynx.

I continued to resist the idea of a diagnostic biopsy, still not sure I wanted even a minor invasive procedure, still unsure I wanted to know. Even if, as I was increasingly certain, I did have cancer, I wanted to try something else. Though the world of alternative treatments looked recondite, quack-infested, sketchily documented, it still seemed to me to hold out promise. Its practitioners stressed building up the body's ability to defend itself rather than attacking it with the full medical armamentarium. The more I plunged into research, the more it began to seem that all sorts of methods at least occasionally worked. I met a woman who claimed to have healed herself of early cervical cancer by retreating to the New Mexican desert with a carrot juicer, and then a man who had gone to the Philippines for supposedly successful "psychic surgery" on a pituitary tumor. On several occasions during my sister's ordeal, psychic healers had seemed to improve her drastically lowered blood counts. And "spontaneous remission" was an accepted, if unexplained (and exceedingly rare) entry in the official cancer annals.

I began to improvise a plan of action. I devised a diet based on my readings in the literature of unorthodox cancer treatment: vegetables with high mineral content, whole grains, megadoses of potassium and vitamin C; no oil, dairy products, salt, sugar, or red meat. My refrigerator, normally a nutritional junkyard of Chinese takeout tins and half-empty Häagen-Dazs cartons, now bulged with enough fresh greens to stock a truck farm.

Within a few weeks, I was feeling perceptibly healthier. Susan, who at the suggestion of an acupuncturist had been applying hot ginger compresses to my aching kidneys every night, exclaimed that my body had become that of a nineteen-year-old boy: The twenty new pounds of watery, gelatinous fat had melted away. "And now, the Cancer Diet," I joked. I took a leave of absence from work. Temporarily freed from the relentless pressures of what I could see had been an impossible job, I began taking long walks, discovering for the first time that my apartment was only a few blocks from a pretty neighborhood of tree-lined streets and old Boston mansions.

I continued to look for alternatives to surgery. I saw an eminent Tibetan physician who claimed to have had some success with cancer using a millennia-old herbal pharmacopoeia that had been tested on cancerous mice at a medical school lab. He took my pulse—his five fingers played my wrist as if it were a tiny pipe organ—and then examined my urine sample by swirling it with a straw whisk and quickly sniffing it, a human lab. "I do not think you have cancer," he said, writing out a prescription in curling flourishes of Tibetan script.

When I asked him about my dreams, he nodded emphatically. "Any disturbance in the 'throat center' produces dreams that seem very real," he said. He added that Tibetan tradition held there were many kinds of dreams, the chief among them being memories of the past, warnings about bodily illness, and, enigmatically, "memories of the future."

"How am I to regard mine, then?" I asked, leaning forward.

"Regard them the same way you regard waking life," he replied. I looked at him querulously.

"As Samsara," he said. "As illusions of hope and fear."

I took the pills he gave me—lovely artifacts wrapped in pink silk and sealed with delicately lettered wax imprints, redolent of incenselike herbs, of ancient, vanishing worlds. But I was not persuaded. I was at last becoming convinced I needed a clear diagnosis, a name, a handle. I was in a game of "You Bet Your Life," where the stakes were becoming impossibly high.

When I asked my medical doctor for the best diagnostician, he referred me to Dr. Wang, a Chinese-born physician who was one of the country's top thyroid surgeons and was known for his accurate "cutting needle" biopsies. As I sat across from him in his office in Massachusetts General Hospital, I was startled to recall the strange dream I'd had the summer before my illness. In it, a middle-aged

Chinese surgeon had operated on my neck and removed a large, needle-tipped bullet.

"Whatever your tumor turns out to be," Dr. Wang told me, "you have a serious physical ailment, and that's something you must leave to real doctors." He added that he was not entirely skeptical about the power of the mind over the body. As a young medical student, he had once studied the unusually steady heart rates of Taiwanese Buddhist monks. "But this is no longer a spiritual problem." Then he uttered the exact words of the surgeon in my dream: "I can take care of this quite easily."

He insisted that whatever the results turned out to be, I had to make a surgical appointment with him on the spot. He was busy, he said; I didn't want to miss my chance. *It's only a precaution,* I reasoned, a little alarmed as I found myself picking a date six weeks hence; besides, it would placate my family and friends, who were beginning to think I was mad to delay treatment. I glanced at the card—the February date fell (appropriately, given her unswerving faith in medicine) on my mother's birthday.

But it was as yet only Christmastime, and I decided I needed a respite from my flailing quest. I spent most of the week with my daughter, reading her stories, taking a deep breath. One evening we hunkered down to watch *A Christmas Carol.* Here was Scrooge, cowering under the sheets, clawing at his bedclothes, trying to avoid the night-spirits' exhibits of his own thwarted life. I was amazed to find myself identifying with him. Scrooge, updated, was a classic workaholic, disdainful of relationship, afraid of intimacy.

"Is there no other way, O Spirits?" he quavers hammily. "Why *show* me this if I am past all hope?"

"Unless you suffer these visitations," the Spirits intone, "there is no hope of escaping your fate." Squeezing Leah's hands, I suddenly began to weep unabashedly—Scrooge was no longer a comfortably distanced caricature.

"Could you die if your tumor is malignant, Daddy?" she asked suddenly, fluent by now in what we had taken to calling "disease-ese."

"Yes, sweetie, but that isn't going to happen, I promise," I told her, striving for conviction.

"Daddy," she overrode me, "if you die, I won't feel completely sad, because we'll have spent my whole childhood together." I re-alized with a start that Leah was already cushioning herself, securing a vantage point somewhere in the future when everything, one way or the other, would be resolved. "But if you die," she added, "I'll be sad for the rest of my life."

When a few weeks later my test results showed cancer—"mixed papillary and follicular cells" was the official diagnosis—I wasn't surprised. My intuitive fears had taken flesh. In a strange way, I was relieved at the certainty. As it happened, another Tibetan doctor had come up to Boston that day, and I drove over to see him. He, too, carefully took my pulse, his head cocked in an attitude of intense listening. "You do not have the signs of cancer," the man said through his translator. I told him the biopsy results, and he gazed at me implacably for a long moment.

"If the Western doctors say you have cancer, perhaps you should consider surgery."

I was taken aback. "Is he saying this," I asked the translator, "because he thinks that I don't have enough faith in his remedies?"

"No," he relayed. "He says it is not a matter of faith. He says he does not believe you have cancer. But the Western doctors say that you do. He says you will have to choose."

"How?" I was thoroughly confused.

"Whatever you do," said the translator, as the healer signaled the end of the interview, "he says you should have Big Mind."

But how big a mind did I need to contain increasingly irreconcilable contradictions? I no longer knew whom or even how to trust. The doctors who, diagnosis in hand, seemed obscenely eager to chop out my vitals? My girlfriend? She was disappearing further into some vortex inside herself, frightened, never sleeping, spending half of every day lying in bed crying, in the throes of what was to become a full-blown emotional collapse.

My dreams? Each night I entered another world that was shatteringly distinct, yet maddeningly ambiguous. The dividing line between waking and dreaming—even between present and future— was becoming fuzzy. One night I dreamed I had a "sacred starfish" in my neck. The next day, paying a spur-of-the-moment visit to the Boston Science Museum, I was suddenly handed a live starfish by a collegiate exhibit guide. "What's amazing about them," he told me, as the moist little creature stirred gently in my palm, "is that they can regenerate their damaged parts."

I thought then of the Tibetan notion of "memories of the future." I thought about hope and fear. I later came across a description by Carl Jung that expressed my predicament exactly: "I felt myself a single eye in a thousand-eyed universe, but incapable of moving so much as a pebble upon the earth." Feeling powerless in the outer world, my thoughts began to turn inward.

I began to read about the so-called "cancer personality," the descriptions of which struck all too close to home. The literature about the cancer-prone pointed to traits like low self-esteem; to a deep-seated need for approval; to relationships that were conditional, predicated on a more desperate than normal need for love.

The psychologist Lawrence LeShan, in his well-regarded handbook for cancer patients, *You Can Fight for Your Life,* had observed that cancer personalities tended to make " 'gigantic claims' against themselves. . . . 'If I can realize these ambitions,' they appear to be saying, 'then others must accept and love me.' " Other studies suggested that the so-called "Type C" stayed interminably in bad relationships, overwilling to please, overly conscientious and self-sacrificing. One study described a leukemia patient who, even though he was deathly ill, would stay up night after night just to sort out his medical bills.

I decided to make an immediate appointment with Dr. LeShan. When I entered his dimly lit basement office, I felt safe for the first time since my ordeal began. Everything about him, the steepled fingers, the owlish gaze, the genial clutter of his study, said *It's going to be okay. I understand. We'll beat this thing together.*

Eager to enlist his help, I rushed through the events of the past months and then, under his gentle prodding, began to describe the last ten years of my life: an unhappy shotgun marriage, a bitter divorce, my lunging, desperate need for success. He stopped me after fifteen minutes. "I don't think it's the death in your dreams we have to deal with, my friend," he said in his kindly but blunt manner. "It's the death in your *life.* It reeks of self-denial."

As he was walking me to the door, LeShan—whose interests in parapsychology had led him to write a book on physics and mysticism—put his arm around me and added, sotto voce, something that pulled me up short. "You have to get out of the trap, out of the iron bars. But somehow the only escape route seems to be blocked.

"You have an inner saboteur," he said, squeezing my shoulder for emphasis. "He doesn't wish you well. You'd better find out who he is, before he completely does you in."

The idea had a creepy ring of truth. But who was the traitor? The part of me that didn't want to get the operation? ("You've always had a death wish," admonished one friend, a former songwriting partner who had just composed the music for *Little Shop of Horrors.*

"If I had some monster-thing in my neck, I'd get it the hell out tomorrow.") Or the part of me that doubted my body's capacity to heal? In either case, I began to see my cancer as a personal message—crude, like a kidnapper's note spliced together from scraps of headline type: CHANGE OR DIE.

But at that point, inner change seemed secondary, ornamental. In the all-too-real outer world, my body was falling apart, along with the rest of my life. Susan had abruptly announced that she was moving back to Boulder. "I'm sorry," she said, in a voice that wafted up from some private abyss. "I'm coming apart." The publisher of *New Age Journal* had invited me to lunch, I assumed to finalize our long-delayed contract; and with little preamble informed me I was fired.

When a friend on the West Coast called and offered me a place to stay north of San Francisco—"When in doubt, California," he suggested cheerily—it seemed, if not a solution to my dilemmas, at least a path of action. Getting out of Boston, with its fast-souring memories and gray, slushy winter, for the inanity of a few aimless weeks of sun seemed perfect.

California was warmly, creamily out of focus. The house my friend had arranged my stay in had a staggering view of Mount Tamalpais. The long honeysuckle dusks were patented Marin County. One day, my host—a genial if overbearing millionaire—announced he was taking me to an Indian sweat lodge ceremony on a friend's property a few hours north.

The old medicine man—I never did get his name or tribe—was a kindly, half-toothless gent in jeans and a worn, red plaid shirt. I liked him immediately. Once we had gathered, he and his son spent the afternoon constructing an airtight cupola out of bent saplings and canvas sheeting. As the sun sank, ten of us ducked our heads and crawled inside. Large, red-hot stones of volcanic basalt were passed in on a forked stick. A sacred pipe went around the circle. As water was ladled, hissing, into the central pit, steam-cleaner blasts of hot mist filled the blackness, searing our lungs.

My sweat poured out in quick rivulets; I felt glued to a naked teenage Mexican girl sitting alongside me, the slippery pressure of her thigh somehow more comforting than erotic. Suddenly, I sensed the medicine man's face near mine. "Where is the sickness?" he asked gruffly. I guided his hand to the spot on my neck. Without warning, he fixed his mouth there and began sucking for all he was worth. I felt the prickling stubble around his lips, as if I were being embraced by an unshaven lamprey. Three times he sucked, spitting out some liquid that sizzled, with an acrid smell, into the fire.

It was a strangely magnificent moment: the intimacy of sweat and steam in the pitch darkness, the feeling of being enfolded in a collective womb, the prayers that crescendoed into a ragged chorus of mutters, murmurs, and yowls, the assurance and tenderness with which the old man went about his work.

That night, I had the first good dream I had had in months: Some grizzled old cowboys had been brawling in a bar and were being led away, blinking in the sunlight, by the police. But before they were driven off in a paddy wagon, they were required to sign "forgiveness clauses" on the deed of some land they owned. Then they were given a Salvation Army–style Thanksgiving dinner.

Waking up, I thought: *Perhaps the disease is giving up its property. Perhaps I can strive for forgiveness.* The next day, climbing a nearby hill with my host's golden retriever, I suddenly had the impulse to try using a gestalt therapy technique I'd read about, to sit and hold a "dialogue" with the disease.

"Why have you come?' I asked aloud, feeling unutterably silly. I was surprised when a voice, strangled and gravelly, seemed to emerge of its own accord from my throat.

"Can't live this way," I heard the voice rasp with great bitterness. "Too cruel," it said. "Too cruel to live."

"I'll change," I found myself saying, glad there were no other witnesses to this dialogue-cum-soliloquy. Then I heard myself pleading. "Please give me my life back."

The voice laughed acridly as the dog gave an anxious whine and looked sidelong. "You wouldn't know what to do with it."

The "dialogue" ended there, but I noticed over the next few days that I was feeling much better. Even so, I was all too aware that the clock was ticking, and my final surgery date, like an artificial barrier reef, loomed in the water before me.

I had been puzzled by the fact that my dreams kept turning to Brazil, a country about which I knew exactly two words: Carmen and Miranda. I thought back to the one in which the circle of Indians and blacks—the racial mixture unique to Brazil—had performed a ritual on my neck by inserting large, empty syringes. One day I found myself describing this scene to Alberto, an anthropologist I knew who had studied purported psychic healers all over South America. He was immediately enthusiastic.

"The best healers in the world are in Brazil," he told me. "The most amazing is named Edson Quieroz. He's an M.D. who does pseudo-operations—or even real surgery—while he's in trance. Sometimes, he just sticks a big empty syringe in the diseased organ and it's cured. Other times he uses a scalpel, no anesthetic. I saw him take out a tumor from a woman who I'm sure would have needed a mastectomy otherwise. Maybe," he said thoughtfully, "he could kill your tumor without removing the whole gland."

I looked dubious. Alberto popped in a videotape he had made on a field trip a few years before. Sure enough, there was Dr. Quieroz, by day a conventional gynecologist, by night a *Spiritist* doctor, digging into a woman's breast with hands and a scalpel, pulling out a bloody mass of tissue. The woman, who was entirely unanesthetized, was shown a few minutes later chatting happily with the filmmakers, insisting that she had felt "only a slight tickling."

I began to think about going to Brazil. I was aching to do something, anything, other than go to the hospital and forever lose a vital organ. Paralyzed by too many choices and none, perhaps I was seduced by the idea of a grand gesture, of getting as far from Boston as I could, of embarking on a healing adventure.

On Alberto's recommendation, I went to Sausalito to talk with a Brazilian psychologist named Edmundo, who had seen Quieroz perform many operations. Edmundo's apartment overlooked the dazzle of the bay and the once bohemian, now desperately pricey flotilla of Sausalito houseboats. An imposing, full-bearded man in his early thirties with two hundred pounds packed on a six-foot-plus frame, Edmundo had the air of someone supremely at ease with himself, his shoulders loose, his arms swinging. "Sit," he gestured with a friendly wave at a couch opposite him. "We'll talk."

I began rattling out my story to him, peppering him with questions. His eyes were gentle and curious. "Once," he said, "I saw Edson remove three large tumors from the breast of a young woman in her twenties. It was very dramatic. She was wide awake, and said that it just felt like he was scratching her with his fingernail. But people who know about him walk on eggs when he's in trance. Because sometimes he'll just pull out his scalpel in the waiting room, pick someone out, and make an incision while they stand there."

For balance, Edmundo added that he had also talked with a few doctors who believed that Dr. Quieroz, who claims to be possessed by the spirit of a dead German field surgeon named Dr. Fritz when he operates, was only using simple hypnotism combined with ordinary surgical techniques.

Midway through our conversation, Edmundo stopped, looking at me with a puzzled expression. "You know, my friend," he said in his lilting Portuguese accent, "when I first met you, I thought, 'Why is he coming to me? He is the big-time editor of this national magazine. He must have people all over the country wanting to take care of him. He must have friends, family.' " He looked at me unwaveringly. "I don't think it was until this moment that I realized: He is completely alone." Tears sprang into my eyes. "How did you get to be so alone?"

For the next five minutes, we sat silently. I felt raw and exposed. Then I got up to go and walked toward the door. "Wait a minute," he said. "We have lots of food tonight. You have nowhere to go. Why don't you have dinner with us?" He gazed at me with disarming directness. But I thanked him brusquely, lying that I had to meet other people for dinner. I was ashamed to have been seen, to confront the fact that I *was* alone, and that to be alone in my condition might betoken something about myself that I didn't want to face.

My surgery date was now little more than a week away. That night, my mind seemed to break with a small, dry crack. Not knowing what else to do, I got down on my knees and did something I hadn't done since I was an eleven-year-old petitioning the stern Hebrew God to help me find a lost orthodontic appliance that had cost my parents a small fortune. "Please, Lord," I said, feeling idiotic. "I need a sign. Something. Anything. I'm lost." After crouching awkwardly on the carpet for a few minutes, I got up and noticed that the kitchen phone with the broken ringer was silently blinking. I picked it up and heard the crackle of an international call.

"My name's Gary," said the voice at the other end. "I'm a reporter down here in Rio. Edmundo told me you were thinking of coming down. I just wanted to tell you that I did a little research on Quieroz and came up with a case he cured of thyroid cancer, just using needles. I could arrange for you to see him next week, if you like."

I decided in a moment. "Is there anything special I should bring with me?" I asked.

The line spluttered.

"What?" I shouted. "Bad connection . . ."

"I said," the man repeated, softly and clearly, "bring your faith."

Two nights later, I was eating a farewell dinner in a restaurant with a friend before my scheduled morning departure. Waiting for the excruciatingly laid-back waiter to return, I called Susan to say goodbye. "I haven't wanted to say anything up to now," she said slowly after audibly inhaling, "but I think what you're doing is crazy. And arrogant. You're refusing to submit to what you know you have to do. Stop playing the tragic hero.

"Submit," she reiterated. "Just go home and get into the hospital."

I was shaken. But the next morning I found myself on a connecting flight to Miami, destination Rio. As the plane rumbled across the continent, I felt like a fugitive from medical justice, as much a man without a country as the guy who lammed out to Brazil after the Great Train Robbery. My flight was late getting into Miami owing to severe headwinds; only fifteen minutes remained to catch the final leg to Rio. There wouldn't even be time to retrieve my luggage. I would have to continue empty-handed. Somehow, it seemed appropriate.

As if in a dream, I got off the plane, aware that I should be moving quickly. I heard rapid Spanish threading the air as I traversed the Miami airport, but I felt as if I were walking languorously on the floor of the ocean, the jostling, tropically colored crowd parting gently before me like anemones.

The sensorium of the busy terminal became oddly muffled. A pressure welled up inside, cottoning my ears, making my sight waver liquidly. As my body moved forward under its own purpose, the surface world was replaced by an undertow of words and images: Leah's frightened face. A smoky-colored sonogram with a tumor-shaped flare of white. A specialist's remark that thyroid cancer could "meander down the laryngeal nerve" toward the vocal cords, like a python coiling insidiously down a branch; or like something less languid— a krait, an asp, killing my voice in an invisible flicker. The friend of a friend who had begged me tearfully to go to the hospital because *his* friend had "run off to some flaky Mexican clinic and died."

What if I went to Brazil and by some strange grace the tumor shrank, only to degenerate years later into a more virulent cell-type? Or if I missed my *real* surgery date, and in the months it would take Wang to schedule a new one, it spread? What if the mysterious Dr. Quieroz decided to operate without anaesthetic, or in the throes of his trance slashed an artery? "He's not *crazy*," Edmundo had reminded me. But how was I to know?

A group of three Brazilian men passed me, tootling festively on paper Carnival horns, going home. When one threw a glance over his shoulder, I had the urge to lunge out and grab him by the arm, pour it all out as they listened in suddenly grave sympathy. Then maybe the gods that clamored only in my dreams might seize them in augury, these loud, careless men in bright shirts, decree through them that if we spent twelve hours roaring south through the night to a place that suddenly seemed dark and unknown, I could truly be made whole.

My reverie was interrupted by a small man with a fussily clipped mustache and a blue airline blazer frantically waving me over. I had arrived at the flight counter. "You have your ticket? You are on this flight? Come *now*, sir. Now. It is leaving!"

Suddenly, I was sweating beneath my trenchcoat. I could hear the plane's engines beginning to thrum and rev. By the time we had hurried to the end of the ramp, I was humid with fear. "Come on, sir, don't be afraid," coaxed one of the blue-uniformed pilots as I stood uncertainly at the door, which now seemed like a surreal final threshold, a point of no return. "Brazilian pilots are the best." The pretty stewardess standing at his arm glanced over at him and laughed throatily.

Without my awareness, my feet took a long adrenaline-charged stride, back away from the door of the plane, then another, and another, like involuntary Simon Says—first a giant step, then two umbrella steps—as I spun and then ran down the ramp from the plane. Bewildered, the little man in the blazer put out a restraining hand as I brushed past him. "I can't," I gasped out to him. "I'm too afraid."

Later, in an airport hotel room, listening to the jets turbine into the night, I felt something inside me compress, grow dense, like a star collapsing inward on itself. A cold, heavy cinder of defeat formed in my belly. The next morning, I boarded a plane back to Boston.

"We weren't sure you were going to show up," said the receptionist in the hospital waiting room a few days later as I signed the papers she placed before me. "You're not just coming in for a strep test, you know." I nodded. "You look too healthy to be here," joked the nurse who led me to my room.

The next morning, there was a knock at the door, and an old Chicano orderly shuffled in, indicating by hand gestures and smiles that he had come to shave my chest. In my disoriented state, augmented by the tranquilizer I'd been given early that morning, I felt I was undergoing a ritual purification. I was overcome with childlike passivity. *Maybe they can make the dreams stop,* I thought. Another orderly came in, loaded me onto a gurney, and pushed me down a hallway into an elevator—*Didn't the executioner in my nightmare take me down in an elevator?* I wondered groggily—and then through the swinging double doors of the operating room.

Dr. Wang was already there, his mask down at his chin, his hairless forearms bare, looking, in his green uniform, like the genial captain of the company bowling team.

He grinned down at me. "How you feel?" he asked cheerily.

"Scared," I said weakly. "Try to cut out as little as you can, okay?"

"Don't worry," he boomed, "We are the experts here." A cold bright lamp loomed above me, a magnesium moon filling the sky, about to shear into its planet. When the anesthesiologist found a vein, I felt a liquid chill run up my arm.

I remember reaching for Wang's hand, craving the yielding pulse of flesh in this room of poised chrome machinery and glaring tile. I felt a sudden dizzy uprush, then a geologic subsidence as I sank, stratum by stratum, into a place of dark and loam. As I spiraled from the light of this world, I was still holding his hand.

I think I half-expected, as some patients claim, to remember the events of the operation, to hear the clinking of the instruments, the o.r. nurses' infield chatter, the hiss of the respirator; to see, from some disembodied perspective, Wang's green-gloved hand reach inside me and change me forever. But there was nothing. I know from my later reading that my limp body was secured to the table with tight straps and raised into a three-quarters sitting position, and my throat was elegantly and exactingly slashed open. After that, the postoperative report notes curtly, "the left strap muscles were transected. The left thyroid was exposed. Lobectomy was done."

I don't remember the moment I woke up. I do remember my first thought: *I'm in Hell.* As a bottle dripped saline solution into my veins, I realized—with the annihilating impact of an epiphany—the meaning of the torture-dream on my daughter's birthday. Here I was, my arms tangled as they had been then in plastic tubes, my throat burning with pain, crying out to a God who could no longer help me. Here, too, were the early puzzling dreams of being decapitated, finally explained by the angry red wound traversing my neck.

I wondered then if the ax-wielding executioner I had dreamed of had not, as I had thought, been the Grim Reaper with his scythe; I wondered if he had been a surgeon.

A few days later I was taken home. Leah had put up a crayoned sign on the door: THE RECOVERY ROOM, embellished with a child's happy-world of bluebirds and suns. But virtually whimpering with trauma, I was unable to put on a brave face. I could feel an uncanny empty space, a uselessly dangling wire, where, hours before, a living organ had still pulsed. I felt inconceivably strange: I had hung my familiar *real* body on a coat rack going into the hospital, but I had somehow picked up the wrong one—a desperately wrong one—on my way out.

Each morning I woke before sun-up from dreamless sleep, my hand scrabbling for the tiny yellow tablet that now sustained my life. My body felt dead, a desiccating swamp with only a few remaining tendrils of vitality. Once Leah, visiting, pulled her favorite stuffed animal, Piglet, from her bag—"He's to keep you company, Daddy, when you're sad"—and to my shame, I buried my face in it, wetting its soft acrylic fur.

Do over! I wanted to cry absurdly. *I didn't mean it.* Like a man who decides to take one last drink before the bar closes and, thus ratcheted one fateful notch toward impairment, smashes head-on into a family of four, I felt I had somehow made a terrible and irremediable mistake.

I discovered that hundreds of letters had arrived, responses to a farewell editorial I'd written in *New Age Journal* months before. "I am moved to see you hopeful, determined, realistic," read a letter from a woman in Quebec. "I find the whole 'new age' a bit insincere, but I really do care what happens to you."

"We are pleased to announce you have been nominated for this year's *Esquire* Register," another anounced cheerily.

Near the top of the pile was one from Susan, containing a Sydney Omarr astrological forecast for the day I was to have been in Brazil: "What had been a promise will now become a reality. You get what you ask for." Just beneath it was an envelope with the hospital's final pathology report. "Thyroid specimen is received fresh in three parts," read the computer printout. "Tumor is a 2.5 cm firm nodule." The words brought me up short. Something didn't jibe. I shuffled through my papers for the measurement from my first test scan months before: "A large nodule measuring 3.5 cm." Against everything I'd been told was possible, the tumor had apparently shrunk in just a month's time. I wondered then what would have happened had I gotten on the plane or, that finally being too grandiosely self-defeating a strategy, simply waited for more clarity.

Have I found the secret saboteur? I thought, wondering how much further the process might have gone had I not intervened. *Myself?*

Dr. Wang pronounced his operation a resounding success, even noting the cancer had turned out to be less malignant than expected. But my body felt freakishly altered. Seeking the solace of the familiar, I flew back to Boulder—crawled back, wept back. One day, I found myself sitting around with the men who had been my three closest friends from what now seemed like another life. I tried to explain how I felt; how when the drug would get low, I could feel life streaming from my body, like the infrared clips of uninsulated houses that were broadcast during the 1970s energy crisis. "Have a drink, man," one said, not unsympathetically. "Entropy's every-where. We're *all* running out of gas."

They treated me kindly, a basket case sent back to them postage-due, but I could tell they sometimes became wearied: *The doctors say you're well, don't they? Rejoice, and get on with it.* Like Philoctetes, whom it is said the heroes of the Trojan War finally left behind on an island because he complained of the never-healing snakebite on his foot, I could tell my presence was growing burdensome.

I spent days on the sunny deck of my friend Rick's house, watching him play the ancient Japanese board game of Go, envying him his life. Where I had written three quick trade paperbacks in a greedy, eighteen-month frenzy, he had taken six years to write a substantial and well-received history of American Buddhism, sticking cheer-fully and penuriously with his small publisher. He had made a life for himself, while I, cleverer, flashier, more ambitious, had somehow let mine slip past. I swung for hours in the backyard hammock watching horses grazing equably in an adjacent field, wondering how I had ever taken it into my head to leave.

But there was still one more journey I had to make. It started with a phone call from Edmundo a few months after I arrived in Boulder. "I'm taking a group down to Brazil," he said simply. "You have to come." I knew it was true; I had to try to find out what might have been waiting for me down there, what the dreams had meant, what might have happened if I had chosen the road that had opened magically, perilously, close to my feet. I still had my ticket and my visa. I needed, needed desperately, to try to close the circle.

It is three in the morning, a humid night in the coastal town of Recife. I stand next to Dr. Edson Quieroz as he removes a large tumor from deep in a man's back. The small white room is crowded with twenty people; two hundred more, some of them women hold-ing babies, still wait outside. The man, his expression ranging from the beatific to the plainly nervous, has been wide awake through the ten-minute procedure. The twangy notes of what sounds like a Brazilian Muzak version of "Johnny Angel" blare from a boombox on the windowsill and ricochet off the tiled walls.

Quieroz, when he is possessed by "Dr. Fritz," moves with the slow, jerkily animated movements of an old horror-movie monster. He

plops the tumor into the hand of the startled woman standing to
my right. An odor identical to freshly cut meat assails my nostrils
before an assistant snatches the tumor away and puts it in a kitchen
jar with a red plastic screw-top. I feel, incongruously, as though I've
stumbled into a cooking class.

I look over at the prostrate man on the operating table; when he
meets my glance, he waggles his eyebrows comically, like Groucho
Marx. Quieroz removes another woman's breast tumor—she, too,
has her eyes open and hardly flinches when he cuts deep into her
skin, which is the lustrous cocoa hue Brazilians call *mulata*.

One of my traveling companions, a surgeon, licensed hypnotist,
and medical history buff, is providing a distracting running commentary. "A conscious person bleeds less copiously than an etherized
one," he tells me calmly as the knife bites again. "Why, in the nineteenth century, the great Esdaile showed the Royal College he could
amputate a gangrenous limb under hypnosis while his fully awake
patient—a soldier, I believe, some kind of war wound—just lay there
and . . ." But now Quieroz, still in trance, motions I am to sit down.
He walks stiffly over to me—Mighty Joe Young—and before I quite
realize what is happening thrusts four enormous, empty hypodermic needles into what is left of my thyroid gland. He taps one with
his finger to drive it in further, like a carpenter hammering a nail.
I squeeze my eyes shut, and when I open them, the linoleum is
splattered with blood. After a few minutes, he removes the hypos.
An assistant offers me a small picnic cup of "blessed water" as I
shakily take another seat. I can't say I notice any effect. It just feels
like giant pins have been jammed into my neck, and predictably,
they hurt.

Later, in my hotel room, I wondered why I had been so anxious
to see a psychic healer who was also an M.D., who used hypodermics
as ritual implements and could, certainly, perform unanesthetized
surgery with a scalpel. It had looked to others like a mad flight
from reality, though I had had a rationale: the off-chance I could
spare a vital organ from what had seemed to me an ultimately
cruder, if cleaner and better lit excision. I was half-consciously
searching for a less sanguinary, less permanently damaging way to
"have an operation."

But I think that Edson Quieroz, classically trained gynecologist
by day, spiritist trance healer by night, was my attempt to find an
archetype—a doctor who merged both the spiritual and the physical,
the shaman and the scientist. I remembered that the night before
my panicky attempt at flight, I had awakened with a luminous vision

still before me: Some implements were being formed from a bright, molten alloy of "healing stone and steel," which coalesced suddenly into an absurdly beautiful, sapphire-blue set of mechanics' wrenches. This, perhaps, was what I'd so ardently but blindly sought: a healer who was at once mechanic and intercessor; not just medicine, but a Grail, a dramatic rite to mobilize the self-healing powers it had seemed to me were just beginning to stir.

Certainly such powers exist. The literature of spontaneous remission contains the occasional cases of terminal diseases mysteriously melting away. Even my own tumor had seemingly, swayed by some mysterious inner process, given up some of its claim. But it was clear to me that whatever I had hoped—that Quieroz could stick me with voodoo pins, resuscitate the small chunk of gland my surgeons had left me, set running again its smashed mechanism— was beyond whatever powers he might or might not possess. I had already made my choice.

I knew then that there was no one to draw back the curtain and show me whether the lady or the tiger had lurked behind it. Ever since surgery, I had felt as if, in one explosive moment of choice, I had undergone a sort of mitosis of fate; that there were somehow two halves of me—one that had gone on, and one that had hesitated and been forever left behind. Months later, I could still sense this shadow-double, whether fool or hero I would never really know, his track diverging in the distance.

But now it was time to try to become whole. I had chosen my path. Now I had to find my way home.

I

THE VARIETIES
OF HEALING EXPERIENCE

What an immense rip
In my life and in all things
In order to be with my entire self
In everything;
In order to never cease being,
with my entire self, in everything.

—JUAN RAMÓN JIMÉNEZ,
Light and Shadows[1]

"WHY EVEN WONDER about whether you made the right choice?" my friends ask with honest puzzlement. "The surgeons took care of the cancer. All you have to do is take a little pill every day. The nightmares have stopped. You did what anyone would have done; you were smart not to gamble with your life." The dreams, they say, were hallucinations, Sirens luring me toward the most dangerous shoals. There's even a medical term for it: oneirophrenia, "dream madness."

But, much as I might wish it otherwise, this interpretation will not wash. No matter how it looks to anyone else, I know I went into surgery in the middle of a mystery, a conundrum I was unable—perhaps even unwilling—to solve.

I had been caught in a war of the worlds: On one hand was the realm of the psyche, a Jacob's ladder from whose upper rungs my medical choices were apparently viewed as travesties; on the other was the domain of scientific materialism, where to be leery of "routine surgery" is to be labeled hopelessly phobic. In my nightmares, I had run, uncomprehending, from heedless blond children twirling butcher knives; from mad scientists in stained smocks who drank blood from victims strapped to surgical gurneys. In the waking world, I talked across polished mahogany desks with the same white-

coated, clear-eyed professionals who, since I was a child, have reassured me they would make it all better.

These worlds spoke different tongues. The doctors had described
my disease as a grim, implacable killer. Based on the terrors that
chased me through the night, I had been more than inclined to
agree. But my dreams, once they had forcibly grabbed my attention,
had in their imagistic dialect portrayed my tumor as "crab-sticks"—
those supermarket items cunningly flavored, colored, and shaped
to look like crab (the symbol for the astrological sign Cancer), but
made only of common fish. Indeed, a second biopsy taken during
my surgery had revealed a borderline, "pure papillary" tumor,
which, though standard protocol calls for surgical removal, only
rarely undergoes deadly metastasis.[2]

Speaking off the record, one leading surgeon recently confided
to me that "probably fifteen *million* Americans are walking around
right now with small papillary cancers. Maybe only eleven thousand
ever come in to see us, and maybe a thousand deaths register nationally every year." Though he was disinclined to go further, it
seemed to me that I had perhaps unduly rushed my rendezvous
with surgical destiny.

The doctors had assured me that the aftereffects of the operation
would be negligible. One had handed me an article by Isaac Asimov
in which the late sci-fi writer had described going gaily into his own
thyroid surgery, "singing at the top of my resonant voice, 'Doctor,
Doctor, with green coat / Doctor, doctor, cut my throat / And when
you've cut it, Doctor, then / Won't you sew it up again?' " Asimov
averred that many years and dozens of books later, he felt "perfectly
fine."

By contrast, my nightmares, a number of them grisly tableaus of
still-living severed heads, had warned me that the personal consequences of the operation might be less blithe. Indeed, my doctors
had neglected to mention that the gland does not just regulate the
metabolism, but affects the delicate biochemistry of emotion. Thyroid conditions have on occasion been linked to disorders ranging
from paranoid schizophrenia to manic depression. When the late
Senator John East committed suicide a few years ago, he left a note,
according to a *Newsweek* story, blaming "disorientation and lapses
of mental acuity" brought on by a malfunctioning thyroid. I recently
spoke to a psychologist who had experienced such severe postoperative mood disorders that she had voluntarily placed herself in a
mental institution.

Contrary to medical assurances, I have found that a human body deprived of this organ cannot be tuned with the precision of a BMW. My feelings, my energy, my attention span have all at times been affected. Sometimes the differences feel relatively minor; at other times, when my thinking is logey, my body vitiated, my moods pendulous, they have felt as awful as my "dream prognosis" foreshadowed.

Over the last few years I've met a number of people who have had the operation. It is partly synchronicity, partly the new shoes syndrome: Walking out of the shoestore, you suddenly notice what's on everyone's feet. I notice neck-scars. I have talked to maybe a dozen people with the delicate white tracery that curves like a scimitar wound, hugging the line of the collarbone.

Many of these people's stories tally with writer Isaac Asimov's favorable experience. For that matter, millions of patients with numberless diseases have had life-saving, even miraculous encounters with modern medicine. In *their* dreams, their doctors may well have appeared as rescuing angels. But as another of my dreams urgently whispered, "One size doesn't fit all." The human experience of disease and healing is as diverse as our fingerprints.

It was after I left the hospital, anointed as cured but feeling sick in heart and body, that my healing quest began in earnest, though I had no idea where to look. I went for a check-up to Dr. Wang a few weeks after my operation and opened the spigot of anguish as much as I dared. He sat me down and squeezed my neck proprietarily.

"This is one of the cleanest jobs I've ever done. Almost perfect." He reached over for a pair of tweezers and deftly plucked a hair from the suture.

"Now, perfect."

He beamed at me, looking for amiable concurrence. But I could only think of a plumber admiring a particularly tidy weld-seam. My inner experience was opaque to him. "You'll feel better soon," he said. "I promise."

But I didn't. Among the Zulu, it is said that the relatives of an afflicted person may ask a healer to banish the spirit that brought the sickness. But if the spirit had also come with a message, the refusal to heed it could cause the patient to be plagued by illness throughout his life. I felt plagued: In curing one ailment, I had been given another one that wouldn't heal. I would have to pharmaceutically be wound each day like a watch: too tight, and I'd tick too fast; too slow, and I'd stop altogether. But the night-messengers, if that is what they had been, no longer pounded on my doors. I dreamed—the images now cloudy, indistinct—of a doctor who performed a "routine eye operation" and accidentally dropped my eye on the floor; try as he might he could not stuff the ruined orb back in its socket.

I felt, in some way I could not articulate, emotionally sightless. I thought of Old Lodge Skins in the film *Little Big Man,* describing his blindness from a neck wound inflicted by a bluecoat's saber: "My eyes still see, but what they see no longer reaches my heart." My life had been voided of certainty, stripped to its existential struts and pinions. Had the doctors saved my life or ruined it? Had my friends cared about me, or simply wished to see the whole episode concluded with dispatch? Had Susan ever loved me? Had my parents wanted me well, or wanted my square peg machine-tooled to fit an acceptably round hole? I had been drawn into a juncture of forces I didn't understand, a vortex that had whirled away body and soul, friends, family, career—the very order of things.

In a private ceremony one night, I immolated all my old magazine files in the fireplace. I had spent too much time, it now seemed to me, pursuing stories rather than inner imperatives, snatching bright gewgaws from other peoples' lives. Yet I clung to the thin consolation that I was still a journalist. I could at least, if only for myself, become a chronicler of the Underneath. Perhaps I could start over among the wounded and damaged, look for a healing path among others forced to travel it.

My experience left me not only with a medical condition, but with questions that were to burn in me for years like acetylene. To be mortally ill in the late twentieth century is to be swept into the confluence of thousands of years of unfinished business between religion, science, philosophy, commerce, politics, and technology. For me, it also meant butting up against what I once considered antique theological questions—higher law vs. casuistry, faith vs. perfidy, appearance vs. reality, fate vs. free will, even good vs. evil—with little more to go on than my own demonstrably flawed intuition.

I carry away a single personal certainty from my experience: To separate *psyche* from *soma,* in any aspect of our lives, even with the most benign intent and soundest rationale, cannot help but be risky business. As it turns out, it is also scientific fallacy. Candace Pert, the neuroscience pioneer who codiscovered endorphins (the brain's "natural opiates"), has argued to former colleagues at the National Institutes of Health that the terms *body* and *mind* are becoming obsolete. In the light of new research, she has urged *bodymind* (a term I will adopt throughout this book) as the only meaningful nomenclature.

I met Dr. Pert five years ago, when she was in town to speak at a healing conference. She was just beginning to venture forth from the autoclaved precincts of official research to more new-age venues, trying out the psychoneuroimmunology (PNI) gospel on an audience more receptive than most of her colleagues. In her flowing orange floral-print dress, slinging her pointer over her shoulder with precision rifle-drill panache, her words ricocheting in breathless spurts, she was like some hip diva of science. The next day, recognizing a kindred glimmer, we decided to play hooky from that afternoon's lectures for a picnic lunch in the mountains.

Though she may tone it down at phlegmier scientific gatherings, Pert—who even in conversation seems on the verge of auto-electrocution from a surfeit of cranial wattage—turned out to be a quintessential Sixties Person, sticking her scuffed boot up on the dash and yelling "Far out!" whenever an idea excited her, which was often. "Emotions exist in two realms," she told me between exclamations about the view from a dizzying curve that sent gravel rattling into our wheelrims. "One is the mind. The other is the realm of living matter. The whole thing's vibrating back and forth. We're actually talking about music."

She hazarded that each neuropeptide—the list of which has burgeoned from five just a few years ago to over five dozen—may "evoke a unique 'tone' that is equivalent to a mood state." I suddenly pictured mind and body as a thousand-octave piano—from the highest glissando of altruism to the middle C of fight-or-flight to bass-heavy autonomic arpeggios—as part of a seamless, interdigitated boogie-woogie.

Growing evidence has shown that consciousness inhabits even the humblest quarters of our flesh. Neuropeptides and their receptors, the so-called "messenger molecules," are suddenly turning up everywhere in the body, flashing on winged feet—in the brain (particularly in the centers governing emotion), throughout the immune system, in organs from gut to gland. They are the bodymind's lingua franca, a web humming with information and intelligence. Our thoughts and feelings are mediated by neuropeptides; some diseases secrete neuropeptides; neuropeptides are key to the healing response.

The richest lode has been found in the limbic system, the "emotional center" linked to those areas of the brain controlling appetite,

rest, temperature, heart rate, sexual impulses, and hormone secretion. Thus the medieval philosophers who postulated the existence
of "Vitall Spirits" that ferried missives between "the panns of the
brayne" and the heart were not far off. A change in body is a change
in mind; a change in mind is a change in body. The Jungian analyst
James Hillman eloquently argued:

> We may no longer make a cleavage between organic pathology
> and psychopathology, following the old Cartesian division be-
> tween physical and mental. Everything matters to soul and ex-
> presses its fantasies, whether ideas in the head or bones in the
> body. . . . Heart, skin, joints, whether congenital, chronic, or
> acute, whether accidental, infectious, or hereditary—each and
> all of these have psychological significance, are metaphors too;
> they are foci of fantasy as well as disease.[3]

From this standpoint, it matters less whether a disease gestates
within the psyche (there are indications that personality is at least
a "cofactor" in some illnesses), or whether it simply has a psychic
impact once it makes its appearance. Disease and healing are not
just physiological processes. They are spiritual detonations.

DISEASE AND TRANSFORMATION

To speak of the spiritual implications of disease raises some justi-
fiably stiff hackles. Illness is an attack on the body by heredity, a
virus, a toxin, an oncogene; a statistical bad hop; an ordeal, unjust
and unlitigiable, sponsored by the Blind Forces of Nature.

"What are you supposed to learn? Are you supposed to learn
something about your psyche?" snapped the paleontologist Stephen
Jay Gould when he was asked about his four-year battle with me-
sothelioma (a disease with only an eight-month prognosis). "It's just
romanticism to look back at something like that and try to find a
good side to it." In her classic book *Illness as Metaphor*, the writer
Susan Sontag, a former cancer patient, reserves especially withering
scorn for "the romantic view . . . that illness exacerbates consciousness."

Still, the interplay of illness, healing, and consciousness has been
observed throughout the history of medicine—has been perhaps at
its very root. Long before Dr. Carl Simonton popularized the role
that mental imagery might play in the healing process, tribal sha-

mans, the world's first psychoneuroimmunologists, were guiding the ill on ritual journeys to the realms of the gods, ancestors, and disease-spirits, yoking the psyche's great powers to the task of getting well again.

Among the hallmarks of what anthropologists call the "shamanic initiatory crisis" is often a period of affliction. From St. Francis to Black Elk to Gopi Krishna, history abounds with stories of shamans and saints whose illumination seemed to go hand in hand with sickness.

The connection between illness and consciousness change does not require strictly mystical explanations. Disease, like any severe crisis, may cause even the most entrenched strategies for living, from work to relationships, to break down. Illness strikes at the core of normal identity (Freud once remarked, "The ego is first and foremost a body-ego"), sometimes catalyzing the breakthrough of deeper aspects of the personality. Symptoms may force our attention in unaccustomed directions, toward areas of the body that contain particular emotional significance. Sometimes the organ that becomes sick has borne the brunt of persistent stress, inner conflict, or festering life issues, its functions either overstimulated or suppressed. Mahatma Gandhi's former physician, Dr. Chandra Sharma, was led to suggest that "an illness . . . is a self-representation of a human being at a stage at which something is demanded of him for the sake of experience."

In addition, certain forms of treatment—for example, drug therapy—can cause altered states of consciousness. A friend undergoing experimental interferon treatment for hepatitis was surprised when the hospital release form listed the possibility that the drug would induce "abnormal dreaming." Physical disorders can trigger secretions that cause everything from depression to ecstasy. There also may be a psychobiology of crisis itself which accounts for the wealth of testimony linking illness and transformation. Some theorists maintain that the stress of illness, accident, or shock induces a hypnosis-like state in which new mental and emotional patterns—even changes in brain function—may be imprinted on the personality.[4]

The shaman's practices of fasting, marathon dancing, piercing the flesh, even chopping off a finger to induce visions, no doubt came from observations by these "technicians of the sacred" that physical injury can trigger altered states of consciousness. Writing about such rituals, the Canadian psychologist Dr. Raymond Prince noted that severe physical stress can "generate appropriate endorphins or other neuroendocrines in such quantities that an unprecedented feeling of cosmic peace and tranquillity is experienced."

These biological substances even may have a healing function. It recently has been found that the release of endorphins not only produces euphoria and pain analgesia, but enhances the immune system.[5] Conversely, immune system components such as white blood cells secrete molecules identical to the pituitary hormones,[6] which also affect emotions. Thinking out loud at a recent conference, Candace Pert hypothesized that peptide T, a neurohormone that prevents AIDS molecules from binding to cell receptor sites, also might be associated with emotions such as love. "We may soon figure out," she said, "exactly which molecules form the bridge between feelings and healing."

FEELING AND HEALING

It now seems to me that in the swirling miasms of my illness, I must have stumbled onto Pert's bridge. In the months following my surgery, I found myself obsessed by the thought of finding others who had traveled yet further, who might be able to tell me what lay on the other side.

I had often heard about so-called healing miracles around the offices of *New Age Journal*, though when it came my turn, the body's self-healing ability suddenly seemed only a chimera—fabulous, enchanting, but as unreal as a paper moon. Reports of patients who get well after the doctor does everything but pronounce them dead have a ring of wistful folklore, particularly when one's own life seems to hang in the balance.

But there are documented examples of such mystifying cures, though they are exceedingly uncommon. One of the first studies (published in 1966) that officially acknowledged the existence of spontaneous cancer remission pegged its frequency at only one case in 100,000.[7] Other writers, however, have speculated that there may be anywhere from ten to a hundred times this number, but that doctors' "reluctance . . . to report cases of apparent regression for which there is no obvious scientific explanation" keeps them from exposing such findings to public scrutiny.[8] In addition, a certain number of "noncompliant patients" walk out on conventional medicine and disappear off the charts—their cures, if indeed they take place, never statistically tracked.

California's Institute for Noetic Sciences has painstakingly compiled some 3,500 references to medically documented cases of remission.[9] They are *rara avis*, to be sure: The co-author, after himself pursuing both conventional and unconventional treatment, died of cancer a year before the study's publication. And a sizeable percentage of spontaneous remissions are years later followed by relapse. But even a single case of remission is the "one white crow" that disproves the thesis that all crows are black. The study, collected from eight hundred medical journals in twenty languages, implies that such quiet, astonishing events may happen more often than we suspect.

When I first began my search—writing letters to holistic doctors, placing ads in health periodicals, putting out the word through my own network of colleagues and friends—I was driven to seek those with "amazing stories," people whose physical recoveries from serious disease were inexplicable. I was sure I would turn up many such instances of entirely nonmedical "miracles." I did not. In our society, the M.D. is our remedy of first resort. Only a handful of the patients referred to me as unusual cures had not undergone at least some conventional treatment, even if that treatment had been finally deemed unsuccessful.

Gradually, I found myself veering away from what was beginning to seem a quixotic pursuit. It dawned on me that what I wanted most to explore was what had baffled me about my own journey: How could disease become a catalyst for profound inner experience? Had the luminosity I had sensed in my illness been merely the delirium of the shipwrecked, mistaking a lambent bit of moon on a dark sea for a white dot of sail? Or was there some way that illness might paradoxically, even heretically, contain its own potential for wholeness?

When, in my dreams, disease had seemed to present itself not just as a marauding destroyer but also as an agent of change, it had seemed absurd, perfidious, a wolf talking its way into the sheepfold. Illness *is* monstrous; it exacts a terrible toll. Two out of three cancer patients never make the five-year mark, a statistic that has stood for fifty years. And the implacable fatality of AIDS can make the cancer victim seem fortunate.

I was surprised, then, when I began to bump into other people who felt as I had about their own illnesses. Many told me almost furtively how their disease had come to represent, as one put it, "a stuckness," something once vital within them that had frozen in place like an old lava flow. Sickness had confronted them with long-tormenting inner demons and unsuspected inner resources. For some, it had been the catalyst that caused them to virtually overturn their lives, switching established careers or leaving long-term relationships. Disease became for them a nonnegotiable demand; an annunciation saying, "There is no time but now; no you but your truest, deepest self. Anything less than the total embrace of life is no longer acceptable."

I realized that what intrigued me most, what I had to understand for my *own* further healing, was how people not only make unexpected progress against illness, but, implausibly, also heal their lives.

MAKING MEANING OUT OF ILLNESS

I learned that most of those who had surpassed their prognoses—securing an abatement of symptoms, the return of function, or a remission that exceeded medical expectations—felt that their attitudes and insights had been integral to their healing process. Perhaps not surprisingly, many were victims of diseases involving the immune system, which is now known to be connected, hipbone to thighbone, with the brain's cognitive and emotional functions.

But I had no way of confirming that these people's inner lives were *the* X factor in their unusual recoveries. Though it seemed possible that their personal experiences might have affected the course of disease, perhaps each was possessed of some special, not-yet-measurable physiological trait. Or perhaps they had, unknown to themselves or their physicians, less virulent varieties of their diseases. (Recent genetic mapping has revealed previously undetected biological differences between more and less invasive breast tumors, a factor that may account for differing recovery rates. The same holds true for certain forms of bladder, lung, and prostate cancers and leukemias.[10]) In addition, most of these former patients had tried therapies like acupuncture, herbs, dietary regimens, or nontraditional medications known to augment immune function or to have antitumoral, antibiotic, or other pharmacological effects.

All in all, any number of unique factors—genetic inheritance, general systemic health, social milieu, exposure and sensitivity to environmental pollutants, nutritional habits, profession, even some quirk in their psychoneuroimmunological wiring—might have proved crucial to their recovery. The problem once again turns upon the inseparability of mind from body, or healing from life.

What, if anything, did these people have in common? Certainly there was no pattern in their choice of medicines, which might have included carrot juice and chemo, psychotherapy and psychic healing, visualization and vincristine. Or in their methods—some had conventional treatment, some used "complementary therapies," and some had explored the further shores of shamanic or spiritual healing.

But each person, some readily, some reluctantly, wound up doing the opposite of what sick people are supposed to do: Rather than simply try to "get back to normal," they embarked, at the most inauspicious time, on a voyage of self-discovery. They managed to cling instinctively to the circumnavigator's faith that the only way home was forward, into the round, unknown world of the self.

What was most striking to me was their willingness to encounter their disease directly, to own it, explore it, grapple with it, speak with it. They decided, as the neurologist Oliver Sacks has written, that "our health is *ours;* our diseases are *ours;* our reactions are *ours*— no less than our minds or our faces . . . expressions of our nature, our living, our being here."[11]

Their stories are not about the white whisper of hospital sheets, the stalactite drip of i.v. units, the murmur of helpless loved ones. They are about a desperate bursting forth of life, the bloody blossoming of hope; about the grunt-work of healing, its crushing tedium, its infinitesimal triumphs; about protocol and ritual, gnosis and diagnosis, technology and poetry. Their experiences provide examples of the many ways people search not only for wellness, but for meaning.

WHAT HEALS?

The meaning some people drew from even the most terrible experiences coincided so closely with various metaphysical doctrines that I began to wonder if it was just the circles I traveled in. Indeed, many *had* come into contact with a subculture of support groups, healing centers, and inspirational tapes and literature that draws heavily on the work of various exponents of new age thought.

But others, like the former brawling, gun-collecting fire chief who told me he had "the inner life of a potato" before healing himself of prostate cancer, did not remotely fit this profile. His quest inward seemingly had arisen *sui generis;* he had intuitively recognized, he told me, that his healing would require, above all, "a deep kindness."

I wondered at what initially struck me almost as pollyannaism in some of these people who still held visas to Hades—butterfly decals plastered on shower doors and fridges (the fire chief), teddy bears propped up on throw-pillows, twinkling electronic music cycling on the CD. But I remembered how I found Pachelbel's Canon, a bit of musical marzipan that has become the national anthem of the self-help movement, uplifting and unutterably poignant when I was ill. Was it my body speaking, the way plants have been shown to grow measurably more robust when irrigated with the music of Mozart than when blasted with rock 'n' roll? Was there something in the ailing bodymind that intuitively sought harmony, even if—in a society bereft of healing icons and rituals—it had to be found in the pop culture cut-out bins?

There *is* some evidence that "positive" emotions like hope correlate with the release of specific biochemicals that in themselves may have specific effects on tissues and diseases.[12] Such observations have led many proponents of self-healing to label traditional virtues like joy and love as healing, and so-called "spiritual failings" like anger and despair as disease-enhancing.

Such philosophical stances can come to resemble what psychologist William James once called "the religion of healthy-mindedness," a philosophy popularized in the early part of this century. According to this doctrine, the only healthy thoughts were, *a priori*, happy thoughts. The "mind-cure" adherents, James wrote, seemed "fatally forbidden to linger over the darker aspects of the universe." He warned that such forced optimism can become a "quasi-pathological" state, wherein "the capacity for even a transient sadness seems cut off . . . by a kind of congenital anesthesia."

And emotional anesthesia is the very antipode of the healing path, according to many of the former patients I spoke with. For them, getting in touch with so-called negative feelings was, to their surprise, a first gateway to greater aliveness. "I'd felt this 'unacceptable anger' toward my whole family for years," one said. "I'm sure that keeping the lid on it, pretending it wasn't there, was *terrible* for my immune system."

Disease created for some a moment that arrives all too infrequently in most lives: when the prime directive was to end compromise and concealment, to become authoritatively, painfully, even crazily the person they really were. If there was one path to health, it seemed closest in spirit to the words of a Japanese shaman: "Healing means to become your real self." The quest for wellness, these travelers told me, was intimately entwined with their search for personal authenticity. Though virtually all had rediscovered the power of "good" feelings and attitudes—joy, forgiveness, faith, trust, love—they had to draw them up deliberately, hand over hand, from their own deep and often dark wells.

I learned that skirting this "dark well" may even be medically counterproductive. In one study, patients who reported suppressing their anger had significantly higher levels of serum immunoglobulin A, a chemical that suppresses immune cell function. Another study has shown that women with metastatic breast disease who exhibited the lowest levels of hostility and the most upbeat mood survived for the *shortest* time. Such patients, writes the psychologist Jeanne Achterberg, "seem bewildered when the same virtues that succeeded for them in the past—kindness, graciousness, a giving constitution, a cheerful outlook—don't work in the struggle against disease."[13]

Achterberg notes, by contrast, that a straw poll she conducted at two institutions for the criminally insane revealed that the inmates, many of whom had committed heinous crimes, had been "unusually protected from cancer, despite poor health habits, such as heavy smoking." Similarly, she observed, the percentage of deaths from cancer for the mentally handicapped was only about 4 percent, compared to 15 to 18 percent in the normal population. As individuals approach normal intelligence, their cancer rates also go up.[14] Is it because the retarded have less frictive inner wheelspinning, more uncomplicated emotional responses, than the "normal" citizen? Does the violent acting-out of the criminally insane mitigate the physiologically corrosive harboring of anger? Does the expression of powerful emotions, even dangerous ones, create a state of autonomic arousal that boosts immune function?

With mind-body science still in its infancy, hypotheses to explain such strange observations are tenuous. All we can conclude for now, Achterberg writes, is that "there is clearly more than one route for the mind to influence the immune system, and not all pathways are pretty."[15]

THE VARIETIES OF HEALING EXPERIENCE

This book is an exploration of pathways, not a repair manual. In *Zen and the Art of Motorcycle Maintenance*, Robert Pirsig noted that even when talking about how to fix something as prosaic as a motorcycle, it was best to tiptoe around specific recommendations. "The chances are overwhelming," he wrote, "that it won't be your make and model and the information will be not only useless but dangerous, since information that fixes one model can sometimes wreck another."

Healing is idiosyncratic at best, a power-sharing arrangement between an individual's physiology, pathology, psyche, emotional history, social context, medicines, healers, and gods. Some people I talked with went off on a quest, some stayed put, tending their own gardens; some found healing within the family, some by escaping it; some healings were dramatic, others gradual. There were different admixtures of Hippocrates's formula, "lysis and crisis," the slow abatement of symptoms or the sudden "kill-or-cure" crescendo. My informants' own definitions of healing changed and evolved over time. For one person, healing was a near-miraculous recovery from an intractable condition. For another, it was finding a personal meaning in an affliction. For yet another, it was ignoring a disability through sheer force of will, like a paraplegic I heard about who had climbed to the summit of Mount Capitan.

I even came to believe it possible that, as one patient insisted, "there are greater things than physical healing. If you look no further than getting rid of what's wrong, you may never deal with what's brought your life to a standstill. The thing you want to heal from may be the very thing you need to focus on in order to learn."

THE SOUL APPROACH

The modern medical strategy is to treat symptoms rather than causes, to fix up the body with as little conscious participation from the patient as possible. The doctor's usual mandate, when confronted with an organism broken beneath the invisible hammer blows of life, is to patch it up and return it to the anvil.

In traditional cultures, by contrast, illness is thought to burst forth from a constellation of disturbed relationships—between body and soul, and between the individual and his family, his ancestors, his community, and the invisible realms—all of which must come into a fresh, dynamic balance to effect the cure. To heal one person, a tribe might participate in a ritual dance, not only providing the patient with emotional support, but acknowledging illness as a complex problem of the entire group.

Often, the patient (or the shaman as her surrogate) had to embark on an Otherworld journey, grappling with disease on a spiritual, emotional, social, and even cosmological level. As Mohawk elder Ernie Benedict once told an anthropologist, "The White Doctor's medicines tend to be very mechanical. The person is repaired but he is not better than he was before." However, Benedict added, "it is possible in the Indian way to be a better person after going through a sickness followed by the proper medicine."[16] Here, the point of getting well is not necessarily to "go back to normal," but to reclaim the soul.

Many tribal societies believe there is a different soul for each strand in life's web—from the soul of our ancestors, to the "bush soul" that ties us to nature; to the part that strikes a spark between us and the cosmos. The Zinacanteco Indians of Mexico's Chiapas highlands believe the soul is composed of thirteen parts, each representing an aspect of life. All must be healthy for the person to be well. If one or more is lost, it must be retrieved through a healing ceremony.[17] Such ancient models of wellness call not just for eliminating our symptoms, but for a thoroughgoing regeneration.

Such metaphors for health speak an inclusive language that our new "biopsychosocial" medicine is learning only haltingly to once again pronounce. Healing literally means wholeness (*holy* and *heal* both derive from the Anglo-Saxon *haelen*, meaning "whole"), with all that implies: bringing the rejected and discarded into the circle; listening with the inward ear for those parts that have been silenced; seeking a deeper, more accurate, more creative engagement with the world around us. Indeed, for some patients, this wider quest may be the only arena of significant action.

But what exactly do we *mean* by healing? Did the woman who felt she had "beaten" her breast cancer and the man who believed he had "beaten" his AIDS—both of whom died over the seven-year period I was writing this book—fail to be "healed"? Or did those who suffered relapses or recurrences? Although they had not banished suffering or lived out their threescore and ten, it seemed to me they had found in the midst of illness—even perhaps *through* illness—a genuine path of healing.

In this light, we might consider several definitions of healing:

Sensitization: Healing implies a restoration of communication with ourselves. According to cardiologist Dr. James Lynch, disease often results when patients "cannot feel in their own bodies" and become "deaf to the language of their own hearts." When we ignore persistent but often subtle messages from within ourselves, we become numb to feedback, in the same way a smoker's lungs no longer cry out in alarm the way they did when he took his first drag from a friend's cigarette. Everything from an unhealthy diet to unsafe sex may follow a loss of inner cues. The first step in healing may be the reestablishment of our lines of "internal communication."

Acceptance of pain: Healing often requires we come to terms with seemingly intolerable truths. A number of patients even noted that at the point when they stopped psychologically resisting their illness—when they "surrendered"—their symptoms began to mysteriously diminish. Steve and Ondrea Levine, a couple who work extensively with terminally ill patients, have the impression that those who tend to heal display "a willingness, a certain nonresistance" to their pain. They are, in the Levines' words, "*with* their illness, touching it deeply, examining it, meeting it with tenderness—me with my pain," rather than being "at their illnesses, their tumors, with a stick—'me against the pain.'"

Finding meaning: Although insisting that illness must "mean something" may seem a form of escapism, there may be a "biology of meaning" that affects the healing process. For example, World War II soldiers who knew their injuries would cause them to be sent home from the battlefield were found to require lesser dosages of painkiller—because, in effect, their wounds *meant* something. The very act of "re-framing" their condition in a different light had apparent physical effects. Healing means, says one Jungian scholar, "the illness is creatively reshaped by successfully combatting it and coordinating it meaningfully into the totality of the patient's life . . . Only then will danger of a relapse be avoided . . . The illness must yield a meaning."[18]

Restoration of balance: According to the Kung bushmen of the Kalahari, we are all born with "seeds" of disease. When our lives fall out of harmony, these seeds find fertile ground. Disease, then, is not just a physical "thing," but a *relationship* between things. Getting well may be less a matter of fighting illness than of counterbalancing it with the healthy aspects of our lives.

Willingness to change: Whatever no longer flows, wrote Milton, "sickens into a muddy pool." All life is constant adaptation. Moving beyond habitual patterns of thinking and feeling is a biological event. Simple changes in life-style can alter the progression even of dire diseases. Dr. Luc Montagnier, the codiscoverer of the AIDS virus, notes that patients who begin to sleep regularly at night and avoid alcohol, coffee, and tobacco may be able to "resist the disease for ten to fifteen years. By then we might have found an effective therapy."

Of course, we may experience the disappearance of symptoms without finding inner meaning. We may experience spiritual growth without being physically healed. (A recent study by Dr. Bernie Siegel of patients who followed self-transformative strategies did not show an increase in breast cancer survival.) Not every disease has psycho-emotional roots, or can be ameliorated through attitudinal change.

If I have learned anything from my own and others' journeys, it is that healing may mean forsaking, once and for all, the misap-prehension that sees good only in what aggrandizes us, beauty only in what is unblemished, wholeness only in what is intact. People who have been through illness's dark passage can occasionally give us a glimpse not only of what it is like to become whole, but of what it is to be fully human.

❧ 2 ❧
THE HEALING PATH:
MAPS FOR THE JOURNEY

Healing proceeds from the depths to the heights.

—CARL JUNG

THE SWISS PSYCHIATRIST Carl Jung discovered a key to healing in a mental institution in Zurich. Through careful, deeply feeling observations of the imprisoned mad, he realized, as one Jung biographer put it, that "every personality had a story. Derangement happened when the story was denied. To heal, the patient had to rediscover his story."

Jung's great contribution was to show how we each partake, wittingly or unwittingly, in the eternal human quest for wholeness. Each of our life stories, no matter how mundane, is a tale of spiritual growth embraced or denied. Beneath the surfaces of everyday awareness, a larger and more inclusive self is ever pressing for realization. Ironically, even inconveniently, it is in moments of deepest crisis that this self may become most insistent, and its story most demanding of realization.

But the crisis of disease seems to us less a part of our story than a desecration of it—indeed, of the act of storytelling itself, as if the book had been suddenly slammed shut, the film wrenched from its sprocket, the play halted in midscene by a theater-fire. In the awful, widening abyss between fear and hope, we long for progress to be restored, for our familiar narrative to resume after a brief interruption.

"Oh, that you would hide me," cries the Biblical Job, suddenly crushed down like a hail-struck blade of grass, "and keep me sheltered till your wrath is past; would fix a time for me, and then remember me!" Like all of us when confronted with illness, Job wants nothing so much as to be transported back to solid ground, where he might banish all suspicion of mortal frailty. Instead, sliding toward what seem to be the gates of Hell, he is, unknowingly, crossing the healing threshold.

Job's story is perhaps the most archetypal of all Western disease narratives. It is usually interpreted as a fable of stoic faith in the face of the incomprehensible Divine, a case of bad things happening to good people. But closer examination reveals a deeper structure, the classic, sequenced ordeal of the shaman, the saint, or the mythic hero: a grave crisis leading to a terrifying departure from ordinary life, a forced confrontation with the profoundest aspects of the psyche, and then, in Joseph Campbell's words, "a penetration to some source of power and a life-enhancing return." Job's odyssey, in the formulation of poet William Blake, describes a series of progressive stages: "Innocence, Experience, Revolution, the Dark Night, and the New Life."

I was surprised to notice how closely my own story-line and those of others resembled the wheeling movement of this ageless cycle. Though the pilgrims were very different, our pilgrimages also seemed to echo other classic itineraries of the spirit: St. John's dark night of the soul; the "metanoiac voyages" (*meta* means "change," *nous* "consciousness") of survivors of madness;[1] Jung's path of "individuation"; Joseph Campbell's "hero's journey"; the shaman's "initiatory crisis"; and other models of breakdown and renewal of the self.

Of course, not all people who become ill have transformative experiences. Suffering is more often *de*formative. Yet illness cannot help but be an initiation of sorts, like any event that yanks us from the familiar, confronts us with forces beyond our control, and sets us upon a course we cannot predict. It marks a dividing line between what we have been and what we may yet become. Observes Jungian analyst John Sanford, "Sometimes an illness, psychological or physical, proves upon closer scrutiny to be an invitation to become a whole person."

But it is not an invitation that makes logical sense: Deficiency is not wholeness. Regress is not progress. A broken glass can hold no fresh water. How can we begin a journey when we can barely walk? Yet it cannot be accidental that in many myths of initiation, the journey is precipitated by an injury to the foot or leg, that part of the body symbolizing our outward progress through life. The centaur Chiron, teacher of the Greek healing god Asklepius, the angel-wrestling Jacob of the Bible, the Fisher King in the story of Perceval—all suffered such wounds, which at once impeded their physical momentum and accelerated their spiritual quest. These mysterious paradoxes of wounding and healing are the sustaining motifs of myths throughout history.

HEALING STORIES

Such myths are not fairy tales, but travelers' tales. Job's story can be seen as a veritable map of the healing path. It begins with a series of devastating personal reversals: the loss of his children, the destruction of his fortune, the tragic wreckage of a good life. These material privations are followed by his physical collapse, much as modern studies have shown that cancer and other immune system–related diseases are frequently preceded by the death of loved ones, the loss of career, or other emotional traumas. The Bible portrays Job's illness (we are told only that it manifests as boils) as the result of God's removing His "protection," allowing Satan to lay a hand upon Job's flesh. This, too, seems a surprisingly modern notion: It is a cornerstone of psychoneuroimmunology (PNI) that a lowering of the body's defenses lets down the drawbridge for pathological invasion.

Job's illness banishes him from the social realm in which he had occupied so exalted a place. Deserted by his friends who not-so-subtly castigate him, Job must travel from despair to acceptance, insight, and finally a direct encounter with a greater spiritual reality, before he returns to the community bearing gifts of wisdom.

Perhaps the story of Job often seems opaque to us because our society has so thoroughly lost the formal myths that in traditional cultures are guideposts to the healing path. Myths contain a level of "truth" that the particulars of case-studies cannot compass. They reveal, beneath the incidentals of character and plot, a deep-woven narrative thread: that of the growth of the psyche. They are a form of shared observation of what happens to people *in extremis,* a way to locate ourselves within an archetypal drama propelled by the secret logic of human development. Fiction instructors often stress to first-time students that all stories that "work," whether exalted myths or trashy potboilers, have this same elemental structure: the journey of a main character from innocence through crisis and loss to hard-won self-knowledge.

Some of our most cherished modern tales are unfoldings of this same healing process. Such seasonal chestnuts as the film version of Dickens's *A Christmas Carol* and Frank Capra's *It's a Wonderful Life* (both broadcast at winter solstice, a time associated in pagan cultures with life's perilous passage into the Underworld), or *The Wizard of Oz* (shown at spring solstice, the time of rebirth), come close to substituting, in our culture, for a collective ritual drama of renewal. If we look intently, they, too, stand revealed as clear formulations of the journey through disintegration to wholeness.

In each tale, we meet the central character in the throes of a **life crisis.** In *It's a Wonderful Life,* George Bailey, husband, father, and community pillar, faces the awful crash of the family savings-and-loan bank into which he has poured his adult life. In *The Wizard of Oz,* young Dorothy's wicked neighbor threatens to take away her dog, Toto (Latin for "all"), who in Frank Baum's original book is her single source of joy in a drab world. Ebenezer Scrooge in *A Christmas Carol* is trapped in an emotionally miserly life that cannot proceed a step further without radical change—an ultimatum delivered by the chain-rattling ghost of Marley, the **herald of the journey.** (Similarly, in many tribal cultures, a vision of a dead relative or friend signals an impending initiatory crisis.)

Each protagonist in these perennial modern tales is also facing a grave **health crisis.** Dorothy has been knocked comatose by debris from a Kansas twister. George Bailey, in *It's a Wonderful Life,* is in the middle of a suicide attempt. The aged Scrooge is faced, unbeknownst to himself, with onrushing natural death. Each crucial juncture is also a **spiritual crisis.** The characters have reached a point in their psychic lives when they must surpass the old limitations that hinder their next stage of growth. George has never reconciled his exalted youthful ambitions with what seems to him a bean-counting banker's existence. Dorothy, in the MGM film, is an adolescent about to leave the charmed circle of childhood forever (while the Dorothy of Baum's book is trapped with two dour, near-loveless stepparents in a gray Midwestern wasteland). The penny-pinching Scrooge has interred his capacity for love and joy in a sepulcher of his own making.

Each narrative begins at the point when the lead character is most mired in personal defeat—the mythic point of embarkation. At first the journeyers try to deny what is happening to them: Scrooge tells himself the hectoring spirits are only "an undigested bit of suet," and then, in a last-ditch gambit of **denial,** tries to summon a constable to toss them out. This stage, which Joseph Campbell refers to as "the refusal of the call," is followed by the "hero's" **despair** at his or her seemingly dead-end predicament. "As a cloud dissolves and vanishes," Job laments, "so he who goes down to the nether world shall come up no more."

But as Dostoevsky observed, "Suffering is the origin of consciousness." The journey proper has begun, inevitably spiraling inward, toward an **encounter with the psyche.** The interior world boldly asserts its sovereignty, plunging the journeyer into what native peoples call a **vision quest.** Dorothy's very arrival in Oz kills the Witch of the East, the direction of sunrise and waking life. Her path then leads west, toward sunset and the dream realm of the unconscious. Job finds himself beset by nightmares—"With dreams upon my bed Thou scarest me, and affrightest me with Visions"—while Scrooge tries to hide beneath his bedsheets from the relentless night-specters who drag him toward self-awareness.

Each character is shocked to find that the psyche, whose existence they had barely suspected, is vibrantly and inescapably *alive,* inhabited by strange creatures whose agenda seems independent of their conscious will. Speaking in part from his personal experience of crisis and disease, Carl Jung describes this stage as "the recognition that the psyche is self-moving, that it is something genuine . . . [Y]ou are not living alone in your own room, there are spooks about that play havoc with your realities, and that is the end of your monarchy."

The monarchy in this case is that of our normally singular sense of identity, the unwavering perch from which we survey the landscape of daily life. Suddenly the ordinary self is thrust into what Jungian psychologist John Sanford calls the "soulscape," a place where "the dream ego is never more significant than any other figure." Each character is humbled to find that their previously viable self-adaptation, the persona they had presented to the world, no longer applies: Who they thought they were turns out to be only one aspect of the great multiplicity of the Self.

The result is a dizzying sense of **identity loss.** In response to George Bailey's panicked question, "Well, who am I, then?" his guardian angel, Clarence, answers, "You're nobody. You have no identity. You were never born." Similarly, Job, bereft of the accumulated trappings of normal life, cries out, "Why did I not perish at birth, come forth from the womb and expire?" The journeyers must relinquish the old self in exchange for what seems a tragic diminution. They are forced to start upon a new path—from scratch, as it were, following a set of as-yet unknown directives.

This paring away extends to the world of others, creating a condition of **social separation.** Job, whose identity, like Scrooge's and George's, is based largely on outer prestige ("the greatest of all the men in the East"), now finds that even those he would "rank with the dogs of my flock . . . do not hesitate to spit in my face." George Bailey's parallel-universe fellow citizens—bartenders, cabbies, cops, the town's once-respectful "little people"—revile him, literally tossing him out on the street. Dorothy finds herself marooned in a surreal landscape, light-years from Kansas, consorting with homeless, outcast creatures. The spirits show Scrooge that his supposedly loyal and admiring colleagues are toadies and cynical connivers. As the ill often discover, beneath the placid surfaces of family and community may lie unresolved and threatening contradictions.

Although the task of negotiating the journey's pitfalls and possibilities ultimately rests with the travelers themselves, they receive unexpected guidance from a **helper,** whose function it is to point out the transformative potential of their catastrophe. The angel Clarence tells George Bailey that his agonizing erasure from accustomed life is secretly "a wonderful opportunity," a final chance to affirm his unique human worth. Scrooge's intrusive spirits replay before his reluctant eyes the long-running tragedy of his life, but they also reveal its still-inhering potential. The Good Witch and the Wizard guide Dorothy and her wounded companions on a path that forces them to draw upon all their inner resources. The helper does not wield the wand that miraculously heals the journeyers, but furnishes them with a sturdy wooden staff to lean on. He or she provides both support and propulsion, pointing to powers they unknowingly already possess.

But to recover their full healing potential, the characters must also uncover the **roots of their predicament.** George Bailey must own up to his well-concealed but heart-devouring resentments over the lost dreams of his youth. The Spirit of Christmas Past shows Scrooge that what by ego's reckoning was an unbroken saga of entrepreneurial triumph was really a pitiable, headlong, and near-terminal flight from love.

At the same time, each character begins to find within him- or herself surprising powers of renewal. The long-buried roots of the crisis, though painful to reveal, are also a primal source of life. By reexperiencing the suffering of the past, the journeyers reawaken to their deeper emotional capacity. Gazing upon the scenes of his childhood, Scrooge experiences both tears of grief and the stirrings of a long-immured joy. He begins his own **rediscovery of aliveness.**

But before the dawn comes the dark. None can escape a shattering **confrontation with death.** The final Spirit reduces Scrooge to a trembling supplicant before his own chiseled tomb. Pursued by the citizens of his shadow-town, George must run despairing for his very life. Job sits in hopeless dejection upon a dungheap. Dorothy's dear friends are smashed, burned, and dismembered by the witch's cruel minions. But these bleak crossroads are also **turning points,** moments of relinquishing an outworn shell. Medieval alchemists called such a stage the *solutio,* wherein the limited self is dissolved as a prelude to a greater synthesis of being. Out of the abyss, a new individuality—or a more creative organization of the old one— begins to emerge. A *metanoia,* or **change of heart,** has been alchemically produced within the very crucible of destruction.

Finally, the characters **return to the world** inwardly changed. Had they made the journey but failed to reclaim their wholeness, it would have been a tragic loss not simply for the self—which, deprived of all hope of integration, could only be impelled toward further decay—but also for society, whose own salvation secretly depends on the healing of the individual.

Even so, the journeyers do not merely return to the place where they began, for they, and normal life itself, have been profoundly altered. Scrooge, restored to the human community as a dispenser of boons, a Victorian version of a **wounded healer,** literally shouts the tidings of his new life from the rooftops. George Bailey is embraced by family and friends, and even showered with fortune (as was Job: "Every man also gave him a piece of money, and everyone an earring of gold"). The power that the evil Mr. Potter wielded over George's town, and over his psyche, is broken. In the book *The Wizard of Oz,* the characters are not only given their long-sought heart, brains, and courage, but are made rulers of kingdoms, the symbolic station of those who have attained greater wholeness.

Not only has healing taken place, but profound and enduring transformation. The psychologist John Sanford writes, "We can never simply return to the condition in which we were before our crisis, without the scope of our personality being reduced." Because the journeyers have shed the encrustations that shielded them from deeper experience, their lives now take on extraordinary coloration. They have become, in effect, **"weller than well,"** for they have obtained something that transcends mere physical health. The Tin

Woodman's new heart is not merely a substitute for the old one, but "a kinder and more tender heart than the one he had owned when he was made of flesh."

THE TIN WOODMAN

The themes of healing and spiritual quest in *The Wizard of Oz* are not incidental but, I would suggest, woven into its very fabric. Its author, L. Frank Baum, had suffered bouts of serious illness since childhood. He had also made a study of Buddhism and Theosophy (whose basic tenet, he wrote, was that "God is Nature, and Nature God"), and believed in reincarnation and its corollary, *karma:* the doctrine that life's purpose is spiritual evolution. Some commentators have pointed out that the Oz books' cosmology so closely parallels that of sixteenth-century Swiss philosopher-physician Paracelsus that Baum may well have been influenced by this eccentric medical pioneer, who wrote eloquently of the influence of the mind upon the body. And the critic and mathematician Martin Gardner has hazarded that the name for the mythical Land of Oz came not, as many accounts have it, from the author's felicitous glance at the O–Z drawer of a file cabinet, but from the "Land of Uz," the home of Job.[2]

It is not farfetched to see Baum's tale as a beautiful allegory for the path of healing. Because I will refer to it so often throughout this book, it might be useful to pause for a moment to examine it more closely:

When Dorothy is snatched up in a whirlwind and deposited in Oz, she encounters a trio of wounded creatures who might be seen as representating an as-yet undeveloped totalilty of being: mind (the Scarecrow), body (the Cowardly Lion), and soul (the Tin Woodman, in search of a heart). All must be healed before the path can come full circle. The Cowardly Lion, for example, has an aggressive, blustery act at complete odds with his inner self—a classic "Type A personality," to whom the Tin Woodman actually suggests, "Perhaps you have heart disease." But it is upon the "heartless" Tin Woodman that Baum has lavished the most poignant narrative care. His creation even shared his own ailments: Baum had a defective heart that left him a semi-invalid throughout childhood, and he once, like the Tin Woodman, suffered a facial paralysis.

The Tin Woodman's pathological predicament is strikingly similar to a pattern I will refer to in coming chapters as the "disease-prone personality": a heavily armored outer persona and a commensurately deprived inner self; an investment of emotional energy outside the self that leaves a ringing hollowness within; and finally, a physical wound that paradoxically awakens the power of authentic being.

The Tin Woodman's personal history is that of a person who has placed all his emotional eggs in one basket. A solitary forester, he has decided he must marry "so that I might not become lonely." He comes to love, "with all my heart," a beautiful Munchkin girl. But she refuses to marry him until he has enough money to "build a better house for her." Feeling unworthy, he resolves to work ever harder to acquire the material things he thinks will secure her love and end his loneliness. But a wicked witch magically turns his somewhat desperate need for love into a self-destructive force, so that one day, "chopping away at my best . . . anxious to get the new house and my wife as soon as possible," the ax blade cuts off his leg. (Here again we see the mythical theme of the leg wound, symbolizing the forced curtailment of the outer life.)

The workaholic Tin Woodman, at this point still a man of flesh and blood, does not see this symptom as cause to slow down. Each time the Witch—who can be seen as not just an external pathogen, but his own lack of self-love—makes him lose a limb, he simply makes an appointment with the tinsmith to doctor up an artificial metallic replacement, then resumes his misguided efforts. The Tin Woodman, not the Witch, is his own worst enemy: He sacrifices his own being for a life of artificiality, trying to attain the love object he imagines will finally make him happy. He lops off in turn his legs, his arms, even his head, all prosthetically replaced with cold, hard metal so he can continue his self-defeating strategy. In a final blow, he literally splits himself in half—a divided self. The tinsmith-physician, who can offer only tools to repair his devastated body, cannot replace his heart.

Ironically, having put all his emotional energy into a labor of passion, the Tin Woodman has become deadened to feeling. "I lost all my love for the Munchkin girl, and did not care whether I married her or not." He has suffered what shamans say is the most serious illness of all: loss of soul.

But he mechanically goes on with his life, literally armored against bodily sensation, his feeling-life atrophied, yet competent and impervious in his tinny persona: "My body shone so brightly in the sun that I felt very proud of it, and it did not matter now if my axe slipped, for it could not cut me." Like Job, George Bailey, and Scrooge, he ascribes value only to his external accomplishments, forsaking his neglected inner life.

But the Tin Woodman's treadmill existence is interrupted by a symptom he cannot ignore: a sudden rainstorm, his own uncried tears falling upon him from without, rusting him where he stands. This "health crisis," a paralysis that stops him in his tracks, forces him at last to take stock: "It was a terrible thing to undergo, but during the year I stood there I had time to think that the greatest loss I had known was the loss of my heart."

This acute sense of loss impels him on an arduous journey. But only later, after he is literally torn apart (an almost universal theme in shamanic initiation as a necessary prelude to greater wholeness), does the Tin Woodman reclaim the soul-world without which life can have little meaning. He at last feels "rattling around in his breast" his "more tender heart." By story's end he has progressed from disease to greater aliveness, from a desperate, need-based existence to an identity based on hard-won authenticity.

BRIAN'S STORY

I vividly recalled the tale of the Tin Woodman when, several years ago, I met a journeyer named Brian Schultz. Brian's apartment in Somerville, Massachusetts—Cambridge's untrendy low-rent twin—was spartan: a black futon on the floor, a few chairs and cotton rugs, the walls decorated with a Chinese acupuncture chart of the body teeming with colorful "meridians," and a framed page from Matt Groening's book of cartoons *Childhood Is Hell*.

Brian was a pleasant-looking man with pale, carrot-colored hair, dressed in the grad student uniform of sandals, tan chinos, and a pin-striped Oxford shirt. But something in the intensity of the gaze behind his oversize hornrims, and the way he walked—a little stiff, his shoulders and torso blocky—suggested a harder knowledge of living.

During the 1970s, in his last semester of Stanford Law School, Brian Schultz's world had been engulfed in a personal holocaust: an obscure, excruciatingly painful degenerative joint disease called ankylosing spondylitis (AS). Overnight, the bright magna cum laude graduate with the world on a half-shell was transformed, by a dire magic worthy of the Witch of the West, into a shambling, pain-wracked semicripple.

No known cause, said his doctor.

No known cure, said another doctor.

These steroids will ease the pain, they all said. *We're sorry.*

Brian's prognosis bore a frightening resemblance to the Tin Woodman's "no-oilcan" predicament. In one extreme historical example of the disease's potential toll, a nineteenth-century victim named J. R. Bass was rendered completely immobile, displaying himself in the dime museums under the moniker "The Ossified Man." In the worst instances, sufferers are unable to move their jaws, a plight that used to mandate the extraction of the patient's teeth to permit nourishment. The ribs can become so immobile that the victim dies of asphyxiation.[3] Though Brian's case was less severe, his doctors warned that his disease could confine him to a wheelchair by his early thirties.

Brian used anti-inflammatory medicines and painkillers for a time, but the steady degeneration only seemed to get worse. The side effects of the medication were making his emotions whipsaw. Suspecting that his treatment was damaging his body's ability to get well, he decided, in what he called "a leap of desperation," to go off his medicines. He immediately experienced a terrifying increase in pain. He hurt unceasingly, and for years barely managed two or three hours of sleep at night. His ribcage collapsed to the point that he felt barely able to gasp enough air to stay alive.

"I had never known how exhausting, agonizing, and final pain could be," he told me. "It was like being strapped down on a table and tortured with icepicks. I was physically, emotionally, spiritually suffocating. I was buried alive." He laughed grimly. "I learned a lot about the architecture of hell."

But Brian clung to what he called a "fragile intuition," the feeling that he might be better off trying to accept his pain than numbing himself to it. He discovered, to his surprise, that "by letting go of a bit of control, I had in some small way transformed my struggle for health. Where before my desire had been to rid myself of my illness as if it were a foreign object, an invader, I now began to treat it as part of me that was calling out to be touched."

From this "tiny, tiny decision," he began to shed "the crushing weight of an entire lifetime of control, of avoidance of pain, of fear of suffering and the unknown. I decided to stop resisting," he told me, "and try to learn how to feel."

Brian began to experiment with unconventional treatments, eventually making regular visits to an acupuncturist and following a rigorous special diet. He noticed to his surprise a small but detectable improvement in his mobility. But he was shocked to discover that his physical progress seemed to open an unexpected floodgate of roiling emotion. Just as the Tin Woodman in *The Wizard of Oz* was rent apart at the very moment he drew nearest his destination, Brian's "despair grew even more intense. Anger and rage began boiling to the surface, and my fear and dread of living grew and grew until I thought daily of suicide. I realized then that my problem was not simply my physiology, but the suffering that had been buried in me since childhood. That was when I had first learned from my parents, from society at large, to suppress my own aliveness. Now, as I stopped blocking sensation, it all came rushing up."

Brian started seeing a psychotherapist who followed the theories of Wilhelm Reich, the influential Austrian psychiatrist who coined the term "body armor" to describe how unresolved emotional conflict can cause physiological blockage. In therapy, Brian set out to confront the traumas of an abusive childhood that had felt "like a concentration camp." He began to see how desperately he had tried to gain his parents' love, and bolster his self-image through academic achievement on "the lawyer track." For the first time in his life, he began to take emotional risks, trying to "pierce the armor" and make honest contact with other people. He felt, he said, "like an autistic kid saying his first words."

Remarkably, after nearly ten years on his journey of recovery, Brian has slowly eliminated his symptoms in what he calls "a complete regeneration." But more than that, he has also created a new life: He has become not the lawyer his parents had wanted him to be, but a licensed acupuncturist—in his words, a "wounded healer."

SURRENDERING TO THE WOUND

Brian's tale is not the happily-ever-after story, neatly packaged between gilt-leather covers, of a hero vanquishing a dragon. Though he has made an extraordinary recovery, he still struggles with deep-rooted psychological pain. His disease, he believes, resulted in part from the rigid defenses he had erected against emotional suffering. "As the defenses that were ossifying me fell away," he says, "the emotions that had literally 'scared me stiff' became available to deal with directly." Healing, as he sees it, is no less than a lifelong practice of vulnerability and openness.

The approach Brian took contradicts many of our notions about the struggle against illness. Medical critic Ivan Illich suggests our society has waged a "campaign against pain" ever since Descartes reduced the "living body experience to a mechanism that the soul could inspect. . . . In this context, it now seems rational to flee pain rather than to face it, even at the cost of giving up intense aliveness." Such an attitude, Illich writes, can only lead to a state of "anesthesia."[4]

In our usual schema, sickness can be seen only as implacably evil; we, the heroes, must be unswervingly good. We fear that to enter into any relationship with disease carries the danger of appeasement, of capitulation to a vicious enemy. To listen to illness, to ask if it might have something to say to us—if it might even be a *part* of us—risks sapping our will to fight for our lives.

Yet the combative attitude can work at cross-purposes to the healing process, as the psychologist Meredith Sabini has observed: "Often the reaction to the diagnosis of cancer is a fierce ossification of the defenses and a determination to fight the disease at any cost rather than be its 'victim.' The imagery surrounding cancer reveals much about this process. One does not simply have an illness, one 'fights the big C'; one does not simply die, one 'succumbs after a valiant battle.' "

From this standpoint, Sabini says, illness becomes "a frantic duel of opposites . . . a battle for selfhood." What is at stake is our freedom to maintain old strategies of existence without changing our relationship to body or psyche; our right—the right of the ego-self—to march ahead with habits, attitudes, and agendas intact. The critique is no less applicable to some new-age approaches—Dr. Larry Dossey calls them "Promethean formulas"—where self-help can stiffen into almost fetishistic exercises in self-control.

This stance, like any attempt to plant the flag of an invulnerable selfhood on life's ever-shifting ground, may be ultimately unworkable. John Sanford notes:

> We are all of us wounded people. There is no such thing as a person who is free from illness, incompleteness, and injury. Some of us can simply hide from our woundedness better than others. When we can no longer hide from our woundedness, we are ready for individuation.[5]

According to many of the patients I talked with, the battle to maintain the "old self" began to seem like one of the linchpins of illness, while surrender improbably became a doorway to recovery. Many said that simply acknowledging the limitations imposed by illness, rather than struggling incessantly against them, felt strangely healing. Carol Boss, an unexpectedly long-term survivor of terminal metastatic breast disease, told me, "We cancer folk are not just shepherds of our strengths, but the custodians of our frailties."

A patient who had suffered from chronic fatigue immune dysfunction syndrome (CFIDS) wrote in a recent issue of a national health magazine:

> I made no progress as long as I wished for my life to return to its prior "normal" state. Only when I realized that my previous life was devastated, and that I had to accept a life as a full-time sick person for an indeterminate length of time, did the progression of my illness begin to slow. When I surrendered the kind of control I was accustomed to having, I could begin to consider the possibility of living differently when I recovered. As I did that, helpful information and intuitions about better ways to feel, think, and relate began to flow toward me.[6]

Such a "letting-go" may even have measurable physiological consequences. One recent medical study noted that a noncombative attitude toward suffering—"a nonrestrictive approach to unpleasant affect"—seems to be associated with improvements in immune system functioning.[7] Another study, conducted at Adelphi University, found that "people who were hiding psychological distress even from themselves" had an elevated risk of heart disease.

Yujiro Ikemi, who wrote several papers on the spontaneous remission of cancer, notes that most instances of such dramatic healings seemed to be accompanied by a "positive acceptance" (as opposed to resignation) of their terrible circumstances. "In our experience," he wrote, "such an attitude toward illness may lead to the full activation of the patient's innate self-recuperative potentials."[8] Similarly, Dr. David Spiegel of Stanford, whose landmark 1989 study demonstrated that women with breast cancer in group therapy survived twice as long as those not in therapy, has suggested that calming the "fight-or-flight" response may liberate more of the body's resources to deal with disease.

But our natural tendency remains to fight against what pains us. We feel we have been expelled from the garden of homeostasis, our body subverted from a wondrous and obedient tool to an enemy agent, dragging us toward the depths. In a culture that celebrates surfaces, speed, and success, disease is an unwelcome, centripetal reminder. We try at all costs to resist our descent, because we believe that once we hit bottom, there will be no return.

PEERING INTO THE UNDERWORLD

Our fear is understandable. Illness is an awful summons, a hellish grinding between millstones. The road to healing has its own stations of the cross. John Studholme, a successful attorney with Stage IV (terminal) lymphoma who had a large tumor near his heart cavity, wrote a poem midway through his healing process:

> I had a universe in me
> in turmoil,
> blasting my guts apart,
> breaking my bones with a new planet in my chest
> I heard my ribs crack in the sky.
> My blood was black from the bolt.
> It left ashes in my heart
> It burned in my veins.
> No shelter from the terror
> of the old flesh and the pain.

His account calls to mind the initiatory agonies described by an Australian medicine man as the flesh of ordinary identity cracks away and the shamanic descent begins: "You will see your camp burning and the blood waters rising, and thunder, lightning and rain, the earth rocking, the hills moving, the waters whirling, and the trees which will stand swaying about. . . . You may see dead persons walking towards you, and you will hear their bones rattle." But, the man added, "if you hear and see these things without fear, you will never be frightened of anything."[9]

Though the idea that a sojourn in the Underworld also might gestate healing is common in traditional societies (anthropologist Joan Halifax calls it a "patterned course"), it strikes us as an alien and even a dangerous notion. Spirituality, particularly as repackaged for the new age, is often a confection of love and light, purified of pilgrimage and penance, of defeat and descent, of harrowing and humility. Nonetheless most journeyers I spoke with seemed to find that healing began precisely where country music lyrics always have insisted: *Deep. Down. Inside.* Or as the Taoists would have it, in *the low, the dark, and the small.* In the broken places.

CRISIS AND TRANSFORMATION

The broken places are a crossroads, containing the converging and diverging lines of our fate. In ancient times, crossroads were places of opportunity as well as the abode of destructive spirits. Hecate, the dark goddess of crossroads, was also, in her other mythic identification as Diana, the moon that sheds light on the night traveler's path. Similarly, crisis may bring with it a strange illumination.

The healing power of crisis is praised in the first aphorism of Hippocrates. At such moments, extraordinary physical resources may be mobilized, as in the apocryphal tale of the mother who, flooded with adrenaline, heaves a car off her pinioned child. Severe stress produces a hypnosislike state that may be the body's way of mobilizing its healing resources. The late Brendan O'Regan of the Institute for Noetic Sciences postulated the existence of a bodymind "healing system" that . . . doesn't manifest unless challenged. Maybe it's a system that can lie dormant until confronted with stress, trauma, disease or illness of some kind. If that [were] so, then it would explain why it just isn't an obvious part of ourselves.

Under crisis conditions, the brain itself may undergo changes. Brain-mapping pioneer Sir John Eccles postulated that in times of physiological stress, heightened electrical activity in the brain's synapses might create new psychological configurations.[10] Psychologist Ernest Rossi suggests that, conversely, any psychological crisis causes "a synthesis of new protein structures that could function as the biological basis of new behavior and phenomenal experience."[11]

Thus, at a juncture of greatest danger, we may come to terms with our ghosts, choose a new direction from a center of radiating spokes, and transform our lives irrespective of the ultimate physical course of the disease.

According to the shaman, transformation *itself* is healing. Though change may be the last thing we are interested in when we are ill— we wish to go back to the way we *were*—the most archetypal stories tell us that the path of healing leads not back whence we have come, but ahead, toward a new beginning. The map of such a route looks like the "open circle" of Zen Buddhism, which symbolizes both the path and its final goal:

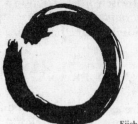

Eiichi Okamoto

Here the wound, the gap, is both entrance and egress. Though we move through the cycle, we do not return to where we first departed, but to a new place of openness and potential. At the end of the story, the person who arrives at the destination is not the same one who began the journey. "Man is born a Specter," said Blake, "and requires a new Selfhood constantly."

Or as a Chinese proverb expresses this same idea: "Changelessness is death." The healing journey is surrender to the process of change. Sometimes the things that go wrong in our lives, including physical illness, may happen when we have refused change at the point it was most called for: when we continue to perform a killing job, ignore the pain of a toxic relationship, perpetuate a self-harming habit; when we refuse to stop what we're doing even when we do not feel well doing it; when we neglect to ask ourselves, "What's the matter?" or turn a sympathetic ear to the reply.

Sometimes illness provides the terrible impetus toward an answer to our deepest existential questions—the ones which in normal life we are reluctant to pose. The story that disease tells, if we listen, may be as much one of the self as of the cells—a story we may have forgotten or perhaps never have really heard. These stories, which in their extremity enlarge the proscenium of the human drama, are often hard to hear: They are too awful, too exotic. But I believe they pertain not just to the ill, but to anyone who has ever collided with his own soul and there encountered a stranger. They show that what people do to make peace with their bodies may be startlingly similar to what they do to heal their hearts.

3

THE TANGLED ROOTS
OF DISEASE

. . . groping in roots, and growing thick in
trunks, and in treetops like a rising from
the dead.

—RAINER MARIA RILKE

To UNDERSTAND a story, we must start at the beginning. But
from its very inception, disease's harsh narrative strikes us as
incoherent. Illness feels like a random act of nature: A bolt of lightning has streaked down at us from a cobalt-blue sky; the blind fates
of biology have scythed our innocent wheat and fed it to the thresher.
Medical science, from its tribal inception to its present technological
apotheosis, has been a project to explain the sources of affliction.

Western medicine has long relied upon a primal axiom: "One
Disease, One Cause." This simple but brilliant tool has led to (among
other marvels) the isolation of disease agents and in some cases their
remedies. Today we know that infections are caused by microorganisms, malaria and African river blindness by parasites, AIDS
from a virus entering the bloodstream. An increasing number of
illnesses appear to be inscribed in our genes. (Most of former president Jimmy Carter's immediate family, for example, died of pancreatic cancer.) Scientists have discovered specific genetic markers
for cystic fibrosis, "elephant man" disease (neurofibromatosis), acute
lymphocytic leukemia, non-insulin-dependent diabetes mellitus,
melanoma, and rare forms of familial breast cancer.

Even Joan Borysenko, the former director of the Mind/Body
Clinic of New England Deaconess Hospital, stresses that the causes
of disease remain preponderantly organic: "You're sick because your

cellar is full of radon gas, your well is poisoned, your father and his father and his father died of a heart disease."

But not all people exposed to a given pathogen succumb to it; not all the inhabitants of toxic wastelands like Love Canal fall sick. Not everyone with the genetic predisposition for a given disease contracts it. Cancers of the same cell type may progress quickly in one person, slowly in another, and halt or occasionally regress in yet another.

"There are people who had the tubercle bacillus in their body for many years," says Dr. Leo Stolbach, a leading oncologist at Boston's Beth Israel Hospital, "and all of a sudden they develop tuberculosis. What happened to activate it? And it's well-known that some people who are carrying the bacillus never get TB. Is the answer in their biology, or also in their minds?"

ONE DISEASE, MANY CAUSES

The idea that the roots of some human illnesses are irretrievably tangled (in clinical terms, "multifactorial") is slowly gaining credence in many medical circles. Medical theoretician Dr. George Engel explains: "[T]he presence of the biochemical defect . . . at best defines a necessary but not a sufficient condition for the human experience of human disease. . . . [I]t constitutes but one factor among many, the complex interaction of which may ultimately culminate in active disease." Medicine is beginning to see that the origin of disease cannot be spoken of without including life-style, diet, social milieu, the environment, and, perhaps most interesting, consciousness and the emotions.

These last categories remain controversial. Once we stray from strictly physical definitions of the roots of disease and allow that there also may be wider soul factors at work, we enter a quagmire. As long as illness is purely the result of random natural forces, we have little role in our ailments or their cure. On the other hand, if the psyche is involved, we are presented with a double-edged sword: On the one side, it may help us use our inner resources to augment the body's healing process; on the other, affliction may become a new-age scarlet A, its victims held accountable for every vagary of their own biology.

Speaking angrily of the latter view, a survivor of testicular cancer writes, "The self-indulgence of believing that I caused my disease by emotional distress or a sloppy life—by not having my 'act together'—is like saying that people are poor because they're stupid and lazy." In the end, he attributes his illness to one brutal fact: "That at times completely impersonal forces bludgeon you, that circumstances overwhelm you, that riding it out is the only course available."[1]

His sentiments are understandable given the glib statements emanating from some quarters of the healing world. "Why did you want to get this disease?" I once heard a new age health counselor ask a patient. In a popular self-help book, an Australian doctor, John Harrison, talks about the "smugness of the multiple sclerosis sufferer who has achieved the incapacity she wanted."[2] "One of the hottest self-healing seminars in the country!" trumpets a fashion magazine article about a "Loving Yourself Into Forever" workshop. "Aging is a symptom of unresolved or limited beliefs," the article quotes the founder, a former drug addict and now a "breathing therapist." "To 'youth' your body, you must be responsible for every cell in your body."[3]

Responsible for every cell in your body. It's the kind of pronouncement that gives both opponents and proponents of mind-body medicine the willies. Not long ago, the *New England Journal of Medicine* published a withering editorial stating, "It is time to acknowledge that our belief in disease as a direct reflection of mental state is largely folklore."[4] But the flood of mail from doctors in response to the piece was surprisingly critical. One accused the journal of thumping the tub for a viewpoint reflective of "the state of psychosomatic medicine 30 or more years ago." Few clinicians, the same letter writer continued, would claim that the mind-body factor superseded all others, but its significance can no longer be ignored.

Discovering a psychological component in an illness, however, does often carry an oddly pejorative connotation. If "plaque deposits" cause coronary disease, one is a certifiable victim of purblind physical forces. But if the mind is somehow implicated, the disease is seemingly transferred into the conscious (and thus moral) sphere, and the person is held subtly to blame. Even as science dismantles the Berlin Wall between psyche and flesh, we are hemmed in by the Cartesian apportionment: responsible for everything that is in our minds, the seat of the rational, intending "I"; but for nothing that happens in the mechanically ticking gearworks of our bodies.

Patients who take a bodymind approach to their diseases must wrestle with this mindset. Poet and essayist Deena Metzger, a former breast cancer patient, chafes at "the new age, exploitative view, as if kids in Africa get yaws from 'bad karma.'" In her own healing journey, she says, she began to distinguish between "What's wrong with you that you brought this on yourself?" and "In what ways might my psyche have colluded with the illness?" or "What was the illness an expression of?"

FELICE'S STORY

"I feel like screaming when people tell me I have arthritis because I'm angry," Felice [not her real name], an attractive woman in her mid-thirties, told me: "I'm angry *because* I have arthritis. Pain infuriates me. I'm a perfectly cheery person when it doesn't hurt." Felice, dressed in trademark New York black accented by fire-engine-red lipstick, pointed to studies that suggest her disease produces secretions that stimulate the amygdala, the area of the brain associated with anger and aggression. Her rheumatoid arthritis (RA) seemed, on the surface, a straightforward accident of genetics: Her mother and grandmother both began suffering from it at exactly the same age.

But looking at other aspects of Felice's family history, the frame of this portrait expands. As a young child growing up in rural Oregon, Felice was a "hyperactive tomboy," an expert tree-shinnier who led her gang of kids on adventures through her suburban neighborhood. Just before adolescence she suffered a bicycle accident whose after-effects had abruptly curtailed her physical exuberance. In this, her profile fit a 1950s study comparing RA sufferers to their nearest unafflicted siblings: One finding was that patients had been "overactive as children but inhibited later in life."[5]

The study suggested that this overactivity in turn stemmed from the channeling of aggressive impulses resulting from "disturbing" childhood events. Only recently, upon entering psychotherapy, had Felice learned what those events were: She began to recall stark episodes of early childhood sexual abuse, the vague memories of which had begun stirring around the time of her first severe arthritis attacks.

Over the course of the past few years, in conjunction with a strict special diet, Chinese herbs, and acupuncture, Felice has begun intensive psychological work to confront the pain and buried rage from her early emotional wounds, whose grievousness had caused unexplained bouts of clinical depression throughout her life. Extricating herself from the latest in a series of blighted romances, she quit a dead-end job, went back to school, and discovered a talent for abstract mathematics that led her to an elite doctoral program. Now passionately engaged in a new life and disease-free for three years, Felice believes that had she not been driven to look for the emotional roots of her disease, she would never have become well.

THE PATTERNS OF DISEASE

How we define a root cause defines the remedy. If the cause is identified as simply an isolated physical disease agent—a germ, a virus, a gene, a hormone—medical treatment will suffice; there is seemingly no need to "treat" the rest of our lives. But the idea of a unitary physical cause may also seem preferable because it allows us to deal with our diseases at a more comfortable distance. We are often reluctant to look too deeply into our symptoms, lest they require us to make fundamental changes in our lives. If a man gets an ulcer from the stress of a high-paying job that is "all wrong for him," he may prefer to coat his stomach with medication rather than to heed his body's message to quit.

If a woman smokes to relieve the stress of a miserable marriage, what is the "cause" of her lung cancer? A genetic predisposition? The histology of oat-cell carcinoma? The smoking itself? Her relationship? How thorough is her cure if she has a lung removed but does not change her marital circumstances, let alone inquire into the personality patterns that permitted her to cling to her longtime unhappiness?

Some researchers believe there is evidence to support the theory that personality may be a factor in disease: Psychologist Lydia Temoshok claims that her controlled studies of melanoma patients reveal a "Type C behavior pattern" (sad as opposed to angry, inexpressive vs. emotionally demonstrative) that is clearly correlated with more invasive tumor growth.[6] Neurobiologist Robert Ornstein states that purely physiological theories of heart disease are not necessarily borne out by clinical evidence. "Cholesterol and heart attacks are not always highly correlated," he says heretically, "but emotional factors almost always are." His remark can be illustrated by the case of a businessman who had his first heart attack at the age of sixty-five. Despite the fact that the man had never smoked, rarely drank, and ate a primarily vegetarian diet, his cholesterol count was dangerously high. The low-cholesterol, low-fat diet his physician prescribed scarcely made a dent in his levels.

A classic Type-A (heart attack–prone) personality—competitive,

ambitious, easily irritated by small daily frustrations—the man discovered to his surprise that, following a happy and relaxing vacation
in Europe during which he indulged himself with Italian ice cream,
Swiss cheese, and other high-fat treats, his cholesterol level precip-
itately *dropped*. Conversely, when he returned to his job in California and resumed brokering another megadeal, his levels rapidly
climbed back into the danger zone. Did his cholesterol "cause" his
heart attack, or was it also his high-pressure life-style? And what
personality factors were at the root of his workaholic behavior in
the first place?[7]

Too often, we attempt to kill off our diseases one by one without
digging down to their intertwining roots: emotional wounds; an
environment filled with toxic by-products; high levels of anxiety and
stress with their associated biochemical effects; nutrient-poor, fat-
and sugar-laden diets (which may have their own emotional and
social causes); etc. I am certainly not proposing that we undertake
to solve the problems of the world before we attend to our own
healing (although if each of us did strive to heal the emotional,
social, and environmental wounds that impact us, the number of us
who became sick would surely decline). But if we insist upon exiling
our diseases from the pattern of our lives, even "successful" treatment can do little more than shore up a life structure that may cry
out for major renovation.

To understand why we are ill, and get clues as to how we might
become well, we may have to look more deeply into how we live,
love, work, and feel—into everything we are. The benefits to our
health could only be considerable. If we begin to strip away layers
of resistance, we draw closer to our own nature, the source of our
healing power. By taking the widest possible "soul approach" to our
illness, we can begin to eliminate the sources of pathology from our
lives rather than merely exile its symptoms from our bodies. If it is
the whole person who becomes sick, it is also the whole person who
becomes well.

LOSS OF SOUL

In Native American healing ceremonies, a pipe is passed around
the circle with the invocation "All my relations," a gesture that affirms each participant's connection to the great web of life—the
"two-leggeds and the four-leggeds," friends and ancestors, totem

and tribe, winds and waters, the personal soul and the Great Spirit. Illness appears, it is said, when these relationships have become sick, subverted; their reconstitution is the ground of the healing path.

According to the shaman, disease may result "when the patient has special talents which he does or does not use";[8] from a breach of taboo; from an intrusion by a "disease object"; from psychosocial factors like "competition, jealousy, greed and lust; witches, sorcerers, and demons; mothers brothers and grandfathers recently deceased";[9] from a "loss of soul";[10] from any falling out of harmony with the larger circle of existence.

In our own culture, the "disease object" is a microörganism; the unhappy "ancestors" our genetic predispositions; the broken taboo environmental pollution, social and familial decay, and other rendings in the modern web of life that have proved so devastating to human health.

But it is "loss of soul"—from the shaman's viewpoint, the centerpole of the disease syndrome—that may be most relevant to our exploration of the inner dimensions of healing. In the schema of tribal medicine, human health is injured not only by something invading the body but by, as Jeanne Achterberg puts it, "the loss of personal power which permitted the intrusion in the first place."[11] (Thus the German physician's typical query, *"Was fehlt Ihnen?"*— "What do you lack?"—reflects a deeper understanding than his American counterpart's "What have you got?")

In contemporary terms, we might translate "loss of soul" as that violation of the sense of self various psychologists have referred to as the "tearing loose of an essential part of one's nature";[12] a "lost intensity of experience . . . a suppression of vitality, creativity, and feeling";[13] "dispiritedness" and depression.[14] The clinical evidence that depression, loss, shock, and grief have powerfully deleterious effects on the immune system is clear, though no study has yet made a direct causal link to disease.[15] For example, University of Iowa psychiatrist Dr. Ziad Kronfol found that the blood of depressed patients showed weaker immune system responsiveness than that of both normal patients and patients with other mental illnesses. A recent study at a Newark hospital revealed that relatives of trauma victims exhibit an impairment in the specific immune components needed to fight cancer. Men who suffered the loss of a spouse from breast cancer were shown to display suppressed immunity for up to two years.

At least one psychologist has suggested that the immune system is the physical counterpart ("biological analogon," in his term) of what we call the sense of self.[16] A recent (1993) article in *Advances* journal proposes that the immune system shares with the psyche "the common goal of establishing and maintaining self-identity."[17] It is perhaps appropriate that the name for the central gland of the immune system—the thymus, located in the center of the chest—derives from the Greek term *thymos,* meaning "soul" or "personality." In light of modern psychoneuroimmunology research, a working hypothesis might be: To wound the self is to wound the immune system.

My Boston doctors insisted that my tumor could no more be an outgrowth of my life than was the Colorado hailstone that cracked my windshield one summer. But their assurances did not ring true. The decade before my illness could not have helped but wreak havoc on the bodymind: a colossally bad marriage; a pattern of overwork that only intensified after the inevitable divorce; and a magazine job that included seven-day weeks, heart- and homesickness, bouts of anxiety, and sloughs of despondency.

Only much later did I begin to question *why* I had so often placed myself in such untenable situations. I started to discern, however faintly, what my family, my colleagues, my body, and my dreams had long been futilely shouting at me: My windmilling through life, sacrificing myself and my relationships on the altar of some abstract greater good, was neither noble nor benign. I can recall—painfully now, though I was proud then of my professional mettle—exhorting my staff that it didn't matter if their feelings got hurt in the rough-and-tumble pursuit of excellence, or if they had to miss dinner with their families night after night. What really mattered were our loyal readers. What mattered was the Good Cause.

Some of my high-mindedness was genuine, I suppose. But probing beneath it, I found an inarticulate notion that if I had five hundred influential names in my Rolodex, five hundred thousand readers on a subscription list—that if I could create a big enough public persona, a homunculus with outsized virtues and tiny sins— I might fill a persistent inner vacancy with the admiration of strangers. Only later did I realize that the devoted readership was a conjured battalion; my colleagues, who began to avoid me at lunch, and the family and friends who chafed at being relegated to support troops were all too real. I had been acting like a self-anointed Atlas. The frightening part of it was, I had no idea why.

THE NARCISSISTIC WOUND

Once, early in my journey, I visited a psychologist who specialized in treating cancer patients. She carelessly let slip a remark that cut deep. "I've rarely met a cancer patient," she observed at the close of our first session, "who didn't show signs of narcissistic character disorder."

Her tone was sympathetic, but I was stunned by what I took as the slur on my character, yet another egregious instance of "blame the victim." A narcissist was a reprehensible egomaniac, a vain, shallow person with no real affection for anyone but himself. I, by my own accounting, was generous and self-sacrificing; I had even taken formal vows to follow the Buddhist bodhisattva path of compassion for all sentient beings. I learned only years later that my problem with the therapist was a linguistic misunderstanding. In clinical lexicon, *narcissism* is not a moral failing but an emotional wound. The narcissist's problem is not high self-regard, but the opposite: a sense, often well-disguised, of crippling inner deficiency.

According to the psychologist Alice Miller, author of the classic work *The Drama of the Gifted Child*, this personality syndrome develops when a child does not receive the "respect, echoing, understanding, sympathy, mirroring" required to develop a healthy sense of self—usually because the parents are themselves too emotionally damaged to provide it. A child in such circumstances, says Miller, is loved only conditionally. He must shape his very being to the parents' needs, forgoing the "expression of his own distress," cutting off in himself "what was alive and spontaneous."

Deprived of the chance to "develop and differentiate his 'true self,'" forced to compensate with an "as-if" personality, such a child's later life is marred by a furtive quest for a lost fullness of being. No matter how outwardly well-adapted or successful such children become, no matter how many relationships or accomplishments they collect, there persists a blight of "emptiness, futility, or hopelessness." Unable to experience themselves fully from within, plagued by a gnawing lack of worth, they are ever compelled to seek outward evidence that they deserve love. Often they construct a grandiose persona which drives ever further from their reach the very thing they most crave.

Here is Narcissus's true plight: He is not only gazing *at* himself in the reflective pool, but tragically, futilely, looking *for* himself, trying to confirm his own existence, as it were, from the outside in. This precise model of personality can be seen in other descriptions of human dysfunction, ranging from "codependency" and "addictive disorders" to John Bradshaw's "toxic shame." Children who are "born in the soil of their parents' alienated split selves," in Bradshaw's words, are unwittingly used as instruments of those parents' unmet "dependency needs," never learning self-love or establishing untainted social connection. Instead, Bradshaw writes, "the child's true self is abandoned and a false self must be created."

This description, in turn, bears a remarkable resemblance to what a number of theorists have come to call "the cancer personality." Berkeley psychologist Meredith Sabini was struck by how many of her cancer patients had experienced an "early lack of nurturance from the mother [which] injured the ego-self relationship." The result, she writes, was a division of identity into a "conscious self that is socially adequate but empty and meaningless, and an unconscious self that is explosive, tragic, tormented."[18]

A CANCER PERSONALITY?

The idea of a "cancer personality," which can be traced back as far as the Greek surgeon Galen, has been the subject of acrimonious debate. The essayist Susan Sontag, a former cancer patient, believes it is an even more pernicious notion than the nineteenth-century equation of illness with sin: "Such preposterous and dangerous views manage to put the onus of the disease on the patient."[19]

Moreover, Sontag implies, the assumptions upon which the theory rests, as well as the research that seems to support it, are implicitly suspect. In her book *Illness as Metaphor* she remarks:

> Investigations are cited—most articles refer to the same ones— in which out of, say, several hundred cancer patients, two-thirds or three-fifths report being depressed or unsatisfied with their lives, and having suffered from the loss (through death or rejection or separation) of a parent, lover, spouse, or close friend. But it seems likely that of several hundred people who do not have cancer, most would also report depressing emotions and past traumas: this is called the human condition.[20]

Sontag singles out the speculations of Dr. Lawrence LeShan as emblematic of an entire body of research that should be "confined to the back yard of folk superstition." LeShan, a New York psychotherapist and author, observed that his patients with cancer seemed to share a psychological syndrome that included "loss of raison d'être" (usually through loss of "the single central relationship"), "inability to express anger and resentment," "defensiveness and constriction," and, most markedly, "despair." Discussing despair, he makes clear that he is speaking of a different clinical syndrome than the usual psychic wear-and-tear, the angst and anomie of modern life. The "hopelessness" his patients felt, he says, extended almost as far back as they could remember. To stress the severity of this feeling-tone, he notes that many told him that "for years they had felt there was no way out of the emotional box they found themselves in, short of death itself."[21]

One of LeShan's first tests of his hypothesis was an attempt to predict the presence of cancer by personality profile alone. He studied a group of twenty-eight outpatients of a Philadelphia clinic, half of them cancer patients and half with other diseases. After examining only personal history records with the "health" sections left blank, LeShan was able correctly to sort out the cancerous from the noncancerous patients in twenty-four of the cases, on the basis of psychological factors alone. (Three of his four "misses" were ill, with, respectively, arteriosclerosis, allergy, and hyperthyroidism— all diseases thought to have psychosomatic components.)

"The odds that this number of correct predictions would occur by chance are less than one in a thousand," says LeShan. He conducted another study, this one with several hundred patients, which revealed a similar relationship between emotional wounds and disease.

LeShan's work has been critiqued by some in the mind-body field from the standpoint of methodology. But research studies over several decades in many countries have supported the idea that a relationship may exist between cancer and emotional dysfunction:

- A study comparing smokers who had lung cancer to smokers with noncancerous lung diseases repeatedly found that the cancer patients' personalities—as determined through carefully structured interviews and psychological tests—had a strikingly "restricted outlet for emotional discharge."[22]
- A British study, of 160 women with an undiagnosed lump of the breast, found "suppression of emotion" in 48 percent of those whose tumors subsequently turned out to be malignant, but only in 15 percent of those later reported as benign.[23] Another American study found "denial of hostility," mem-

ories of childhood emotional deprivation, and difficulty
maintaining close relationships in breast cancer patients.[24]

- Researchers at the University of Rochester found they could
predict with high accuracy which women out of a group
whose Pap tests had revealed "suspicious" cells would later
be shown to have cancer. Most of the women found to have
malignancies reported having responded to major life up-
heavals with emotions of "despair and futility." Most who did
not report this same degree of depression and hopelessness
in the face of difficulties turned out to have relatively benign
conditions.[25]

Art McGrary, a fifty-year-old former fire chief, was a stoic front-
liner always willing to take as much heat as he asked of his men.
"The point," he told me, "was to 'eat the most smoke' and never
complain." But his face, bluff and lived-in after twenty-five years
spent fighting "every kind of conflagration known to man," still
twists in childlike pain when he talks about the "old-country" mother
who "never gave me the love I needed."

"She was completely disapproving," he says. "The highest praise
she could come up with was, 'You'll pass with a push.' "

His father was scarcely more help. "Whenever I'd try to do something with him, he'd get drunk. We'd try to go fishing together, and
he'd get plastered and fall in the water. I just wanted him to say,
'You're all right, a pretty good guy.' But I quit trying after a while."

As an adult, McGrary's romantic relationships were driven by a
desperate search for love. "When someone cared for me, or I
thought they did, it became the most important, the most supreme
thing," he says. When marriage or the relationships crashed, he
would be gripped by "pitch-dark despair, like the world had ended."
He can count "at least a dozen times" he seriously contemplated
suicide.

His career became the Everything to which he could give his All.
McGrary, who also worked on a county bomb squad for several years
("I'd rush into any place someone else would run away from"), now
characterizes his life strategy as one of "overcompensation. I identified myself with two words: fire chief. My career was the value of
my *being*." His jury-rigged life, built on shaky emotional foundations,
held up until he was finally forced into retirement. Not long after,
he was diagnosed with prostate cancer.

I was surprised at how often the same patterns appeared[26] in the
patients I interviewed: emotionally abusive, unavailable, or lost par-

ents; futile childhood strategies to win their love; an outward adaptation of stoicism and/or grandiosity coupled with low self-image; a series of compulsive, need-based relationships; compensating through outer achievement and/or addictive behaviors; finally a severe crisis when the things which were supposed to substitute for a sense of self—things in which emotional investment had been total—inevitably failed to live up to their billing.

THE WOUNDED CHILD

We can glimpse similar "case histories" in the modern healing myths described in the previous chapter. The Spirit of Christmas Past reveals the young Scrooge as the only boy in boarding school whose parents did not fetch him home for holidays. A stoic "little adult," the lonely child tells a friend with false bravado, "Father and I talked it over and we decided that swatting away at my books would do me more good than being home—Christmas and plum pudding and turkeys are for *children*." But he breaks down in bitter, very childlike tears the moment his friend is out of earshot.

In the movie *It's a Wonderful Life*, George Bailey's father tells the unusually responsible boy, "You were *born* older," a comment that entirely misses the point: George has been *made* "older," well-behaved to the point of self-abnegation. He has been called upon in turn to take care of his younger brother (for whom he repeatedly makes sacrifices we would usually consider parental); his employer; his alcoholic, befuddled Uncle Billy; his own father, whom he eventually must replace as paterfamilias; as well as an entire dysfunctional town.

In *The Wizard of Oz*, Dorothy's emotional deprivation is even more severe. In Frank Baum's descriptive passages, the unremitting grayness of her life takes on a quality of incantation: The great prairie is a "gray mass with little cracks in it"; the house was "as dull and gray as everything else"; Auntie Em's eyes, cheeks and even lips are "sober gray"; Uncle Henry is "gray also, from his long beard to his rough boots." Stern Uncle Henry "never laughed" and "rarely spoke." Auntie Em was "thin and gaunt and never smiled"; her only response to Dorothy's merry laughter is to "scream and press her hand upon her heart." Could there be two more emotionally desiccated stepparents for a lively little girl?

DEBBY'S STORY

Like Dorothy, Debby Ogg suffered the loss of her real parents early in life. The story of her unusual recovery—without conventional treatment—from lymph-node cancer was made into the CBS-TV movie *A Question of Faith*. Debby had lost her mother to breast cancer when she was seven, and her father to a heart attack five years later. Debby described herself as having been, prior to her multiple tragedies, a "lively, feisty, rebellious kid. I wasn't at all girlish by societal standards, but very assertive, with a real mind of my own."

But in the wake of devastating emotional losses, she reined in her exuberant individuality and "began getting very, very busy fitting in." By the time she reached high school, she was student-body vice president; in college, she was the high-achieving, perpetually cheerful vice president of her dorm. "I was a very popular girl, and more importantly, I was in control. I was afraid to have any needs. Until I had my own daughter, I didn't realize how extreme my childhood deprivation really had been. I'd always thought that I must have deserved what had happened, that I'd essentially killed my parents, or they'd left me because I wasn't lovable. This was the black thought that functioned continuously inside me, a black enormity too big to deal with, so I tried to pretend it wasn't there. I was afraid if I ever hit bottom, I'd never come up."

I was surprised at how uniformly the journeyers I interviewed reported serious childhood losses and traumas. One melanoma patient recalled "mopping up blood from the floor" after parental battles royal. Brian Schultz, the ankylosing "Tin Woodman" described in the previous chapter, remembered that "it wasn't just the aberrations of an otherwise normal family. Once my father picked up a knife and threatened to kill my mother, and I had to restrain him. I was nine at the time, and I was afraid he was going to kill us both. My mother would get drunk and then hint to me she might take the car, drive off, and never come back, or worse, kill herself. In order to survive, I learned to stuff down my real thoughts, feelings, and perceptions. They were just too dangerous."

The childhood emotional privation among these patients was so consistent, it was almost like an equation: Parental love was a quantum that mysteriously appeared and vanished, leaving ephemeral particle trails in the cloud-chamber of the heart. If the child molded herself to her parents' needs—became a confidante, peacemaker, lover, punching bag—she could receive the affection she thirsted for. If she did not, she risked rejection. Her inner feelings—her longing, her discomfort, her anger, her grief—were unwelcome realities that could drive the parent away. Since emotional abandonment to a child is synonymous with death, she was boxed in, forbidden indefinitely to feel what she felt.

DEFERRAL OF AUTHENTICITY

Such a childhood places a person on a poignant trajectory of incomplete development. The inner self is denigrated and hidden away, the outer self—the "brilliant disguise"—serves as both cover-up and caricature of authentic being. It was a strategy the people I spoke with had hit upon so early, so instinctually, that they often did not become aware of it until illness supervened. "It's astounding," says Debby Ogg, "that no one—not even me—knew I was just a shell of someone."

Similarly, in *It's a Wonderful Life* young George Bailey constructs a grandiose fantasy-self who will someday explore the Coral Sea, have a harem, make a million dollars. Later, as a young man, every fiber straining toward escape, he plans to "shake the dust of this grubby little town off my feet, build airfields, skyscrapers a hundred stories high, bridges a mile long!" By constructing such monuments, he will at once create incontrovertible evidence that he exists, and cover up the pain of his inner erasure. In the typical all-or-nothing thinking of such personalities, he hankers after unassailable bigness. When he instead winds up diverting the energies of his soul into job, home, and the duties of family and community, he feels defeated. Seesawing between fantasy and abnegation, he has lost the authentic self which can dream an attainable dream. There is a kernel of truth in the taunting words of his archenemy Mr. Potter, who slyly accuses him of being "a warped and frustrated *young* man."

Lymphoma patient John Studholme was also a striver who filled his outer life with achievement and service to others. He became a lawyer, married, had children, and began what he now sees as an obsessive climb through the thicket of the world. Like the fictional George Bailey, John was civic-minded to a fault: He joined groups, clubs, and committees as "a way to get ahead." He usually became a leader, his success so seemingly effortless that a wealthy neighbor once offered to back him for a run for the U.S. Senate.

During his cancer journey, however, John took a Meyers-Briggs personality test and was surprised to find that he was an "introvert, in the ninety-ninth percentile. I was more in the category of the poets than the politicians! I had done the 'right' things all my life, but they were wrong for *me*."

He began to see he had spent his life scaling life's visible peaks but somehow never had managed to conquer the invisible vales of self-worth. He remembers that when he was a young lawyer with wife and baby boy, "the present didn't even exist for me, didn't seem rich enough or secure enough. I wasn't satisfied with our quaint little low-rent carriage house, with the beat-up roadster with cracking leather seats I'd picked up for a thousand dollars, with my first child, with my youth."

Four years later, after his twin boys were born, John bought a house, paying the banker with a wad of bills wrapped in a red ribbon. "I was doing everything I was supposed to," he says, "fathering, cooking, changing diapers, putting my nose to the grindstone." But something continued to gnaw at him from within. "Consciously, I thought I was great to be doing all this. But I also felt a constant need to get away. I'd hop in my old Porsche and head off, anywhere. My male friends thought I had lovers, sexual destinations. To me it was just the thrill of traveling, of rounding into those curves with the sound of that tight little engine behind me. But it was escape. In my family, and in all those groups—God knows why—I felt responsible for everyone else's happiness but mine. Flying along the road was the only time I felt alive."

John remembers turning forty, still making road trips, now shimmering through the desert in a new Alfa Romeo, "feeling I was better than the sad men and women I imagined stuck in their own dull lives. I thought I was onto something." Looking back, he says, "I think something was onto me."

On a visit to a friend's ranch in New Mexico around that time, an old friend innocuously asked him how he was faring. "I'm in that group of locusts called lawyers," he burst out miserably, surprising them both with his vehemence.

When she asked about his family he said, "You know, marriage, kids, and career, the end of passion." He realized that he had reached a frustrating plateau, "bored with my career and life, with continually trying to be all things to all people." The following morning, "I woke up stiff and sore from the inside, all over my body, as if I'd played football on a gravel field. When I left, I still felt invulnerable, the provider, the rock, the mountain, always coping regardless of the weather. But a few months later, I was diagnosed with Hodgkin's disease, Stage Four-B."

John, like George Bailey, was the "good son" who had learned to readily give himself up for others. He, too, chose a profession that involved saving people from their own mistakes, defending them in their helplessness, ignoring his own needs. Though John was well paid for his troubles, George's cinematic cri de coeur—"I feel like if I didn't get away, I'd bust!"—could have been his own.

The fictional George Bailey is about to bust from his own pent-up selfhood, a condition not ameliorated by marriage, children, or business success. It seems appropriate that George's rampage through the family home preceding his suicide attempt—kicking the carefully arranged furniture into splinters, howling in rage at his wife, his children, even his children's schoolteacher—was triggered by his son's innocent question, "How do you spell 'Frankenstein'?" In the movie, George has become his own Frankenstein's monster, a creation cobbled together from the expectations of others, lurching through the house he had once told his fiancée he "wouldn't live in as a ghost."

THE ALPHABET OF DISEASE?

"The frustration," exclaimed the Buddhist sage Longchenpa, "that comes with the fatigue of traveling the road of fictitious being!" But what a physiology of "fictitious being" might look like, if there is such a thing, we can only speculate. Does a "divided soul" make of what should be smoothly meshing biological systems a cacophony of grinding, clashing gears?

To an extent that most of us have not yet truly grasped, the body seems to be incised by our emotions, the way a river meandering over the same ground eventually cuts out a canyon. Our bodies are continents on which our ways of thinking and feeling, our habits of living—the grinding tectonic plates of chronic stress, eruptions of rage, steady streams of anxiety—over time create a distinctive landscape.

At least one neuroimmunologist suggests that particular emotions seem to correlate with the release of specific biochemicals that can have specific effects on certain parts of the body. "The brain, as the organ of emotions and attitudes," writes Dr. T. Melnechuk, "seems to be in a position to dispatch appropriate mixtures and amounts of . . . neurotransmitters and hormones to particular sites."[27]

The members of the Therapeutae sect of ancient Alexandria, whose medical practices were held at the time to be marvelously effective, believed that particular diseases arose from specific "pleasures and desires and griefs and fears." The Nei Ching, a centuries-old Chinese medical classic that provides the theoretical basis for acupuncture, proposes that certain emotions affect certain organs— anger injures the liver, for example, or fear the spleen.

In the Chinese view, however, illness comes not only from the emotions themselves but from the inability to *transform* them, causing them to get "stuck." Pathology was seen not only as a case of "good" and "bad" emotions, but of fixation—when, in the words of the Nei Ching, "grief, fear, pity, joy, and anger cannot change into those that are secondary to them, and thus cause man to become gravely ill." Emotions had to *move* if human beings were to remain healthy.

In contrast to this psychologically sophisticated approach, the "metaphysical counselor" Louise Hay's recent book, *Heal Your Body*, addresses the emotional factors of disease in terms as simplistic as a rebus. Thyroid problems are said to be caused by "humiliation," arthritis by "deep criticism of authority," and leukemia is a case of "brutally killing inspiration." Such literal-minded formulae seem of little more utility than Sidney Omar's astrology column in the local paper.

But is there any more evidence for the more scientific-sounding lexicon of "Type A" (heart disease-prone) and "Type C" (cancer-prone) personalities? Psychologist Lydia Temoshok believes she has identified thirteen "nonverbal characteristics" that differentiate the Type C behavior pattern, which she has found in several studies to be correlated with thicker, more invasive tumors than non-Type C patients. Hers and other studies single out cancer patients as people who have trouble meeting their own emotional needs. "He never thinks about himself," murmurs one of George Bailey's townsfolk. "That's why he's in trouble."[28] George resembles no one so much as the patron saint of cancer himself, Peregrinus Laziosi (1260– 1345). A member of the Servite order in Siena, Peregrinus was so tireless in his service and devotion to others, it was said that he never sat down. Constantly on his feet, St. Peregrine developed a cancer on his foot. (Fortunately, the night before the foot was to be surgically amputated, he dreamed his cancer was healed by God, and miraculously the cancer was gone in the morning.)

As opposed to the self-sacrificing Type C, the Type A is said to be a hard-charger who manages to be first across the finish line, only to collapse as he triumphally bursts the tape. He is said to have an emotional makeup dominated by anger, hostility, and impatience—"fighting with time, fighting with others," as one clinician summed up. According to the internist Redford Williams, author of *The Trusting Heart* and a behavioral medicine specialist at Duke University Medical Center, "Type A people appear to react as if they're always running from a grizzly."[29]

Type A's also show physiological anomalies, among them a more pronounced "fight-or-flight" response to emergency, particularly in adrenaline secretion. Such physical reactions can cause the sort of arterial injuries that lead to arteriosclerosis and heart attacks. In addition, Type A men who score high on the Cook-Medly Ho scale, which rates "hostility, cynical mistrust, and anger," show a more pronounced testosterone response, a hormone that increases arteriosclerosis in animals. A research team at North Carolina's Bowman-Gray School of Medicine discovered that even Type A *monkeys*—monkeys that strive for dominance over their peers—exhibit accelerated formation of artery-clogging plaque.[30]

But cardiologist Dean Ornish told me he believes it is time to look past the standard portrait of so-called Type A behavior—"hostility, cynicism, and self-involvement"—and search for the deeper pattern of which these traits may be only symptoms. "The real question," he said as we sat sipping tea one day on the balcony of his home in the Sausalito hills, "is *why* are these people hostile, cynical, and self-involved?"

Ornish's place was a virtual treehouse, a double-decker aerie alive with the din of chirping birds. An electric guitar—a gold-topped Les Paul classic—was visible in the corner of the living room. "I've been memorizing a solo from this rare Jimi Hendrix performance of 'Red House,' " offered the cardiologist, confessing cheerily to being a Type A himself.

His long, tapering fingers looked as if they could scuttle as nimbly through one of Hendrix's searing glissandos as through the innards of a heart, this latter a skill he acquired under the tutelage of surgical superstar Dr. Michael DeBakey. It was during his time with DeBakey that Ornish first noticed how many coronary bypass patients were coming back for second and even third operations. Subsequent studies have shown, he says, that within five years, half the patients who have had bypass surgery return: Their arteries simply clog up again.

"The real issue lies further back in the 'causal chain' that leads to chronic stress and then to heart disease," Ornish said. What stood out among the heart patients he treated, he told me, was a tendency to develop a "pretended self" that played itself out in arenas such as money, power, fame, sexual conquests, possessions, where no victory could ever be sufficient. "They feel they are unlovable, and the only way to get love is to somehow buy it with these outward tokens. Of course, they're left worse off than before. Not only do the outer achievements fail to deliver self-esteem goodies or end their deeper loneliness, but now they've backed themselves into a position where they must keep up a constant false front."

Ornish, who obtained the first documented regressions in coronary artery disease patients using only diet, exercise, meditation, and group therapy, offers as a poignant example a heart patient who had boasted of being a former Olympic athlete. In order to "maintain his persona," the man continually drove himself to the limits of his physical conditioning. Finally, in what became a terrible object lesson for his fellow patients, the man died on an exercise machine, competing against a video game of a rowing race. Only after his death was it discovered that his Olympian résumé had been a complete fabrication.

THE DISEASE-PRONE PERSONALITY

It is hard not to notice in Ornish's description a parallel to the "cancer personality," which raises the possibility of a connecting principle, a theoretical Rosetta stone for different disease syndromes. Certainly, an increasing number of *physiological* linkages have been suggested: Candace Pert speculates that AIDS, multiple sclerosis, Alzheimer's, and even schizophrenia may include similar immune system anomalies. Others have suggested patterns in the etiology of rheumatoid arthritis, lupus erthmatosus, and Hodgkin's lymphoma. Dr. Arthur Samuels, a UCLA hematologist and cancer specialist, has noted that similar mechanisms seem to produce both cancer and heart disease: "chronic stress, a predisposed personality type, and chronic hyperactivation of neural, endocrine, immune, blood clotting and fibrinolytic systems."[31] Prolonged stress creates excessive clotting, which can lead to heart attack and strokes. This same clotting can also create "fibrin cocoons," which can shield cancer metastases from T-cells and other body defenders.

The stress hormone cortisol, which figures in both cancer (by weakening the immune system) and heart disease (by beefing up the production of adrenaline), also has been linked with depression and feelings of hopelessness and helplessness. These same two emotions were noted in a small—seven patients—preliminary study (cited in the quarterly of the Albert Einstein College of Medicine) that found "major depressive illness between nine months and two years prior to the diagnosis of AIDS." Prior to symptoms of AIDS, "These people all had a remarkably similar set of family psychodynamics. . . . As adults, they felt helpless because of life stressors [that seemed] out of control."[32] What seems to emerge from all of this is a consensual description of a disease-prone personality which contributes to an as-yet unmeasurable extent to a host of human ailments, particularly those with immune system correlations. Dr. George Solomon, a professor of psychiatry at UCLA who has studied AIDS survivors, has coined the embracing term "immuno-suppression-prone personality pattern."

The deepest roots of this personality appear to be an early lack of appropriate nurturing, which may start as early as infancy. Even rats deprived of handling in infancy grow up with weakened immune systems. Says researcher Dr. Steven Heisel, "Early conditioning of lymphocytes [white blood cells] makes a life-long difference." This may be one reason that some people do not become ill under circumstances that topple others. But at whatever point in childhood the wounds are incurred, they are later reinforced by self-defeating life strategies (each with its own physiological consequences and perhaps predispositions), by self-destructive habits, and by chronic stress. Like probing fingers of molten magma, the disease-prone syndrome will find the weakest spot through which to erupt to the surface.

HEALING THE SPIRIT

The weakest spot may be the very construct of the self. "The original emotional wound may explode upwards, shattering the personality," suggests Meredith Sabini, "or it may drop into the body. Either way, it's got to find expression."[33] Another Jungian psychologist, comparing schizophrenia and cancer, has suggested that "malignant diseases and regressive psychoses could be seen as alternative biographical expressions of illness proneness," stemming from the same underlying "pathology of alienation."[34]

Some descriptions of schizophrenics' life-histories sound remarkably similar to the "cancer personality" (and indeed, to what I am calling "the disease-prone personality" in general). Dr. John Perry, a Jungian-oriented psychotherapist who founded an innovative clinic for schizophrenics in the 1970s, observed that most of his patients had parents whose own emotional woundedness had kept them from loving their children "wholeheartedly . . . with full acceptance." As a result, patients came to see themselves as "faulty, undesirable, unworthy, and unpromising." To compensate for these painful feelings, they clung to fantasies of being "superlative, more than human, a genius, or a person of momentous importance to the world." They tried to bandage the wounds of their "unlovability and . . . crushing insignificance" with a hollow shell of "absolute mastery." Finally, says Perry, this fragile, inherently unstable construct had to crack, frequently with the shattering of a key adult relationship. The shaky scaffolding of the self would collapse into ruin.

Perry came to believe that in some cases this process was actually part of a person's "developmental crisis"—an attempt to "reorganize the self, and resynthesize and reintegrate along new lines." Such a crisis could, after a period of chaos, lead to a more wholly constituted identity. But this could only occur, he theorized, if the underlying agenda of the original crisis was addressed—to dethrone the "power principle" that had previously governed the person's relationship to himself and others. In this case, the crisis could function as a means by which the "Eros Principle of relating and loving and allowing intimacy" could be restored.[35] (Recall the Tin Woodman's touching self-diagnosis: "I have no heart, and I cannot love.")

Dr. Dean Ornish, a longtime student of yoga teacher Swami Satchitananda, speculates that heart disease may really begin with a basic sense of emotional and spiritual aloneness: "If you feel separate, spiritually cut off, you get a sense that you are lacking. With that comes the idea that if only I had more . . . *blank*, then I'd be more okay, and then people would love me and *then* I wouldn't feel so isolated. It's a kind of subliminal circular reasoning that leads to a series of behaviors—workaholism, for one—that create even *more* isolation."[36] Lawrence LeShan claims that the cancer syndrome, too, is characterized by a greater than normal "sense of aloneness," an unbridgeable gap between self and other, a feeling of being the pawn of fate in a "cold, clockmaker's universe."

The healing of human alienation is generally thought of as a spiritual rather than a medical task. But Dr. Meyer Friedman, the physican who first studied and described Type A behavior, says that a factor he refers to as "spiritual need" is the main predictor of heart attack.[37] The Type A's hostility, he told me, "arises from a lack of self-esteem that has slowly eroded aspects of the personality. I'm finding that Type A's often seem to have lost those parts of the self we associate with right-brain functioning—the ability to appreciate music, to 'get into' a painting, to read poets who use metaphorical language, and especially to empathize with others."[38]

Friedman added that the Type A syndrome is marked by what he calls "an atrophy of the fundamental spiritual function—the ability to transcend oneself." In a related study, University of California at San Francisco psychologist Larry Scherwitz discovered that people who overused the word *I* or *my*—who felt a need to constantly reinforce and cling to an isolated identity—were twice as likely to have heart attacks.[39]

"The kingdom of heaven—and healing—is love," says Friedman, who is in the midst of a thirteen-year, three thousand–person study to see if "Type-A counseling" can prevent heart disease. "I work on trying to restore people's love for themselves and for other people, whom they tend to treat as objects or acquisitions. I tell them, 'We're going to start a tiny sapling of caring in the midst of these huge trees of habit. Then we're going to watch it grow.' "

Almost all the journeyers I interviewed discovered that new life can grow from the same painful roots that may have contributed to their disease. For if some disease springs in part from an early-thwarted need for love and relatedness, a soul-growth denied, then the roots of illness are, paradoxically, the very roots of life.

So it is that in our contemporary healing myths, the characters return from their sometimes lonely journeys affirming the power of love. George Bailey realizes not only his own self-worth, but embraces (and is embraced by) family and community. Dorothy utters her famous epiphany: "There's no place like home." Scrooge renounces the Power Principle, acknowledging at last his own never-quenched yearning for love, and is snatched at the last possible moment from the cold grasp of entropy.

Perhaps there is much that bears contemplating in Thomas Mann's controversial formulation: "Symptoms of disease are nothing but a disguised manifestation of the power of love; and all disease is only love transformed." This may be, symbolically if not literally, the subtext of the healing odyssey.

"If I can find the story disease is telling," says poet and breast-cancer patient Deena Metzger, "then I can find the healing story."

❧ 4 ❧
THE HERALD:
THE UNHEARD CALL

For God does speak, perhaps once or even twice,
though one perceive it not.

—JOB 33:14

LIKE ALL STORIES, the story of disease begins in advance of the telling. Though illness seems to burst suddenly upon us from secret depths, it may have quietly announced its presence long before we were willing to pay attention.

Lawyer John Studholme realized something was terribly wrong with his body during an eight-mile dirt-road marathon near the mountain town of Gothic, Colorado. Looking back on it later, he says, my body had been "shouting loudly at me at full volume" for months before the race. He had been having chills and night sweats that had left his sheets "as wet as baby's diapers." He had been uninterested in sex and frequently "bone-weary." On his fifth mile that day along the ridge of the magnificent Elk Range, "the colors too bright, my senses too heightened," he was puzzled that he seemed to have lost the usual spring in his legs. "I blamed the altitude, my biorhythms, whatever. But I knew inside that something wasn't right." Five months later, John's doctor discovered a softball-sized lymphoma tumor in his chest.

Sometimes, however, the signals of illness are far more vaporous— an intuition, a feeling, a nightmare, or other subtler alarms sounded by the bodymind. Samantha Coles [her name and characteristics have been changed], an art professor, remembers a specific sense of foreboding that had been with her for years. By her reckoning, she had devoted most of her life to "looking good on the outside." A tan, lanky testimonial to Florida sunshine, a "beach kid" who grew up thumbing a ride to the ocean every day, she was also the child of two physically abusive parents. Like many children of troubled homes, she had become by default an expert at coping, staying protected, depending only on herself. Always a "perfectionist and performer," she had confirmed the seaworthiness of her personal motto—"Be strong, don't take help, never cry, never trust"—from the storm-tossed decks of several disastrous relationships.

A talented painter, she had landed a university teaching post while she was still in her early twenties. Her only conscious, inescapable anxiety centered on a simple mole on her left thigh:

> I had lots of other moles and freckles, but this one, I don't know why, really bothered me. I was always putting something over it, sort of keeping it from the sun.
>
> This went on for ten years before I finally went to a doctor and said, "I think there is something wrong here." I'd also started having a lot of dreams where my teeth were falling out— just crumbling!—which for some reason felt like the worst thing that could possibly happen in the entire known universe. These dreams were so real, I'd get up in the morning and check to see if my teeth were still there!
>
> The sense of utter horror in the dream was the *same feeling* I had about this mole. It seemed really bad, poisonous, something I had to get off my body.
>
> But when I went to the doctor and told him I wanted him to remove it, he refused. He didn't think it was anything serious. He told me to come back only if it changed. Well, a year or so later, I scratched it and a bump grew out of it within a couple of days. And I go, 'Aha, *now* the doctor will listen.' Three days later I had an appointment, and a week later this little blemish was diagnosed as a late stage of malignant melanoma.

CRIES AND WHISPERS

To medical science, an intimation is a particle without weight or mass. Traditional societies, however, accord dreams and subtle warnings far greater gravity. Siberians believe that when the guardian power they call Sila rouses itself to intervene in human life, its first messages are gentle, delivered to "little children innocently at play" to whom Sila speaks "in a soft voice like a woman's." The children then tell the shaman, who knows he must heed the warning to avert catastrophe.[1]

According to anthropologist Ruth Inge-Heinze, one reason severe illnesses are rare in some Asian tribal societies may be that for them even a bad dream can be a respectable medical complaint. This way, she says, serious disease is headed off early, "because the conditions leading up to it are nipped in the bud. The community and the family have home remedies for feeling unwell and not knowing why."[2]

In our culture, to enter a doctor's consulting office because we are having nightmares or just "feeling strange" would be viewed as sheer hypochondria. We assume that what is "in our heads" probably has little connection with what's in our bodies. But according to Chinese medical philosophy, mental premonitions may be a sign that the body is no longer able to communicate with itself. When we become too imbalanced, says the Nei Ching, "the Tao no longer circulates warnings against physical excesses."[3] Perhaps at this point only dreams can speak, as the flesh has become mute.

One former patient told me that for a year before she discovered she had advanced lymphoma, she had been having dreams that ended with a disembodied voice frantically shouting "Help me! Help me!" *Help who?* she wondered. *With what?* On the surface her life was fine. What was the source of this plea? From what province of being did it hail? She could only respond with bafflement.

Like an infant who cries without being able to point to the source of its distress, the body is often inarticulate. Unlike a parent, who becomes attuned to the nuances of her baby's distress signals, we often turn a neglectful, incurious ear to the urgent phonemes of the bodymind.

For several years before I was diagnosed with thyroid cancer, my girlfriend told me I was giving elaborate lectures in my sleep, sometimes for hours at a time. "It sounds important," Susan informed me. "You shout and wave your arms around. But I can't understand a word."

I begged her to try to record me. Not a person to be roused gratefully from a good sleep, she agreed to park a tape machine by her pillow, but that plan flopped: every time she turned it on, she said, I instantly shut up. Once, she told me exasperatedly, "You opened your eyes—which was terrible because I could tell you were still fast asleep—and said to me indignantly, 'I was talking to myself!' Then you turned over with this smug little smile."

It was cute, but a little ominous. Some part of me, some unknown doppelgänger, was clambering onstage every night to babble, mutter, and rant while I slept unawares. Whatever he had to say was apparently his little secret.

At the time I was working on a book on the history of the nuclear era, harrowing, sardonic work that had produced some sixty manila folders of grim minutiae: statistics of how many times our bombs could reduce their cities to radioactive carrot sticks; or, somehow more awfully, the code name for the first French A-Bomb ("the Blue Gerbil"). One night, nearing a deadline, I had a terrible dream:

> *I am playing in my garage, assembling, as I used to when I was a kid, a "spaceship" made of scrounged junk—baby buggy wheels, radio knobs, appliance cartons. I step back to admire my handiwork, but realize with a gasp of horror that I have unwittingly constructed a real atom bomb. I lunge to defuse it, but it is too late. At just that moment, it throbs to life with a low, malevolent hum. All I can do is stare in horror, feeling the weight of the millions of lives about to be obliterated by this thing the size of a shopping cart.*

I awoke gasping, like a man whose head has been held underwater, feeling the suffocating presence of pure evil. The menace that lingered in my bedroom was so palpable that, for the first time since childhood, I left the nightlamp on so I could get back to sleep.

In the morning I chalked it up to the dire stuff I had been wading through: atomic-father Robert Oppenheimer sepulchrally intoning for the cameras, "Now I am become death, the destroyer of worlds," after Hiroshima; Teller's eerie, triumphal cry, "It's a boy!" when his H-bomb at last flashed on. But the nightmare's sense of unmitigable disaster was unlike any feeling I had ever experienced. Had I been wiser, I might have realized that a dream so searing is a personal message, not a newsclipping; that a bomb in the house is a bomb in the body; that something not out-there but in-here was armed and ticking.

Seemingly prophetic nightmares had continued desultorily to trouble my sleep during the two years leading up to my cancer diagnosis. During my first month in Boston I had dreamed:

> *A tidal wave is about to engulf the house of the former editor. I'm pointing up at it, screaming—it is poised, as awesome as the final scene in the film* The Last Wave, *to drown the world. I can see dolphins, crabs, and various other marine life caught up in this rearing, mile-high wall of seawater.*

The next day, the same editor had called unexpectedly to ask if I wanted to spend the weekend with her and her husband at a beach house they had rented. I had been impressed at this synchronicity, but assumed the dream had only symbolized my anxiety about taking over the magazine, where each new deadline was a looming natural disaster. A few days later, though, I received a mailed-in submission, a Montana woman's memoir of her father, describing the last sculpture he had created before he died of cancer—a roiling, frozen wave filled with meticulously crafted sea creatures.

Years later, watching *The Last Wave* again on video, I realized how appropriate my dream-reference had been. A lawyer defending an Australian aborigine against murder charges begins to have disturbing visions of a wave that will destroy the world. At one point, exasperated at the aborigine's indifference toward the white justice system, he shouts, "You don't understand—you're in desperate trouble!"

The aborigine gives him a long look. "It is you who are in trouble. You no longer know what dreams are for." Later, the lawyer cries out to his minister father, "You explained away our dreams, and now when they return, we don't know what they mean!"

THE LANGUAGE OF DREAMS

Not knowing what my dreams meant, I dismissed them as curiosities, oddities that could sometimes perform such parlor tricks as promising an unexpected weekend at the shore. But dreams that symbolically point to illnesses yet unseen are well known in psychological literature. Aristotle observed that "since the beginnings of all events are small, so, it is clear, are those of the diseases. . . . It is manifest that these beginnings are more evident in sleeping than in waking moments."[4]

The human body echoes with whisperings. Unknown to us, who find it a laconic stranger, it is a regular Chatterbox Café, absorbed in a constant dither of cross-conversation. We are just now beginning to discover the built-in early warning system housed beneath our skin. Psychobiology researcher Ernest Rossi proposes that "the immune system can function as a sensory 'organ,' signaling the central nervous system about noncognitive stimuli such as bacteria, tumors, viruses and other toxins within the body."[5]

In this, he holds with Freud, who once cited with favor a colleague's remark that during sleep the mind "is obliged to receive and be affected by impressions of stimuli from parts of the body and from changes in the body of which it knows nothing when awake." This phenomenon occurred "owing to the magnifying effect produced upon impressions by dreams."[6]

Perhaps my earlier nightmare about hot coals burning my throat was in this category. At the time, my thyroid gland, directly adjacent to the larynx, had unbeknownst to me contained a good-sized tumor. Had subliminal physical sensations been translated into mental images? But then why had the dream been so hellishly alight, so fraught with strange symbols and unsettling ritual?

Jungians call the dream the client brings to the first session with the therapist the "presenting dream." Such dreams often turn out to be particularly significant, as if the psyche, knowing it will at last have a chance to be heard, produces an image that at once expresses the crux of the disorder and augurs the likely outcome. Similarly, we should not be surprised if our first dreams of illness contain clues to both the origins of sickness and the prospects for healing.

Such dreams might be placed in the same category as Joseph Campbell's "herald," the figure who summons the hero to embark, however reluctantly, upon the journey. These figures, Campbell writes, represent the "unconscious deep," in which we find the "rejected, unadmitted, unrecognized, unknown or undeveloped factors, laws, and elements of existence." It seems clear to me now that my dreams were not only foreshadowing the onset of illness, but highlighting deeper "soul issues" I had long avoided—a rolling series of *tsunamis* that now threatened to inundate me.

DEENA'S STORY

I was fascinated to discover several other cases in which a powerful dream that seemed to reveal an illness also addressed a central psychospiritual issue in the dreamer's life. Deena Metzger, poet, essayist, and former breast cancer patient, provided me with one such example.

I visited her one afternoon in her elegantly ramshackle house at the end of what may be the last dirt road in the overdeveloped L.A. basin. A fence was hung with bright ceramic masks. A nearby stump, circled by colored stones, had a delicate salmon-and-gray whelk stuck in one cleft. A brick patio overlooked a staggering view of the dry Topanga canyon lands. Dogs, one a pure white shepherd-wolf mix named Isis, after the Egyptian goddess of healing, loped around the property. Everything was silent but for the drifting wind-chimes and the buzz of a single fly.

Metzger had been a fearless radical in the hothouse early days of the women's movement—once, she remembers with a bemused laugh, losing her college post for "reading an outrageous political-sexual poem." Her firing made her a cause célèbre in an academic freedom case. One night, finding herself standing before a rally of two thousand people at a fundraiser, "the persona of the public warrior just sprang fully clothed and armored out of my head!"

Later, as a teacher in three different colleges, she began puzzling over why so many young women she knew were getting cancer. Not long afterward—a few months before discovering that she, too, had a breast tumor—she had an unforgettable dream-vision. Deena had visited Chile just before the coup that brought military strongman Augusto Pinochet to power; now she dreamed that she had been kidnapped by the Chilean secret police and dragged away to a house of interrogation:

> They take off my blouse and give me only a piece of plastic, like the kind that dry-cleaning bags are made of, to cover myself. I am put on a torture table, the door opens, and this ugly, obese woman enters. I recognize her as the concentration camp matron from the documentary Night and Fog. She's going to torture me by delivering electric shocks to my genitals. Now the odd thing is, the name of the secret police in Chile, the acronym, happens to be D.I.N.A.! This dream was visually so vivid, the story so clear, I knew it meant something important, but I wasn't sure what.

The fat, ugly woman is a creature of the Underworld, the hidden realm of "night and fog." Deena's genitals are going to be "shocked" in the attempt to wrest a secret from her which she has sworn never to tell. But it was not until many years later—after a successful operation for breast cancer and prolonged psychotherapy—that the "shocking" secret was revealed to her: childhood violation.

Upon learning of the suppressed events that had secretly manipulated her adult existence, things began to fall into place. "It was why I always felt I had to cover up the intuitive side of myself—because intuition is a path that might have led me to stumble on this hidden truth." Having to hide the truth from herself all her life created what she calls "the split" in her being: "I had to create a masked self, split off from the experience, because the memories would have been intolerable. I realize now that my sexually crusading outer behavior was a smokescreen—a way to both tell the story and conceal it, to know and not know. Everybody considered me the most outspoken person that they knew, but all the time I was covering up, even from myself."

It is fascinating that in her nightmare Deena is being tortured by D.I.N.A.—by *herself*. *She* is the "secret police" whose job is to both reveal the truth and suppress it; she is the secret-keeping victim who is being forced both to tell and deny.

When I ask Deena if she thinks there was a root, a psychological nubbin, to her disease, she nods vigorously. "The silence. The cancer is made of silence."

An equally extraordinary case is that of a British mystic named Edward Thornton, author of an obscure work titled *The Diary of a Mystic*. In midlife, Thornton began to have abnormally vivid and inexplicable dreams: In one, his head was being shaved "after the manner of a monk"; in another, he was in an operating room in which Christian hymns were being sung.

> Then on May 9, 1948, I dreamed I was in a room where an operation was to take place, before a class of medical students. . . . Then on September 23, 1948, I had the following dream: I was going the round of solitary cells in a prison with my brother, whose job it was to awaken the various inmates by chopping their foreheads with an axe. Each occupant was found kneeling in the classical Christian way at a prayer-desk, with his head resting on a block. As we entered the last cell my brother gave one chop at the slumberer's forehead and immediately awakened him. I felt that I was the one to whom this had happened.[7]

Shortly thereafter, Thornton was diagnosed with a brain tumor. Exactly one year after his first "operating-class" dream, he found himself in the hospital awaiting surgery: "A male nurse arrived and shaved off my hair, and shortly before nine o'clock I was wheeled to the operating theatre. . . . The operation lasted about five hours, and when the bandage was removed from my head, I discovered that my skull had been cut right down the middle, thus fulfilling in the outer world the head-chopping dream which I had experienced."[8]

I found it fascinating that in Deena Metzger's, Thornton's, and my own dreams, despite our differing psychological histories and diseases, our illnesses and their treatments had been prefigured in such significant ways. Like Thornton, I had woken up in the hospital after a surgery I had symbolically dreamed about on several occasions as a "decapitation." Metzger had dreamed of being on a gurney and having her chest covered, as is customary in breast surgery, with a sheet of plastic. (In her dream, however, it was a "plastic dry-cleaning bag," itself symbolically interesting: Such clear plastic would serve to reveal, not conceal, what is within; dry-cleaning is a process for removing evidence of serious stains, as well as a kind of "chemotherapy"; and unattended children have been known to suffocate soundlessly in dry-cleaning bags.)

What was particularly interesting, however, was the element of ritual sacrifice that appeared in all our dreams. In shamanic initiations, a symbolic dismemberment of the body is a necessary prelude to spiritual reconstitution. One scholar explains that Egyptian priestly texts specified, "A dissolution or sacrifice of the old body must occur; it is to be tortured or fire tested, or the like." Shamans talk of dream-visions in which their heads are cleaved open and their brains taken out and "washed," or their eyes plucked from their sockets and impregnated with gold dust, enabling them to perceive the deeper order of things.

According to Robert M. Stein, a Jungian psychologist, the underlying agenda of the healing sacrifice is the surrender of whatever impedes the greater stream of our life: We must relinquish a part of ourselves, perhaps an entire pattern of identity, which we have cherished and clung to even after it has become an obstacle to our growth. We may be asked to face a painful truth, heal an ancient wound, realize a suppressed potential, or change a relationship. As Stein points out, the roots of the word *sacrifice* come from the Latin *sacer*, sacred, and *facere*, to make: "That which must be given up, far from being discarded, is the very thing in need of transformation and renewal."[9]

For example, the dream-image that began my journey, the "boiling out" of my brains, is suggestive of what Jung called the *sacrificum intellectus*, a partial abdication of the evaluating rational intelligence in order to free the unconscious to speak. Tibetan yogis drink sacramental liquor from a skull-cup to symbolize, among other things, a relinquishment of the limiting logical faculties.

I always had been told I was "too smart for my own good," too adept at rationalizing, too skilled at complex yet often obfuscatory reasoning that often hid a reluctance to act. In the dream I refer to, my brains are being vaporized, hissing from three holes drilled in the top of my head, a burnt offering to heaven. (I was interested to read several years thereafter of the work of the late Australian psychiatrist Ainslee Meares, who has obtained several documented and dramatic spontaneous remissions teaching patients with advanced cancers a technique he called "atavistic meditation." This involved a "regression of mental function" characterized by "mental stillness and absence of intellectual activity." Meares theorized that such a state permitted the "self-righting system of the body" to function unimpeded.)

In all three of our dreams, too, the "target organ" seemed to hold specific psychological significance. For the highly religious Thornton, the location of his brain tumor symbolized the seat of Athena, *sapiens sapientae,* divine reason, for whom he had always felt a particular affinity; for Deena, it was her sexual organs, the site of trauma as well as liberation; for me, it was the source of my voice.

For in my dreams, the "target organ" was not the thyroid gland but the larynx, the organ of self-expression, long an area of ambivalence in my life. I had literally and figuratively suppressed my voice for as far back as I could remember. Chronically shamed in childhood for being a rather oddball kid, I had developed a false persona that had left me with a nagging suspicion that I could never tell the whole truth. Later, in my early teens, distressed that my voice wasn't cracking and deepening as fast as my friends', I began trying to force it lower. The result was a strangled-sounding tenor that fooled no one, but which once adopted proved an iron cage: I had to keep up the pretense—it seemed for years—lest my fraud be discovered.

My dream also suggested a psychospiritual remedy: the destruction of my voicebox by fire, which traditionally purifies. Perhaps the dream was saying that the "false voice" needed to be burned away so an authentic one could emerge from the ashes. Exaggerated as this hypothesis may sound, I have even wondered whether, if I had heeded the call for inner healing, a psychological "sacrifice" might have replaced the cruder surgical one I was later to undergo. Had the psyche been stating, in the most urgent terms possible, use it— properly, honestly, feelingly—or lose it? When a sickness has meaning for the psyche, the Jungian scholar C. A. Meier notes, it has the "inestimable advantage that it can be vested with a healing power." The Greeks, he explains, believed that the god who created the illness was the same one who could make it well, thus allowing for the possibility that illness "contains its own diagnosis, therapy, and prognosis."[10]

Thus heralds of illness may, if we pay them sufficient heed, announce the nature, origins, treatment, and psychological significance of illness all at once. They may point to a way to approach disease that may lead to a greater wholeness, regardless of our choice of treatment or its eventual outcome. Though Joseph Campbell describes the bearer of tidings as "often dark, loathly, or terrifying, if one could follow, the way would be opened through the walls of day into the dark where the jewels glow."

WHEN THE HERALD CALLS

The herald, Campbell adds, appears at the moment when, unknown to the hero, "the familiar life horizon has been outgrown; the old concepts, ideals and emotional patterns no longer fit; the time for the passing of a threshold is at hand . . . marking a new period, a new stage, in the biography."[11]

In my talks with former patients, I was frequently struck by the fact that illness often seemed to announce itself at a critical moment of life-change rather than at a point of stasis. People were poised to accept a promotion, get married, finish a project, end a relationship. Sometimes it came at a nadir of life, a juncture when everything that could go wrong was going wrong.

As I noted earlier, my dream of the "throat-burning ritual" and the physical symptoms that soon followed came as I was putting the finishing touches on my crowning effort of nearly two years, a prototype issue for the magazine's new direction. It was a moment of profoundly mixed significance. On the one hand, I had accomplished, earning some laurels, what I had set out to do. On the other hand, my efforts had failed to reap any of the emotional rewards I had been subconsciously laboring toward. The day that I left my office for the last time, I had reached into a bag of fortune cookies I kept around as tie-breakers in editorial meetings and cracked one open. There was no printed scroll. For the first and only time in my life, my fortune cookie was empty. I had helped bring a magazine into being, but I had inadvertently erased myself.

Psychologist Meredith Sabini notes that before the eruption of disease, "There may have been many years of satisfactory adjustment in life, including having one or several central relationships or roles which bear heavy libidinal investment." But then something turns sour; the carefully arranged centerpiece of life begins to crumble, and along with it the unsuspectedly fragile sense of self. It is sometimes at this moment that the herald makes its appearance.

ERNIE'S STORY

With his sandy hair, salt-and-pepper mustache, and boy-devil grin, Ernie Scharhag bears a passing resemblance to the jazz singer Mose Allison. Nearly a decade ago he was diagnosed with nonspecific nodular lymphocytic lymphoma and presented with a maximum prognosis of five years. Ernie's life until then had been a series of steeplechases after dreams whose real-world obstacles he could never quite hurdle. He had started out as an ambitious and talented science student, getting a job as a professional chemist while he was still in college. He married, had a baby girl, and then dropped out to follow the hippie trail, buying a tract of land in a small Hispanic-populated town in northern New Mexico. He lived a few happy years there, supporting himself by farming his land and selling Indian art and jewelry, "getting a real feel for the kinds of lives the Indians led, for their worldview and spirituality."

But his growing family needed more money. They moved to Albuquerque, where Ernie quickly landed a high-level job fabricating humidity-sensitive crystal for a probe on the first space-shuttle mission. Soon he was a partner in a company that designed printed circuit boards for satellites. He also fell in love with his partner's girlfriend. The two lovers soon ran off to Phoenix, where, after an idyll that lasted until the money ran out, Ernie was forced to take a new job. "I found myself in sweltering hell, selling commodities in a stockbroker 'boiler factory' for a man I hated." The more money Ernie made, the more he hated himself, but over a few jaw-clenching years he had amassed a small fortune. He decided to retire young and pour all his energy into building "the love nest of my life for my girlfriend, complete with the cedar fence and the swimming pool."

Working at a furious pace, Ernie compressed a year of remodeling into a few months. But once again, ultimate happiness eluded his most diligent efforts. His girlfriend began having an affair. He was overcome with the feeling that his life had been "a gigantic mistake. I've given up my wife and kids, thrown everything away, for what?" One night, drunk and crying during a visit to his ex-wife, he had a sudden realization. "I just knew, on a cellular level, that I was going to die soon. I kept telling my ex, 'I'm gonna die, I'm gonna die.' I was so blotto that I didn't even know what I was saying. Then two days later, the same horrible feeling just overwhelmed me."

The final indignity, he says with a self-deprecating smile, was being robbed and beaten by a disturbed Vietnam vet he had befriended. The man had waited behind the door until Ernie arrived home from a screening of the movie *Gandhi,* and then leaped out and knocked him nearly unconscious. "All I could think was, gee, Jeannie's not going to like this blood on the white carpet."

The portents seemed to him unmistakable: The time had come for radical change. He decided to give up everything and move to Colorado to pursue his early love of Buddhism. He felt free, exultant—he had at last broken the cycle, and was ready to begin again. But within weeks of his arriving, he discovered he had cancer. "I wasn't all that surprised," says Ernie. "My *karma* was overripe."

JOY'S STORY

In a number of cases, the illness was discovered at a moment when freedom suddenly beckoned, when the ice had begun to thaw and old patterns were falling away. Alexis de Toqueville once observed, "It is not always when things are going from bad to worse that revolutions break out." Rather, it is when a repressive regime long tolerated without protest "suddenly relaxes its pressure," allowing long-pent-up energies to erupt.

Joy Ballas-Beeson had just decided to get a divorce after what she calls "a represssive marriage to a traditional Greek man." One of the reasons she had married Dmitri, fifteen years her senior, was that men her own age seemed "too childish"; Dmitri was a man she could look up to. But things began to go wrong from the beginning. His parents promptly arrived from Greece and gave every indication that they intended to stay with the new couple indefinitely. Joy, it was given out, would be expected to teach school to support the extended family; Dmitri would go to college, while his parents would take care of the baby.

Joy soon rebelled against the imposed arrangement. Things came to a head in a pushing, screaming donnybrook. Joy's new father-in-law barricaded himself in his room until Dmitri drove the fuming old man to the airport. But in winning the battle, Joy lost the war. Only twenty-five, guilty about the intrafamilial chaos she had created, she began to press down her real feelings and submit to her husband all the more. Joy recounts that Dmitri, sensing his advantage, became even more controlling and manipulative. Eventually, he induced her to give up the love of her life, elementary school teaching, to work in his struggling restaurant business. But no matter what she did, she could never please him.

> I skipped my twenties trying to be as old as he was. I became more of a possession and a business partner than a wife. We had a ten-acre farm outside of town and a restaurant. We worked eighty or a hundred hours a week in the restaurant, plus I had to drive our teenage kids around, and when it was a slow period I got an extra job to help out. It was a ridiculous life: Work, work, work and then . . . get to work!

At last, she demanded a divorce. Around the time of the proceedings, Joy became involved in a variety of metaphysical study groups. Previously unknown new vistas began opening in her life:

> I kept doing "releasing exercises" and zapping Dmitri with unconditional love. It was a tremendous relief to me after all those years of suppressed anger. But, during the year after I was divorced, I suddenly lost my job and then got rheumatoid arthritis that progressed very rapidly through every joint in my body.
>
> The timing was so strange! Here I am, finally taking steps to resolve things, and at that moment *everything* goes wrong. I think that sometimes it's like when you pull the cork out of the champagne, it squirts out from all the unreleased pressure, foaming everywhere. All that energy that's released has to go someplace. Maybe symptoms are like that foam.

JACOB'S STORY

Even when illness seems an errant stroke of fate, it may fit into the pattern of a life in wholly unsuspected ways. Dr. Jacob Zieghelboim remembers sensing from the time he graduated from medical school that he would only pursue his profession for twenty years. "I would mention this to people occasionally," he says, "but they could only say—humoring me, no doubt—'How strange.' "

He couldn't help but agree. Jacob's trajectory had been a smooth, well-planned ascent into the stratosphere of the medical world, where he was ensconced as a highly respected UCLA oncologist. When he discovered he had lymphoma, in a single lymph node in his neck, his reaction was one of incredulity: "I was doing great professionally. I was a happy person. The kids were fine, healthy. I felt sexually attractive, my marriage was good, I was popular. Moneywise, I was very comfortable. In fact, I'd just gotten a grant from the government to leave work to do research for a few years. I thought, isn't this ironic? I *work* with head-and-neck cancer and here is a cancer on *my* neck! It seemed so bizarre."

Though a dread disease had suddenly (and potentially, terminally) interrupted his life, Jacob was baffled by his own response. "I felt *excited*. Like something amazing, incredible, was happening! It was like this adventure. I suddenly felt free to call my own shots."

During his treatment, he began unexpectedly to examine what until then had seemed a life as unblemished as a California plum. After undergoing successful treatment, he went back to work, but the pieces no longer seemed to fit together. The chairman of his department, an idolized longtime mentor, was oddly unresponsive. "He seemed to feel that nothing had happened to me. As if I had gone on a vacation, and now it's business as usual. He said, essentially, 'You've been treated, you're fine, just get back to work.' But I knew something *profound* had happened, something I needed to figure out."

That's when Jacob Zieghelboim, rising medical star, suddenly crashed to earth. Work, marriage, what he calls his "polarization of the human aspects of myself," were suddenly thrown open to inner scrutiny. Long-forgotten passions from his youth began once again to draw him—his childhood fascination with the workings of the mind, the articles in *Planet* magazine about mysteries of the unexplained he used to devour in his native Venezuela—all of which had been shelved, with great finality, by the ambitious young medical student. Now he was changing, feeling urges to color outside the lines, straying into new yet oddly familiar territory.

He was due for a sabbatical that he had felt too busy to accept. Now he decided to take it, beginning what was to become a protracted period of veering-off—attending self-development workshops, exploring various meditation techniques, eventually even traveling to China and Tibet. Living today in an airy, Spanish-style house, and defining himself as a "practicing psycho-oncologist," Jacob views the moment his illness appeared as "the last chance I would have ever had to get off the railroad train."

Leaning back in his padded black leather chair, he says, "I'm incredulous now at how restricted I was. I think if I hadn't changed at that exact juncture, I would have remained on dead center for the rest of my life."

Though the first inklings of disease are by no means always synchronous with the ripening of psychological issues or the call to self-discovery, the herald can provoke, as Campbell says, "the awakening of the self." It is supremely ironic that we may only begin to knit together the strands of our lives when they seem to be unraveling, perhaps for the last time. It may even be that, as the philosopher P. Manly Hall once remarked, "If a life is going outwardly contrary to its inward need, nature will not permit this disaster without making some effort to correct the situation." Sometimes disease, either by default, attribution, or the mysterious inward workings of the soul, becomes a message that is simply too terrible to ignore.

5

THE SYMPTOM:
THE VOICE OF THE
BODYMIND?

The gods have become diseases; Zeus no longer rules
Olympus but rather the solar plexus, and produces
curious specimens for the doctor's consulting room.

—C. G. JUNG[1]

THERE IS NOTHING more shattering than being betrayed by our
bodies. Job manages to bear up under catastrophe—the destruction of his flocks, his children, and his social status—but when
Satan demands, "Skin for skin . . . put forth your hand and touch
his bone and his flesh," and God sends an affliction of boils, Job
crumbles.

A symptom expresses an ultimate human vulnerability. It is evidence that we can be invaded; that our body is no longer—and
perhaps never was—entirely our own; that though we may consider
ourselves primarily psychological beings, we are ever subject to the
purposeless whims of blind matter. Something dumb, brute, and
disabling has sunk its barb into our flesh, and our natural tendency
is to try to rip it out.

Ironically, the symptom may be the result of ignoring far quieter
knocks at the gate. As the narratives in the last chapter show, we
are used to dismissing the cries and whispers emanating from the
psyche as insubstantial, their messages as unsubstantiated. The herald may have appeared to us in many guises, spoken in many voices,
before revealing itself in our flesh.

The symptom, too, is a herald—or perhaps more accurately a
harbinger—of a systemic pathology extending beyond the place
it first appears, perhaps even beyond the body itself, into the family,

the society, the environment. A symptom is more than an announcement—it is a collision of intersecting forces. In antiquity, says C. A. Meier, the symptom was considered "an expression of the consensus point between the outer and the inner." Chinese medicine views it as a product of "intercommunication of internal and external systems."² The word derives from the Greek *syn*, "together," and *piptein*, "to fall." Disturbances in life, in the body, may have been present for days, months, or years before "falling together" into an obvious symptom.

The body can damp down such disturbances for a time, in the same way a living lake can absorb and purify a certain volume of industrial effluents, or greenery can recycle excess carbon dioxide. But at some point, the natural capacities of any environment—outer or inner—are stretched beyond the system's ability to adjust, and a breakdown occurs. An overt sign of imbalance—a stomach cancer, a die-off of river pike, a bloom of red algae—appears at last, seemingly out of nowhere.

GEORGE'S STORY

"When we get the symptoms of a cold," George Melton observes, "we run down to the drugstore to get Contac to suppress them so we can go back to the behavior that gave us the cold in the first place. But if we don't listen to the symptom that first taps on our shoulder, we may get a much harder one later on."

George's speaking style, as relentless and mellifluous as a rushing brook, has served him well as an inspirational speaker. He has barnstormed the alternative healing circuit, delivering a patented lecture that credits inner work, diet, and other holistic therapies for his current state of health. When I talked to him, he was in remission from ARC (AIDS-Related Complex):

> I didn't wake up with AIDS. I woke up with "the crabs" a long time ago. But I didn't know it was a message. Even if I had, I would have been afraid to look inside because I was convinced I'd only find out how wrong, bad, and awful I was.
>
> So I went down the drugstore and got some A-200 to get rid of it. Then I got gonorrhea, so I ran to the doctor and took some pills to get rid of that, too. Even if I'd *known* it was a message, I wouldn't have listened. I would have assumed it was about my homosexuality, and all the negative

parental and social messages that go along with that, and just shut it off.

Then I got syphilis and so on and so on, till one day I woke up with AIDS. AIDS was something spoken by my body in the language bodies speak, which is symptoms. And it said, "Stop trying to kill the messenger and respond to the message," which was that I'd been living self-destructively for a long time. AIDS was the one disease my body manifested that couldn't be cured with a pill. It forced me to go beyond the physical and find the things inside me—the self-hatred and fear—that I had been dying of for a long time.

Certainly, not all AIDS patients feel this way. Many are enraged by perspectives such as George's, which they regard as infuriatingly glib. Indeed, the skeptic might well view George's diagram of his illness as pure confabulation. Like a pagan trying to ascertain which god is responsible for the calamity that has befallen him, or a tribe blaming an eruption of Mt. Pele on a broken taboo rather than plashings of igneous rock beneath the Pacific floor, George is searching for human notions of purpose in a universe of random collision. His belief that his symptoms were a personal "message" seems on a par with the solipsistic eighteenth-century notion that a melon has ridges to facilitate its division at the family table.[3] His reasoning might be interpreted at best as a way to dignify an ineluctably bad situation, to find a handhold on a slippery slope; or at worst a form of denial and a delusory attempt at control. Nonetheless, I found that his attitude was echoed by many patients who had exceeded their prognoses, who had come to see their symptoms as organic outgrowths of their lives, and so as mandates for change.

MARGARET'S STORY

Margaret Green's [a pseudonym] first symptoms of ovarian cancer appeared two months after she had been given a clean bill of health by her gynecologist. It was June, and she was preparing to remarry her ex-husband, Kent. Their first union had been disastrous. Kent was charming, handsome, athletic, and a dead ringer for Margaret's idolized older brother, whose tragic death had devastated her. Unfortunately, Kent had also turned out to be an abusive drug addict.

Margaret, the child of an alcoholic, had left him after ten months and made a successful new life for herself. Kent had joined a small religious community and "found Jesus." But then, a few years later, he abruptly appeared again in her life—clean and sober, he insisted. He was going into the construction business with his brother in the Bay Area. He loved her. He had changed completely. Wouldn't she join him and rebuild their lives together?

Margaret, after some deliberation, decided to take a chance on hope. She had done well in real estate in her two-year, Kent-free interim, but she agreed to sell her house and move north of San Francisco to be together.

That summer began "two months of the greatest stress I'd ever known." Her money ran out as if from a sieve; by August, it was nearly gone. "Soon," she told me, "I'm selling all my beautiful clothes for groceries, my carefully built-up credit is kaput, they're threatening to repossess the expensive new car I'd bought myself. We can't even afford to drive across the Golden Gate Bridge because it costs a dollar!"

But money troubles were the least of it. Her dream of reconciliation began rapidly curdling into nightmare. She recounts: "Kent, because of his beliefs, says he can't have sex with me until we're married, at which time we're supposed to start immediately making babies for Jesus. I began to see I'd allowed myself to become trapped, boxed in, and once Kent realized he had me, he became physically abusive again.

"And I just felt . . . this is finally *it*. I've created it, I've made my bed, I have to lie in it. I'm going to have to stay with him the rest of my life."

Margaret was too proud to turn to her friends, who had all vociferously opposed the planned remarriage and had drifted away when they couldn't change her mind. "They would have written 'I told you so' in big letters across the sky. All my bridges were burned. I felt hopeless, trapped—there was no way out."

Then, one morning while showering, she found a lump. In the two months since her last completely normal exam, her ovaries, which were to be Kent's baby-making factories when he finally gave up his punitive celibacy, had suddenly become "huge." She was rushed into surgery. Though she was told there was an 80 percent chance that her tumors were benign, she instead woke up to a total hysterectomy—the tumors had been cancerous. Looking back from a distance of several years, Margaret muses, "Getting cancer was the only thing that could have gotten me out of that corner, short of divine revelation. It got me out of marrying Kent. It got me out of having his children. It even got me out of financial stress—there was a clause in my car insurance that said if I got sick, the company had to cover the payments. In some weird, horrible way, it was freedom."

Whether Margaret's inner conflict in any way contributed to the growth of her cancer cannot be determined, though a number of researchers have put forth the controversial hypothesis that some tumors may be seen as a "somatic expression [of an] existential crisis."[4]

The psychologist A. David Feinstein has reported on two patients in whom "a tumor of the female reproductive system revealed conflicts over a decision regarding childbearing." One was a nineteen-year-old gay woman with a three-centimeter tumor in her right ovary for which surgery had been recommended. The patient spontaneously had an extraordinary catharsis during her first group therapy session, replete with wild bodily movements, shouts and screams, "resembling at various points an exorcism, death wails, and childbirth." Later, after a "dialogue" with her symptom, the young woman came to see her tumor as, in Feinstein's words, "an expression of an inner desire toward becoming a mother, a wish she had been suppressing in the service of her homosexual identity."

The woman afterwards wrote in her journal, "Being a heterosexual meant having babies. Having babies meant being heterosexual. Being torn about my sexuality created what felt like a tear in my body. A wound. The wound was my ovary. My struggle manifested itself in a tumor."

Two weeks after her pivotal group therapy session, the tumor (it had not been biopsied, so there is no way of knowing if it was cancer) failed to show up on a scan. Five years later, she remained disease-free. Feinstein takes pains to stress that the emotional conflict and its subsequent resolution did not necessarily *cause* the tumor and its healing. But the inner work done by the young woman enabled her "to discover meanings associated with her illness, which assisted her in integrating the experience."[5]

CAN SYMPTOMS SPEAK?

There is a story told in the Korean Zen tradition: One morning as he is getting dressed, the hard-working prince of a powerful kingdom notices two red, painful spots on his thigh. Assuming them to be the bites of a poisonous insect that had burrowed into the royal bedclothes, he scolds his chamberlain, orders the silk sheets burned, and without a second thought begins his routine of palace duties.

But later that night, readying himself for bed, the prince beholds a chilling sight: The two bumps on his leg have turned into a pair of furiously darting eyes! Only with great difficulty he falls into fitful sleep. The minute dawn breaks, he flings aside his coverlets to inspect his leg. To his horror, not only are the eyes still there, but now, beneath them, a pair of rhythmically flaring nostrils! Terrified lest anyone discover his affliction, he binds his leg with a silken bandage; ignoring the faint sound of labored breathing (the nose seems to inhale each time he does), he attends to the affairs of state.

That evening, at a ceremonial banquet for his vassal-warlords from the outlying districts, he makes a pretense of merriment. But the assembled guests are startled by a muffled shout from beneath the table. The prince clamps his hand over his leg, nearly losing two of his fingers in the process: His symptom has grown a mouth!

Hastily excusing himself in the ensuing hubbub, he runs at full tilt to his private quarters, summons the court surgeon and, swearing him to silence, forces him to operate and cut away the face. A miracle cure! For several months, life returns to normal. But one day, as the prince leads his elite horse cavalry in a wheeling close-order drill, a furious scream erupts from nowhere: His symptom has returned with a vengeance. The prince's mount shies and rears, landing him in the mud. His men, hearing the secret face's strange cries, break ranks. Rumors begin to fly through the capital that the ruler is possessed by demons.

A second clandestine operation is performed, and a third, but to no avail. The face relentlessly reappears. Now unable to leave his room, the prince spends his days receiving magi and astrologers, muttering old frauds all, while the kingdom falls into disarray.

Finally a grizzled monk in frayed saffron robes barges unannounced into the prince's chambers. Brushing aside the handwringing courtiers, he informs the prince of a stream that lies off in a corner of a distant province, protected by Kwan Yin, the goddess of compassion. Its miraculous waters heal all wounds. Equipped with the monk's scrawled map, the prince sets out with a small company of imperial horsemen. After an arduous journey—during which the face, despite being swaddled in layers of muslin, continues its loud, inarticulate bawling—the party arrives at the sacred stream. Eagerly the prince leaps from his horse and removes a silver chalice from his gold-embroidered saddlebag.

He unwraps his leg and is about to pour the holy water on the hated face to silence it forever, when its mouth stops shouting.

"Wait!" it cries out. "All this time, you have never even looked closely at me nor tried to understand a single word I have said. Do you not recognize me?"

The prince, gazing closely, suddenly recognizes a distorted likeness of his own face, its eyes filled with a pain long unacknowledged. At the sight of it, the prince begins to weep, and as he does so the face begins to soften, the eyes growing limpid, melting into those of Kwan Yin herself. "You had no heart of compassion," she says. "No sword of self-insight. How else could I summon you to your true nature?" Now the courtiers, decamped at a curious distance, heard the sound of two voices talking, long into the night, about the secret suffering that had been disturbing the prince's sleep long before the face had appeared. When the sun came up, the prince had been healed—though a single eye would occasionally reappear and look around, just as a reminder.

A charming folktale, certainly, but scarcely a practicable healing protocol. The idea of symptoms as some visible text of the soul seems cruel and superstitious drivel, a throwback to Hieronymous Bosch's sixteenth-century canvases where sinners would suffer the bodily anguish befitting their moral state: A knight whose failing was anger is depicted being ripped limb from limb; a chronic gambler is missing his hands. We are rightly repelled by such views, in which the victim is blamed for the ailment; where a humped back announces a deformity of character, or leprosy a secret rot blooming in the soul. Yet we sometimes sense that, beyond naive ideas of a symptom as punishment or an exact symbolic rebus, the body may in some cases articulate, as do dreams themselves, an unspoken truth.

Certainly, that the body responds powerfully to our thoughts and feelings can scarcely be doubted. "The soul's passions all seem to be linked with a body," wrote Aristotle, "as the body undergoes modifications in their presence," a fact apparent to anyone who has ever had an unseemly fantasy about their junior high school English teacher and then blushed.

Still, a heart-pounding daydream is one thing, a disease quite another. The issue of whether a specific symptom may sometimes "express" a specific emotional pattern is a thorny one. It *has* been demonstrated that emotional events and acts of imagination can affect specific musculature, alter electrical potential, biochemistry, and immune function. Nor does it seem too far-fetched to suppose that the messenger molecules which latch onto various body sites with an exact lock-and-key fit might convey messages of emotional distress to our organs. But medical science has a lengthy task ahead to ascertain which biological conditions may be affected by our feelings, by what means and to what extent.

There are, of course, any number of apocryphal-sounding stories linking disease symptoms to a variety of emotional conflicts. Claims Leslie Weatherhead in his study of healing and religion:

> I have known a case of blindness caused through a refusal to "look ahead"; of abdominal disease because a patient "couldn't stomach" a certain situation; of bronchial catarrh that was cured when a patient "got something off his chest"; of anorexia nervosa due to a patient being "starved of love"; of disease of the esophagus brought on because a patient could not "swallow" the facts of an emotional situation.[6]

Weatherhead's formulations may well strike us as too pat, his anecdotes impossibly vague. But the idea of symptoms as bodily inscription is a persistent one. Aristotle defined human emotions as "words [*logoi*] expressed in human flesh." Indeed, in such phenomena as the stigmata of religious adepts, the body becomes positively literate, a stage on which might be enacted—as with the purported German stigmatist Therese Neumann—the Passion Play with all its bloody stations of the cross. When spiritual leader J. Krishnamurthi was about to heed his own spiritual call, his body suddenly manifested mysterious, goiterlike swellings at the site of each of the seven Hindu *chakras*.

Accounts of stigmata—the Korean prince in our story was also, in effect, a stigmatist—have long been curios of medicine. Today there is renewed interest in this phenomenon by mind-body theorists, for here are the most graphic illustrations (literally) of how the mind can seemingly write upon the flesh. Michael Murphy, in his encyclopedic work *The Future of the Body,* cites the case of Marie-Julie Jahenny, a nineteenth-century peasant girl on whose skin the words *O Crux Ave* appeared with an image of a cross and a flower.[7] Murphy suggests that such cases show "the great specificity with which the human body can dramatize highly charged issues."[8]

Stigmata, he points out, were not always skin markings, but sometimes significant physical wounds that were on occasion rigorously examined by medical panels. The laceration on nineteenth-century stigmatist Gemma Galgani's hand, according to the testimony of one attending doctor, "as a rule was very deep, and seemed to pass through the hand—the openings and both sides reaching the other."[9]

Murphy quotes psychoanalyst Sandor Ferenczi, who explained stigmata as the effect of "localized, converted excitement," which "masses at parts of the body which could be easily placed at the disposal of unconscious impulses."[10] It is a formulation strikingly similar to Alfred Adler's theory of disease as an "organ dialect" in which, as the psychologist Alfred Ribi explains, particular organs are predisposed to "react especially sensitively to psychological conflicts . . . If the conflict is projected onto the body, the 'inferior organ' reacts. If over a period of time the conflict cannot be transferred out of the projection into the psyche, where by nature it belongs, then the organ begins to show damage, which finally becomes irreparable."[11]

Carl Jung suggested that a simpler instance of mind-body language—blushing—pointed to the presence of a psychological complex with an intense "feeling-tone." Such a complex, he said, has "a certain amount of its own physiology. It can upset the stomach. It upsets the breathing, it disturbs the heart."[12] Doctors Laurence Foss and Kenneth Rothenberg maintain that blushing, a bodily "symptom" produced in response to the specific emotion of shame, shows that the human being is the only animal that "possesses a corporeal 'language for dramatizing the mental.' . . . Diseases of choice have to be reperceived in part as enacting a drama whose text is the body."

They suggest that, particularly in the case of chronic "diseases of civilization," the body may become an avenue of communication when other means of social and personal expression have become blocked. "In infomedical terms, when normal transmitter channels are closed off, psychosocial signals can be redirected along physiological channels and so translated into biological language."[13]

REROUTING EMOTIONS

In his film *Hannah and Her Sisters,* Woody Allen sputters to his girlfriend, "I don't get angry. I have a tendency to internalize. I . . . I grow a tumor instead." Though most of us would take it as merely a sardonic punch line, the tendency to "somaticize" unacceptable emotions is a trait I noticed in many of the journeyers I spoke with.

Arline Erdrich related, "I had one of these screaming mothers. The minute you ask them a question they don't listen, just start yelling at you. I could never counter that. It intimidated me. Every time I would try to express anger, my throat would close up so badly I would start choking."

Arline, whose advanced lymphoma began in the lymph nodes in her neck, remembers that the only time her mother ("a punitive person" who would whip her with wet towels) paid attention to her was when she was sick. "So whenever I was at a low point, I would almost consciously 'create' a fever and swollen glands. At least she would come and take my temperature."

Joy Ballas-Beeson, whose onset of rheumatoid arthritis was described in the last chapter, also had a lifelong difficulty expressing anger. During her healing journey, "I went in and yelled at my boss— something I'd never done in my life—and immediately broke out in these incredible hives which lasted for weeks."

Many researchers have noted psychosomatic cofactors in rheumatoid arthritis. Victims often have the sort of traumatic childhood in which emotions and memory become split off from consciousness. Ernest Rossi suggests the following model: "Neural activity that is usually associated with emotions is not experienced in the higher cortical pathways of mind, but is instead shortcircuited through the hypothalamus and its direct associations with the autonomic, endocrine, and immune systems."[14]

We might even speculate that a tendency to "reroute" or "somaticize" emotions might not only predispose certain persons to certain illnesses, but, given their apparent ability to influence the body with the mind, might also make them better "self-healers." For example, Niro Asistent, who believes her unusual remission from ARC (AIDS-Related Complex) had an inner component, told me, "When I was eleven and didn't want to go to school, I was able to paralyze my legs. The doctor would come and find them *literally* paralyzed, no reflexes at all. They would do all kinds of tests, but it was mysterious to them. Then, after schooltime, when I got bored and wanted to go out and play, I would just be able to walk again."

I, too, can recall half-consciously avoiding school and other childhood pressures by becoming ill. I had severe allergies and suffered frequently from asthmatic bronchitis, both classic diseases of children in emotionally troubled families. Asthmatic conditions have been related to disturbances in the parent-child relationship, particularly when a child is prevented from "speaking for himself." Asthmatic children's symptoms have been shown to respond strongly to what one researcher not wholly facetiously called a "parentectomy"—the removal of the child from the parental environs for a few months. Studies have shown this may produce dramatic symptomatic improvement in otherwise incurable cases, even when dust samples from the home were brought along and the child secretly exposed to them.[15]

Asthma has also been called "inner crying." The near-inability of some asthmatic patients to cry has been noted in some studies. One researcher has suggested asthma represents a regression to a "primitive speech mechanism," noting that crying is the basis for the respiratory control later employed in true speech.

Speech and self-expression had been painful issues in my own life. My parents claim, I suspect apocryphally, that I uttered my first sentence at seven months. As a child, I was congenitally gabby, a trait not welcomed at home or in school. My report card in fourth grade, under "citizenship," noted pointedly, "Marc's problem is that he talks incessantly." The year of that report card, I was taken to the hospital for the removal of my infected tonsils, a routine procedure in the fifties, but one which, as Ivan Illich points out, a child often experiences as "emotional aggression: . . . incarcerated in a hospital, . . . he learns that his body may be invaded by strangers for reasons they alone know."[16]

Looking back on the experience, I believe I subconciously experienced it as a punitive assault on my voice itself. I remember forming a decision that I would try to behave more like a "normal" kid. I began to damp down what I now saw as my excessive energy, tried not to "think so much about everything," spoke less, became watchful. This push-pull between self-expression and silence, the struggle between energy (the function of the thyroid gland) and its suppression, became a life-long motif. Always afire to express myself, I found within me a built-in flame retardant, a powerful inhibitory mechanism against bringing forth "unapproved" thoughts and feelings. When I finally got to *New Age Journal,* a suppressed desire to speak loudly, to make my presence felt, had poured forth. As is so often the case in illness, my symptoms "fell together" at a juncture of danger and opportunity, when a difficult psychosocial history was condensed into a single moment.

SYMPTOM AS HEALER, SYMPTOM AS SLAYER

Raymond Berté, professor of rehabilitation and a gifted amateur singer, developed a rare throat cancer that led to the surgical removal of his larynx. The cause, he believes, was in part his relationship with his father:

My father would confront me when I was playing with the other children. He would berate the hell out of me in front of all the other kids. "How come you're the only one I can hear? How come you have the biggest mouth on this street?" When he wanted to get my attention from a distance, he would let out a piercing whistle. . . . It would absolutely freeze me in my tracks. I would turn, and he would reach up and grab his own throat like that (Ray put his hands around his neck) and the message was, "I'm gonna strangle you!" . . . When I was being led into surgery, I heard a frightened little voice deep inside of me saying, "You won't have to listen to me anymore, Daddy."[17]

In this case the throat was a "target organ," the site of greatest psychological resistance, the place in the body that had became both the bearer of repression and the site of the struggle for emotional liberation.

In fact, even the timing of Berté's disease, as we have seen in other cases, seemed to show up at a moment when the self-strangling fingers of repression were beginning to loosen. Berté "used to get off on singing. Oh God, I didn't give a damn if anybody else enjoyed it. I used to thrill myself; I'd give myself goosebumps. . . . They say that a lightbulb shines brightest just before it burns out. The best singing I ever did in my life was just before I got the cancer."[18] It was almost as if, just when he was discovering a renewed sense of authentic being, his internalized forces of repression rose up with commensurate authority.

Again, Berté's experience evokes the concept of "falling together"—of body and mind; of inner and outer self; of individual and society; of immune system and pathogen; and in some ways perhaps even of health and illness. For our symptoms have a Janus-like quality, facing outward to the world and inward to the soul, expressing both deficiency and potential, both disease and the need for healing.

Jungian analyst James Hillman suggests that the disease site is precisely the part of our bodymind where we feel the most vulnerable: "where we are most exposed, we expend most efforts to conceal." But for the same reasons, the site of the symptom also may contain the potential for greater life. The place of vulnerability, says Hillman, is also an opening: "In your symptom is your soul, could be a motto."[19] He points out that Adler believed bodily symptoms were doorways into the undeveloped parts of the personality. Adler suggested that symptoms' "organ dialect" or "organ jargon" could "furnish us with inexhaustible material" about our central emotional conflicts, once they had gained our attention.

This paradox often has been remarked upon by psychologists and physicians alike. The symptom is at once an attack on the life of the body *and* an expression of it. Abraham Maslow, speaking from a psychological viewpoint, asked, "Does sickness mean having symptoms? I maintain now that sickness might consist of not having symptoms when you should."

In the eighteenth century, before the idea developed of "fighting" fevers with aspirin, an elevated body temperature was considered a sign not of the disease, but of the resistance to the disease. Indeed, elevated temperature is now being recognized as a brain-initiated strategy to combat pathological agents. In a balletically intricate choreography, the body responds to bacteria by releasing chemicals called pyrogens (literally, "heat-causing") into the bloodstream to kill off the offending microorganisms. Perhaps, then, the earlier medical canon had it right; fever is " 'an affection of life striving to break away from death.' . . . *Februare* is to expel ritually from a house the shades of the dead."[20]

Psychologically, a symptom may represent an attempt to throw off the dead hand of the emotional past—a last-ditch effort to both exorcise and express the deepest personal pain. The site of the symptom may be the place where the issues of transformation are focused most poignantly, most pressingly. Whether one sees the symptom as the product of some unconscious "purpose," or merely attributes a symbolic meaning to a biological accident after the fact, seeing it as a resonant event may provide a powerful healing tool. Jung notes that symptoms, "on account of the introspection and concentration bestowed on them . . . are precisely the places of the most potentiality."

Several anecdotal cases of cancer that seem to be related to the need to "give voice" to the self appear in medical literature. A psychiatrist who has studied spontaneous remission cases relates the case history of a thirty-two-year-old patient who had witnessed his own father plan the murder of a beloved relative. After the crime was committed, the son was overwhelmed with fear that he would be called to testify against his own father in court, and eventually repressed the entire incident.

Around the same time that this psychological trauma occurred, the man developed throat cancer. But during an intense psychotherapy session the night before he was to undergo surgery to remove the growth, he broke down and recounted the entire episode, weeping and trembling as he relived his long-buried emotions.

Within four hours, he finished the first meal he had been able to eat without pain in a week and subsequently canceled the surgery. Within four days, the tumor had completely disappeared.[21]

The oft-cited Japanese researcher Yujiro Ikemi, who made a study of spontaneous remission, relates the case of a Shinto preacher, "taciturn and self-punitive by nature," who developed cancer of the vocal cords. In a moving conversation, the president of his religious organization told him he was an "invaluable asset" to the church and should continue to preach. He did so, the hoarseness disappeared, and he was cured of his cancer in less than a year.[22]

In these two cases, a surrender to the unacknowledged potential embodied by the symptom seemed to catalyze a healing process. Mind-body researcher Ernest Rossi suggests that "tuning in to a symptom with an attitude of respectful inquiry rather than the usual patient stance of avoidance, resistance, and rejection" can give the patient access to "signals from those parts of the personality that are in need of expressive development."

From what I have observed, when people submit to these interrogatories, disease may begin to look less like a mysterious monster than a part of their own substance. Our monsters—the word derives from the Latin term for a portent of the gods—as often as not reveal us to ourselves.

THE HEALING DIALOGUE: ALBERT'S STORY

The Jungian analyst Albert Kreinheder was stricken with crippling rheumatoid arthritis at what seemed to him a high point in his life. Every joint in his body became so painful that he was unable to get up from bed or put on his coat without assistance. He had to crawl up and down steps and "worm" his way across the floor. His dry bones grinding against each other caused pain that not even two dozen aspirins a day could touch. After exhausting every possible avenue of therapy, "including physicians, chiropractors, nutritionists, masseuses, and tarot cards," Kreinheder decided that the only thing he could do was to try to "talk" to his pain.

His dialogue was at first the cry of a vanquished innocent to a mindless, tyrannical oppressor. "You hold me tight in your grip. I am terribly frightened by you. I have no control over you, no access to you, no power to influence you."

"Pain" responded to him that its only purpose was to show its superiority: "I have a power beyond your power. My will surpasses yours." But then, the "conversation" took an unexpected turn. Pain declared itself to be not just a petty tyrant, but "he of whom there is no other. I want to be with you closely in your thoughts at all times. That is why I press you in the grip of my power and make you think only of me. Now with my presence in you, you can no longer live the same way and do the same things."

Suddenly Kreinheder discovered a meaning in his disease: "Our wound is the place where the Self finds entry into us." His arthritis was no longer experienced simply as pure anguish, but as an aspect of the "larger personality." His illness was a "window," and "a positive sign showing potentials for growth. . . . Either we grow with the individuation urge, or it grows against us." Although he had, in effect, given up the fight—not in resignation, but in "intimate involvement" with his "companion of pain"—his disease slowly went into remission.

In another dialogue, Kreinheder was told by a "guide" figure who arose out of his imaginary landscape:

> The paradox is that the wound is also the treasure. The physical misery gets your attention. But then if you go deeper into it, there is much more to it, memories and imagination and . . . psychic images that come with the symptoms. The symptoms open you up. They literally tear you open so that the things you need can flow in. . . . With every symptom there comes also a symbolic content, and it is the task of the soul to expand itself so it can include the invading images and symbols. . . . The disease always carries its own cure and also the cure for your whole personality.[23]

AMPLIFYING THE SYMPTOM

One of the principal exponents of this heretical way of relating to symptoms is Arnold Mindell, a Zurich-trained American psychologist now living in Oregon. Mindell discovered his technique through a client who lay in the hospital dying of stomach cancer. When the man, who was only intermittently conscious, told him he was in unbearable pain, Mindell impulsively urged him to "make the pain even worse." The man distended his disease-swollen stomach until it felt ready to burst, finally shouting out, "I just want to explode, I've never been able to really explode!"

At that point the man realized he had never given full vent to his powerful but long-suppressed emotional life. Mindell came to believe that this stunted vitality had become "somaticized and was urgently expressing itself in the form of a tumor." Though the man had been given a prognosis of imminent death, following this emotional catharsis his condition unexpectedly improved. He was discharged from the hospital and eventually worked in intensive therapy with Mindell, aiming at further emotional "exploding." He died three years later, having greatly surpassed his prognosis and, far more important, his previous capacity for aliveness.

Mindell also describes the case of a little girl who was dying of a rapidly growing tumor on her back. She asked him to remove her supporting corset so that she could "fly away to a beautiful world." Mindell was afraid that this fantasy might presage or even hasten her death, but nonetheless he encouraged her to lie on her stomach and make flying motions with her arms. She delightedly "flew away" into a vividly imagined universe of planets and clouds, but soon she began to cry, protesting that she would like to come back to earth for a while and not leave until she was ready. In the weeks and months following this session, the little girl improved rapidly and could soon remove her corset. At last, Mindell claims, her tumor disappeared.[24]

We cannot base our hope—or our fate—on anecdotes that could be classed under the rubric, "The Mysterious Case of the Vanishing Tumor." But Mindell, after working with hundreds of physically ill people, has come to believe that

> the body's symptoms are not necessarily pathological; that is, they are not just sicknesses which must be healed, repressed, or cured. Symptoms are potentially meaningful and purposeful conditions. They could be the beginning of fantastic phases of life, or they could bring one amazingly close to the center of existence.[25]

He surmises that the symptom may be "the part of you that is trying to grow and develop in this life . . . your wise signaler. When it signals to you in the body, we call it a symptom. When it signals to you through a dream, we call it a symbol."

Mindell's technique, which he calls "amplifying the symptom," is based first on self-exploration. He advises patients to focus intently on a symptom: "Forget what you think is wrong with you and experience it as a scientist investigating the unknown." As the experience intensifies, Mindell reports a "channel switch" seems to take place: "When situations become too extreme or painful in one perception channel, when they reach their limit or edge, the experience switches suddenly and automatically." Mindell has observed that at the absolute limit of the bearable, the pain will transform into seeing, hearing, moving, or other cognitive modes. If a patient attends to the images, voices, music, dances, or stories that emerge—by talking to them, expressing them, entering into a creative engagement— then a healing process may begin; if not a physical one, at least a journey toward those "dream[s] that [are] pressing for realization."

Mindell's approach would be recognizable to members of any shamanic culture. Essie Parrish, a renowned healer of the California Pomo Indian tribe, began having unusual visionary experiences in early childhood. At the age of thirteen she noticed that something which felt "like a tongue" had begun to grow in her throat. The strange obstruction continued for four years until it began to dangerously constrict her breathing. When the tribal medicine man's interventions were to no avail, her alarmed relatives called in a white doctor.

"The white doctor didn't recognize it; he told me that it was probably diphtheria. But I knew what it was. It told me for what purpose it was developing. It told me, 'Power is developing.' " She refused treatment. Finally, the "tongue" began to sing to her, to teach her healing songs. When it had finished growing, not only did she get well, but she was able to use "the doctoring power in my throat" to heal others.

What traditional cultures consider an illness does not always correspond to Western disease categories; conversely, what Western doctors consider pathology is not always viewed as such by indigenous peoples.[26] And of course, the meaning of a symptom, if indeed we can talk in these terms, can be easily misread. Mindell's work is controversial, and he has been privately accused by some colleagues of potentially dangerous excesses in applying his theories.

How literally such ideas can be taken and to what extent they can be put into practice will continue to be debated. Certainly, when it comes to footnoting the text of the body with the right medical correlations, most laypeople are functional illiterates. An AIDS specialist at UCLA described for me a patient who had been elated that his lymph nodes were reducing in size, which he saw as his body's signal that a cure was in progress. "What he didn't realize," she said, "was at that point it meant that his immune system was losing all ability to fight the virus." Psychotherapist Selma Hyman relates the story of a cancer patient who reported a wonderful dream about a litter of "pretty, silky" kittens who were pregnant, a condition symbolized by the "lumps on their backs." But the symbols that the patient found so pleasant in the dream in fact presaged a poor outcome: She developed fatal metastases in the bones in her back and spine.[27] Here again the double-edged character of a symptom is metaphorically represented. In the dream, the patient herself was also pregnant, a symbol, like the baby kittens, of potential rebirth of the self. But pregnant, immature animals also strongly suggest the nature of cancer: embryonic, nonfunctional, immature cells which nonetheless "give birth" and multiply.

Similarly, in Thomas Mann's *The Black Swan,* an older woman comes to believe she has miraculously begun menstruating again, when in fact her bleeding is a symptom of the cancer that finally kills her. At the same time, however, Mann shows how this perception enables her to meet her death more peacefully.

In another example, this one from the late Norman Cousins, an erroneous interpretation of a symptom had physically as well as psychologically salubrious effects: A hospitalized man overheard his doctor saying that his heart had a "wholesome gallop." This, unfortunately, is a medical term that describes a dire cardiac condition. But misunderstanding it to mean that he was "healthy as a horse," the patient enthusiastically rallied and made a miraculous recovery.

The intersection between symptom ("to fall together") and symbol (from *symballein,* "to throw together") is neither well-marked nor well-lit, and is fraught with a certain danger. How can we decipher the street signs when we are strangers in a strange land, barely speaking the language? We are left, in the end, with at best a sense of direction—that we need both medical truth and psychological truth in order to heal. Writes Albert Kreinheder:

> Doctors who cut people open have to believe in the reality of the flesh and the blade and the one-to-one relationship of virus to blood to cell to lymph node. . . . But we patients need our fantasies and our dreams and our mythologies. Let him see it his way. . . . But let me also see it my way. My way is not a delusion. It is my experience, my reality, my psychological truth.

And it makes me well. I could have been dead three times in the last ten years if I didn't have this "psychological reality" to pull me through.[28]

The Greek *symptoma* means "anything that has befallen one," as in a blind accident. But Freud, among others, did not believe all accidents were blind. Sometimes (as Joseph Campbell paraphrases him), they are ". . . ripples on the surface of life, produced by unsuspected springs, and these may be very deep—as deep as the soul itself."[29]

By making a symptom our own, we bring it within the charmed circle of awareness. By making relationship, acknowledging and analyzing it, we may augment our healing potential: We open ourselves to what analyst Robert Stein calls "this third mysterious power which transcends both psyche and soma." By taking a soul approach to our illness, we become awakening participants in the ongoing drama of healing.

6

DIAGNOSIS: THE POWER
OF NAMING

*Perhaps the immobility of the things that surround
us is forced upon them . . . by the immobility of
our conception of them.*

—MARCEL PROUST,
Swann's Way

I F A SYMPTOM is the final, irrefutable call to the journey, then
diagnosis is a Rubicon. Until named, a symptom is still private,
personal, wholly owned. Afterward it will fit into institutional medical space, be translated into social lexicon, hold different subjective
weight. A diagnosis is an initiation, a rite of passage from which one
emerges with a new name and title: The Patient with Disease X.

Just as we may have denied the heralds and harbingers of disease,
we may be reluctant to translate their still indecipherable commu-
niqués. Most of us share a subliminal fear that to utter a disease's
name could be to summon, as in some necromantic ritual, its terrible,
still unpronounced specter into full being. Like Scrooge trying to
dismiss his Spirits as a dyspeptic "blot of cheese," we may try to keep
our symptom within the bounds of the commonplace as long as
possible. A woman's discovery of a breast lump, according to Jane
Cowles, can precipitate

> a kind of breakdown in her processing of information. . . . Al-
> though she has all the information she needs to take some sort
> of rational action—she knows she has a breast lump and she
> knows it could be cancer—somehow she can't do anything about
> it for the moment. . . . Some psychologists have postulated an
> average time of four to six weeks before a woman can suffi-

ciently marshal her weakened emotional resources to call her
doctor. Even educated women have been known to live in a
crisis state for five years or more—living with the lump—before
they seek medical attention.[1]

In psychological terms, denial; in mythical terms, refusal of the
call. If the formal summons is never acknowledged, perhaps we can
remain as we are, and delay or evade our departure. "Even after
my lover tested positive for AIDS," Niro Asistent told me, "I resisted
going in for my diagnosis. I thought, I am not the kind of person
to have such a disease. Absurd! The day I finally went to get my
results, I first sat in the car, waiting. It was November, one of those
blue, clear, crisp winter days. My senses were sharpened. I felt this
connection with the trees, as if I could feel them breathing clear
through the earth down to their roots. I remember saying to myself,
'You'd better look around, because when you come out of that building you are going to be different.'

"Then finally I said, 'Come on. Stop fooling yourself. You know
you have AIDS. What are you going to do about it?' "

No matter how prepared a person may feel, no matter how braced
for bad news, the moment of diagnosis engenders shock. One San
Francisco oncologist makes a practice of tape-recording the diagnostic session because he has found that so many patients unconsciously resist hearing him. Most of the patients I spoke with,
however, remembered the moment (if not the precise content) of
diagnosis with pristine, frozen clarity. Even in cases of non-life-
threatening illnesses, it was as if a little death were taking place, an
end to ordinary identity, a formal break with personal history.

Mark Pelgrin, who chronicled his final struggle with cancer in an
extraordinary work, *And a Time to Die,* experienced a floodgate of
long-suppressed emotion: "Who was it who told me once: 'Little
boys don't cry!' . . . For a moment I hovered on the verge of tears.
Then the walls came down, like Jericho, and it seemed as though I
cried for hours and hours. Little boys MUST cry, for crying is a
kind of prayer. . . . I started crying for myself . . . for delights in the
future of which I had been robbed."

On the other hand, many patients described feeling an almost
eerie sense of calm. Jacob Zieghelboim noticed with surprise, "All
my colleagues at work were very distraught about it, but I didn't
feel emotional at all. I felt, this is amazing, something incredible is
happening, some kind of weird adventure. I know it sounds inappropriate, but I felt a sense of freedom."

When John Studholme was told that he had Stage IV-B lymphoma, with one "huge" thirteen-inch tumor in his chest and tumors throughout his lymph system, "My doctor, the nonpatient, the non-victim, was crying. It was my turn to be humorous and stoic." Says another patient, "I was taken aback that I wasn't lying on the floor crying and kicking my legs in the air. 'That's the kind of guy you are,' I was telling myself. 'You don't react right away. It'll hit you and all hell's going to break loose.' "

Such strange equanimity may be what psychologists call "inappropriate affect," a displacement of feeling, an organismic response to shock. The impact is delayed, only to hit later with gale force. Ken Purcell [not his real name], an AIDS patient, remembers, "My first response was, 'So that's how it is.' No trumpet and no fanfare like on the soap operas. I was just sort of numb. I told my lover, Rick, and he started to cry. All I could think was, 'Thank God my mother isn't alive.' But a few days later, I was driving along and started weeping. Suddenly everything came so clear."

But Ken, too, felt strangely liberated. He had begun his career as an art professor with a fervent idealism about "combining art with learning and healing," eventually rising to department head at a small midwestern college. But in the years leading up to his diagnosis, he had begun to feel his accomplishments were "empty and meaningless. I had this high position within the system, and all it meant was my plans, proposals, my authority were being sniped at from every direction. I felt immobilized, prevented from doing this very heartfelt thing that I'd spent years climbing the ladder to attain. I'd started having these out-of-control episodes where I'd teach, then go home and get chattering drunk and find myself screaming, 'I want to die!' This went on for two years."

When he was finally diagnosed with Kaposi's sarcoma, he remembers thinking, "Well, this is the opportunity you've been waiting for. The worst has happened, so there are no restrictions anymore. You can look death in the face, quit the crap, and finally do what you want with your life. There's nothing to lose."

Carol Boss had just moved to northern California after burning out as a yoga instructor in the New York State prison system. Her friends had thrown her a big going-away party—someone had even led a horse into the room—in honor of her new beginnings. Everyone told her that she looked radiant, and that was how she felt— lit up with possibility. That first warm, eucalyptus Christmas on the Coast, she had taken a trip to the country with a group of friends to meditate on the meaning of the coming year. But during the retreat, she discovered a frightening symptom: "I was taking a shower, and my left breast looked somehow different. I felt it, and the entire breast was hard like a rock! It had been fine a few days before, nothing at all. I looked great, felt great, never a better time in my life. Later in the day, sitting in a hot tub, one of my friends who is a nurse-practitioner said, 'It couldn't be cancer, it just doesn't show up suddenly like that.' Ironically, I was scheduled to go to a seminar called, 'Conscious Living and Conscious Dying.' I held off going to the doctor and went there instead."

When Carol finally went for a diagnosis, "The medical people couldn't move fast enough." The doctor told her she had inflammatory carcinoma—one of the most rapid and uniformly deadly varieties—while she was still lying on the biopsy table. "He gave me a few months at best. It was a moment I'll never forget, looking back at the operating table, at the pool of blood on it, knowing the blood was mine and that I had cancer. You change gears, and the world seems to change, too. You know that nothing is going to be the same again."

But paradoxically, there was a "shift in consciousness," as if for the first time she had been plunged fully and unalterably into the present.

> All my life, I'd been a self-improvement freak. I'd had a rough childhood, lots of traumas and emotional damage, and I'd done everything I could imagine to try to heal it—workshops, Reichian bioenergetics, Esalen psychotherapy. But no matter what I'd done, I still felt this self-rejection, like I still wasn't as together as the next person.
>
> From the point in time I had the biopsy, I dropped it all. It was like, I'm here, now, this is how I am, and I'm as together as I'm going to be. I'm not married? Okay. No children? So what? Not quite successful, fulfilled, doing as well as I should? *Fine.* All of a sudden, I felt good about my life, about how I'd lived. It surprised me. The biopsy was like a graduation day, as if I were walking into the real world, no more rehearsal. If I'd ever learned anything in my life, this was where I would have to see what it was worth.

The period of shock is "an early opportunity for healing," says San Francisco psychotherapist Virginia Veach. If the patient can find a supportive setting with a caring friend, nourishing food, a shelter from the storm, she suggests there is a chance to come to grips with an enormous life transition before embarking on what is too often a bewildering rush to treatment.

WHAT'S IN A NAME?

A diagnosis *implies* treatment—not only implies it but determines it, for each disease has a corresponding medical protocol. Aristotle held that a proper medical name was the gateway to a cure. From a name—scientifically derived, experimentally validated, and laboratory-tested—prognoses can be given and a specific treatment prescribed.

But are scientific diagnoses the only way to describe our encounter with disease? Our system of classification (or "nosology") is in part a cultural artifact, a product of history and philosophy as well as science. It is not simply "objective truth," but one way of conceptualizing, interpreting, and containing a complex human phenomenon. A diagnosis, no matter how sophisticated, remains, in the words of philosopher Michel Foucault, "a region of description around the grayness of things."

Shaped by three centuries of Western thought, from Descartes's mind-body separation to Newton's world of discrete, caroming objects, a modern diagnostic label treats key questions as foregone conclusions: Is disease a thing or a process? Is its "natural history" inexorable, or have there been instances of reversal? Does it reside only in a particular organ, or is it merely the most visible evidence of a wider systemic disorder? Is it purely physical, or is it affected by interactions with the mind? Each of these usually unasked queries has enormous implications, not only for diagnosis but for the treatment that will inevitably follow from it.

Ted Kaptchuk, a scholar of Chinese medicine, points out that Eastern and Western diagnoses are based upon different logical structures. "The M.D. asks, 'What X is causing Y?' The acupuncturist inquires, 'What is the relationship between X and Y?' " Western physicians look for a single disease agent, which they isolate and then try to control or destroy. Chinese doctors examine the whole individual, body and mind, searching for a "pattern of disharmony."

For the patient, these diagnostic biases have very real, practical consequences. In his book *The Web That Has No Weaver,* Kaptchuk cites the hypothetical cases of six different patients who go to their doctors complaining of severe stomach pain. In Western medicine, all would likely be sent to the hospital for upper-gastrointestinal-tract X-rays or an endoscopy and be diagnosed as having a peptic ulcer.

A Chinese doctor would painstakingly question and examine each patient, taking into account his emotional temperament, the cast of his complexion, his sleep patterns, voice, tongue, skin, food cravings, pulses, frequency and type of elimination. (These are the "four examinations"—looking, listening/smelling, asking, and touching.) Each person might then be diagnosed with one of six different diseases—"damp heat affecting the spleen," or "deficient yin affecting the stomach," or "disharmony of the liver invading the spleen," etc.—each of which would mandate a different treatment.[2]

Chinese medicine has shown that these poetic-sounding diagnoses can resolve many of the same endocrinological, neurological, and pathogenic conditions treated by Western science, even though their system does not recognize many known anatomical structures and postulates some that are as yet unverifiable. Additionally, since the entire organism is taken into account, the body is often strengthened and tonified on a long-term basis.

Western medicine, too, once considered a wide range of indices to diagnose illness. A Hippocratic diagnosis took into account not only overt physical symptoms, but race, sex, locale, climate, water supply, social and political conditions and customs, overall constitution, mode of life, personality, and such details as

> talk, manner, silence, thoughts, sleep or absence thereof, dreams, scratchings, tears, stools, urine, sputum, vomit, earlier diseases, sweat, chills, coughs, sneezes, hiccoughs, breathing, belching, flatulence, hemorrhages.[3]

But by the nineteenth century, patients' idiosyncrasies came to be viewed as not only irrelevant to a new standardized medicine, but so "accidental and fortuitous" as to impede accurate scientific understanding of the disease-entity. Neurologist Oliver Sacks calls this "the madness of the last three centuries . . . which reduces men to machines, automata, puppets, dolls, blank tablets, formulae, ciphers, systems, and reflexes."

Today, a new generation of physicians is beginning to question this legacy, and to revive more venerable forms of inquiry. Yet most conventional diagnosis still tends to discard personhood in a misguided attempt to boil a case down to its bare, manipulable variables. The patient's life history and personality—as well as the living bodily context of the disease—become secondary to laboratory specimens and instrumented read-outs. The individual is evaluated, but scarcely encountered. To my hospital internist, I was little more than a stick-figure version of myself, a connect-the-dots simulacrum drawn from a sheaf of papers on his desk. This one-dimensional sketch—drawn up in service of time-and-cost efficiency as much as science—tends to supplant other ways of knowing.

It is a long way from Hippocrates's early maxims for fledgling diagnosticians: "You can discover no weight, no form nor calculation to which to refer your judgment of health and sickness. In the medical arts there exists no certainty except in the physician's senses."[4] The Greek founder of modern medicine might have been hard-pressed to recognize today's clinician: "a biological accountant engaged in input/output calculations," in critic Ivan Illich's words, who often functions as little more than an adjunct to flask, slide, and microscope.

THE EFFECTS OF DIAGNOSIS

The effect of all this upon the patient cannot be overestimated, for diagnosis sets a trajectory, looses an arrow of inevitability. Illich writes:

> His sickness is taken from him and turned into the raw material for an institutional enterprise. His condition is interpreted according to a set of abstract rules. . . . Diagnosis always intensifies stress, defines incapacity, imposes inactivity, and focuses apprehension on nonrecovery, on uncertainty, and on one's dependence upon future medical findings, all of which amounts to a loss of autonomy for self-definition. It also isolates a person in a special role, separates him from the normal and healthy, and requires submission to the authority of specialized personnel.[5]

CAT-scans, bone marrow tests, lymphangiograms, myelograms, electroencephalograms, sonograms, laparoscopies, biopsies, "blood work"—the amazing, sometimes painful phalanx of diagnostic techniques is rapidly deployed on the patient, who may in turn feel violated, vivisected, objectified.

The doctor's "professional judgment," his power of interpretation, has great import for the patient. Indeed, in the court of clinical evidence the doctor takes on the stature of a judge; his or her smallest remarks become verdicts of destiny. Mark Pelgrin describes his first visit to the surgeon: "The silence became more intense, for suddenly I realized this was Jehovah speaking. This was the man who contained in himself the words that would make my future intelligible or unintelligible."

Naming, as the Biblical Adam knew, is a subsidiary act of creation. Words shape perception; how a thing is named defines how it is perceived and, in some sense, what it *is*. Hindus refer to the world as we see it as *namarupa*, "name-and-form," implying how tightly bound a thing and its label are. A label is also a presumption of dominion, a ratification of control. He who names, lays claim. Jungian analyst James Hillman remarks about the realm of psychotherapy,

> [A]s soon as the move is made of professional naming, a distinct entity is created, with literal reality. On the one hand I am protected from this "thing" by separation from it; it now has a name. But on the other hand, I now "have something." . . . Moreover, the therapist has become the very God who by bringing the condition is the only one who can take it away.[6]

THE POWER OF PROGNOSIS

A story is told about Pablo Picasso's famous Valentine's Day portrait of his last wife, Jacqueline. A worshipful forty-five years his junior, Jacqueline was described by a friend of the couple as a "highly susceptible girl." Picasso, who sometimes boasted that he could "predict" his wife's state, once by way of demonstration drew the image of her face "imposed on a shocking-pink network of lines like a fever chart. When a day or two later Jacqueline obligingly ran a temperature, the artist took pride in having foreseen it. 'You see, I'm a prophet,' he claimed, not entirely in jest."[7]

Similarly, when a diagnostician paints a graphic, often worst-case picture, suitably bolstered with statistics, his remarks may unwittingly acquire similarly "prophetic" powers. Norman Cousins observed that there may be a sudden worsening of cancer patients' physical condition immediately following diagnosis. He speculated that this might be due to the emotional depression that diagnosis can engender, which in turn could have a negative effect on the patient's immune system (though he acknowledged that some of these instances might have to do with the natural progress of the disease).

Jeanne Achterberg suggests, "Images are so readily translated into physical change that dying from having been given a feared diagnosis by a credible physician is just as feasible as a hex death is to a cursed Haitian." Her remark is reminiscent of the observation by one medieval medical observer that a mental image "doth so imperiously command our bodies . . . that it works on others as well as ourselves." Clergyman Robert Burton's seventeenth-century treatise, *The Anatomy of Melancholy,* cites an account by a Jesuit missionary in China: "If it be told them they shall be sicke on such a day, when that day comes they will surely be sicke, and will be so terribly afflicted, that sometimes they will dye upon it."[8]

AIDS patients particularly feel the weight of this medical sentencing. Niro Asistent says, "The moment I was diagnosed, my symptoms seemed to intensify very quickly. In three weeks, I became really sick. My energy level was so low it sometimes took me forty-five minutes to get out of bed. Instead of having night sweats only once in a while, it would be every night with chills all day. After the diagnosis, all those things suddenly became multiplied by twenty."

When an internist told one journeyer over the phone that he was HIV-positive, he "just went blank. At that time AIDS was splashed in the news a lot. It meant the most destructive thing there is, death. Channel Seven News here had a running count each night. One hundred percent fatal. My ego felt paralyzed, while all the rest of me was going Alert-alert-alert, you're-gonna-die you're-gonna-die you're-gonna-die, whattaya-gonna-do? whattaya-gonna-do? whattaya-gonna-do?"

George Melton, the ARC-patient-turned-inspirational-lecturer, says ironically, "When I was a kid, missionaries used to come to my church from Africa. They would talk about how voodoo doctors would cast a spell and people would die. And I would think, 'Isn't it great that I live in America where these things don't happen?' I think the hysteria and fear around AIDS is as much a part of the disease as HIV. I've watched people get diagnosed and decide to party themselves to death, or just pull the blinds and wait to go. When I got my diagnosis, I sentenced *myself* to death."

TO TELL THE TRUTH

There is a famous story of a man condemned to death by a king. But the man announces that, if the king will but spare his life for a year, he will teach His Majesty's horse to fly. The king, intrigued, grants the short reprieve. Turning to face his jeering detractors, the man says: "Who knows? In a year's time, the king may die. The horse may die. I may die. Or maybe the damn horse will fly."

In what might be seen as clear instances of denial, George Melton and other journeyers took a similar stance vis-a-vis their own death sentences. Their attitudes were in some ways vindicated—not only by their own long-term survival but by changing medical opinion. Though AIDS remains a nightmarish affliction with a near-total mortality rate, two doctors at the National Institute of Allergy and Infectious Disease wrote recently that the disease, "once viewed as an automatic death warrant, is now in the process of becoming a chronic, potentially long-term treatable illness."[9]

To be fair, it should be noted that doctors often feel they must guard against "building up false hopes," and so present the patient with worst- or at best average-case scenarios, and rarely with exceptional ones. One doctor confided to me, "Sometimes we're scared to be optimistic. I'm trying to protect *myself* as much as I am the patient from disappointment. When I see a malignancy, I think of a guy I just treated—an engineer, two kids, a beautiful wife, everything to live for—who died. And the better the doctor, the more hopeless the cases he tends to get referred to him, which means that more of them die, which in turn adds to his pessimism."

The Houston oncologist Adan Rios says, "We too often don the black gown of a judge and take away hope, hope that all of us will one day need. When the approach to the terminal patient becomes so formal and rigid, it is as if we doctors are forgetting that the time will come when we ourselves will be talking to another doctor and saying, 'I don't know what is happening to me, I feel terrible, I think I'm going to die. What can you do for me?' "

The way doctors approach the patient with a serious illness still varies greatly today from country to country. In Japan, cancer patients are almost never told their diagnosis. A leading Japanese physician explains: "Human beings react very strongly to the notion of death. We should let the patients spend the rest of their short lives without anxiety."

On the other hand, writes Michael Lerner, program director of the Commonweal health retreat in Bolinas, California, "Studies have shown that most cancer patients who are not told of their diagnosis still know that they have cancer. The failure to tell the patient of the cancer diagnosis may be worse, for the patient may infer from the silence that the disease is completely hopeless and be struck by a feeling of helplessness. . . ."

Former cancer patient Ernie Sharhag, for example, remembers instantly intuiting the truth. "When I saw the doctor's face after I got out of the biopsy, I knew right away. He had Death written all over him. He was kind of humbling himself the way doctors do when they have bad news. Sure enough, it was nonspecific nodular lymphocytic lymphoma. He gave me five years at most, no cure."

REFUSING THE VERDICT

Ernie, however, rebelled against his diagnosis. "The doctor told me all I could hope for would be to suffer through chemo, get shorter and shorter remissions, and then finally die. *If I've gotta die,* I thought, *I'm going do it my own way.*" Ernie's healing path led him to cut short his course of chemo and embark on an exotic route of cure, which we will hear of later. After I first met Ernie, I called his oncologist to ask him about his patient's apparent recovery.

"Oh, no," the doctor said confidently, after I pointed out that Ernie's last scans had revealed none of the tumors he had when he had left the doctor's treatment. "He can't have recovered. The disease will cycle, perhaps, but he *will* be dead in five years." Ten years after the doctor's pronouncement, Ernie is still very much alive.

A surprising number of other people I spoke with refused to accept their medical verdicts. As Elisabeth Kübler-Ross points out, "Denial, or at least partial denial, is used by almost all patients." Psychologist Richard S. Lazarus claims that "illusion and self-deception can have positive value in a person's psychological economy. Denial buys preparation time. A temporary disavowal of reality helps the person get through." Lazarus quotes Don Quixote in *Man of La Mancha*: "Facts are the enemy of truth."[10]

The journeyers I spoke to almost uniformly affirmed a belief that there was a deeper truth than the harsh facts proffered by their doctors. Psychologist Glenda Hawley in her excellent (unpublished) study of sixteen unusual cancer survivors noted that almost all had "paradoxical" responses to their diagnoses: "They were not denying they had cancer and that cancer was often a fatal disease, but they did not accept that it was fatal for *them.*"

Joy Ballas-Beeson, after undergoing a series of lengthy procedures, was finally diagnosed with rheumatoid arthritis. "I remember one doctor—he was an older man in his sixties—finally telling me, 'It's so severe, it's come on so quickly in every joint in your body at a relatively young age, you will most likely wind up crippled for life in a wheelchair.' He gave me some kind of remission percentage, like ten percent, but said it would probably keep coming back, worse and worse. I got mad. I didn't yell, but I just said something like, 'Shit, I refuse to believe this.' And I never went back."

George Melton says, "Death wasn't the issue for me. Helplessness was. The diagnosis that something in my body was killing me and there was nothing I could do about it was too bitter a pill to swallow. You can say I was in denial, but a little voice in the back of my head just didn't buy it. It said, 'This isn't true. It just isn't true.' "

After fire chief Art McGrary was tested for prostate cancer, he went to the laboratory and finagled his own copy of the complete pathology report.

> I just marched in and asked for it. I wasn't about to wait for my doc to tell me—he'd been telling me for months I just had kidney stones! When he told me I needed immediate surgery and then radiation afterwards, depending on how the bone scan went, I told him to go fly a kite. He was rather a young man, and he said, "You're signing your own death warrant."
>
> Well, I've faced death an awful lot of times. Nobody wants to die. But prostate cancer hits you at a different level. I was only fifty-one, and I felt, maybe irrationally, that having my prostate out would be like being castrated. The standard procedure is to remove the prostate and then, if the disease continues, treat you with female hormones. If it continues on, they remove the testes. Even with all that, the doctor was only giving me a thirteen- to eighteen-month prognosis anyhow. Thanks a lot, you know?

After an arduous emotional and physical journey through the murky world of alternative medicine, Art managed to beat his prognosis. "I went back to the guy after three years and told him, 'I'm still here.' He couldn't find any evidence of the disease. Still, he pulled out his plastic mockup of a prostate and immediately started talking surgery."

SURVIVING THE PREDICTIONS

Of course, Art is an exceptional case, and his doctor's concern—and alarm—were understandable. We cannot infer from Art's case and a few others like it that there is an established basis for discounting a physician's diagnosis. Many pathologies have been studied for nearly a century, and it is hard to deny that in many cases their timeline seems nearly immutable.

Nevertheless, the determination to recover which these patients evinced could not be fairly perceived as simple denial. Most of them had accepted the possibility, even the likelihood, of death. "Hope is dope," one told me. "It can become just another way to gloss over your real feelings." Instead, theirs was a sort of heuristic belief, a "What if?" proposition that affected the tangible choices they made about their lives.

But scientific certainty is difficult to resist. The blizzard of statistical prognoses ("a cloud of figures . . . like a call-board on the stock market," wrote Mark Pelgrin) can freeze any unseasonable shoots of optimism the patient may try to nurture—especially when there is already something within us that feels skeptical of repair. Common sense seems to whisper that once something is shattered, it can never be made new. One cannot hurl a wineglass to the floor and then, as if running a film backward, make the pieces magically coalesce again. A demolished building cannot be reconstituted from dust and rubble. "If He breaks a thing down," Job laments, "there is no rebuilding; If He imprisons a man, there is no release."

Every doctor described to me in great detail how my tumor could progress—invading arteries, spreading to lungs and bones, degenerating into a less differentiated cell type. Not one volunteered— or even seemed to know—as detailed a physiological picture of how a tumor could regress, become inactive, calcify, or even be resorbed by the body, though all these have been known to occasionally occur.

I was up against my own fatalism as well. Lawrence LeShan has commented on how many of his cancer patients seemed to have had, even before they became ill, an exaggerated sense of Moira, the Greek term for the imprisoning web of destiny; of the "cold clockmaker's universe" of Galileo and Newton; of being enmeshed in a blind mechanism that took little account of their fears, hopes, and dreams.

It is sometimes hard to keep in mind that prognosis, the stockticker of the disease trade, is not based on immutable fate. It starts from a particular reference point—*now*—that is constantly shifting. The present moment is a fulcrum; if one element in a situation changes, the sum and sequence of what follows is less easy to predict. The epidemiological analyses upon which prognoses are based are averages. Diagnosticians rarely include in their calculus the measure of the whole human being—psychospiritual outlook, health of relationship and family life, willingness to undertake special regimens, perhaps differing immune system competence, all of which may alter an illness's course.

Prior to my own diagnosis I had any number of vivid dreams that seemed to address the question of whose prognosis to trust: the doctors', that my disease would only continue to grow and eventually kill me, or my own sense that I might find a gentler path of improvement.

One dream depicted the issue of the reparability of the body in graphic terms:

> *I am driving the first car I ever owned, a classic 1949 Studebaker. But it is in terrible shape: Its brakes are gone. Its steering mechanism barely works. The main problem seems to be a ball of partly congealed "jelly" located at the juncture of the steering shaft and the axle. I wonder despairingly if I will really have to junk the car, for the engine is still powerful and the interior has been mysteriously reupholstered with shimmering blue fabric.*

At the time I found my dream indecipherable. But looking back years later, it seems achingly clear. My beloved Studebaker Champion was a 1949, my own birth-year, when in a sense I first clambered into the driver's seat of my body. The engine, the animating lifeforce, is still vibrant. The "interior" is the beautiful deep blue traditionally associated with healing and spirituality. It was a redemptive image that something damaged might be renewed. The dream faced me with an agonizing choice: Was the deterioration of my organ so far gone it would have to be "junked," or could it somehow be repaired?

IS THE COURSE OF DISEASE FIXED?

In some ways, our medical views have not changed much from those of the nineteenth-century physician who wrote, "The author of nature has fixed the course of most diseases through immutable laws that one soon discovers if the course of the disease is not interrupted or disturbed by the patient."[11]

The subtext of this statement is astonishing: Diseases, like Descartes's universe, have been set in predictable motion by God Himself. The patient is somehow extraneous to the disease. In such a formulation, she becomes little more than a beclouding variable in the otherwise pristine unfolding of an inexorable natural process.

Even today, in an era of real-time scans, diagnosis and prognosis still tend to be drawn following the conceptual gridwork of nineteenth-century pathological anatomy, when the doctor's gaze saw little more than what critic Michel Foucault has described as "a flat surface of perpetual simultaneity . . . coincidence without development . . . one plane and one moment."

Despite the medical insights made possible by this isolated view, it remains profoundly flawed. Within a given diagnosis there are many planes and many moments. Dr. B. A. Stoll goes so far as to suggest that it is "impossible to use a statistical probability derived from a large clinical trial in order to predict the likelihood of either cure, tumor regression, or long survival following treatment in the cases of a particular patient."

The statistical uniqueness of the person is a worthwhile diagnostic consideration. The great physician and teacher Sir William Osler once remarked, "It is more important to find out what patient has the disease than what disease the patient has." Some studies indicate that the same flu virus may behave differently in a person with a competent immune system than the same "objective" microbe does in a person who is run-down. Cancer cells also may behave differently in a bodymind that is under chronic stress, poorly nourished, and emotionally devastated than in one more balanced.

According to one recent study, for example, normal mice implanted with lymphosarcoma cancer cells were able to partially or totally contain tumor growth. But when the animals were experimentally put under stress known to increase secretions of corticosteroids, the tumors grew. If the growth of tumors in mice can be affected by stress, how much more so in human beings, with their complex psyches and intricate bodymind pathways?

The "disease entity," in other words, often does not exist as a simple object, independent as, say, a stone by the side of the road. It exists in relationship to the larger organism, which is ever in motion. Medical scholar Eric Cassell notes, "The idea of structure itself is an artificial one. Structure is what you see under a microscope. . . . But what you see under a microscope is not what is happening in sick people. Nothing in nature holds still like that."[12]

I found an appropriate metaphor in a recent article about a public school experiment in open enrollment that took place in Arkansas. Administrators were afraid the policy would encourage all the "bad" kids to flock to certain schools, where they would fatally infect the educational process. Instead, they discovered that children who exhibited emotional, behavioral, and learning problems in one school *did not display the same characteristics at the new school.*[13] These supposedly incorrigible children changed their behavior in response to a healthier environment.

Of course, the blind machinations of cancer cells cannot be compared to the miraculous responsiveness of human beings. And though an increasing number of medical studies are in progress to determine the effects of psychosocial cofactors on the outcome of disease, evidence remains largely inferential. But though they lacked any hard data, the patients I met often drew strength from their own raw observations. Arline Erdrich says, "I saw others with the same disease I had, people with fewer symptoms than me, and they ended up dying. I also saw people with far more serious conditions than I had survive. I had to ask myself, Why is this happening? If it's all chemistry and biology, then anyone with Stage Two-B should be just like I am, alive and thriving, and anyone with Four-B, predicted as absolutely fatal, should not be around at all. But sometimes it was just the opposite."

It also may be that there are highly significant differences in disease types that cannot yet be diagnostically measured. M.I.T. biologist Maurice Fox suggested in the *Journal of the American Medical Association* that there is good evidence for the existence of cancers whose cell-types are malignant but whose behavior is biologically benign, a dilemma that he says "introduces major ethical and clinical problems." Fox also observes that the mere identification of a breast-cancer cell-type "does not permit a prediction of the likelihood that a lesion will follow the sequential steps believed to characterize the natural history of breast cancer. Some lesions may rarely, or never, make the transition to metastatic disease; others may appear and disappear in the normal course of events."

One ethical problem is the possibility of opting for too-radical treatment on the basis of a diagnosis. Every year, thousands of American women in their thirties and forties are given so-called "prophylactic mastectomies" for diagnoses of fibrocystic breast disease, even though this condition only rarely leads to breast cancer.[14] ("Fibrocystic disease," says Dr. Susan Love, director of the Breast Clinic at Boston's Beth Israel Hospital, "is a 'garbage term' that has no meaning—clinically, microscopically, or any other way. It can mean twelve to fifteen different things.")

Small cancers of the prostate are routinely treated with surgical removal of the organ, chemotherapy, or radioactive "seeds." Prudent treatment is understandable: 36,000 men in the U.S. die of the disease annually. But an estimated one out of every three men over fifty carry—and their bodies often keep contained—microscopic prostate cancer lesions. And in a recent Swedish study that followed early prostate cancer patients who would have undergone surgery or radiation in the United States, but were instead treated only with hormones *if* the cancer spread, the patients' survival rate was actually three percentage points *higher* than those who were treated more aggressively. It was found that less virulent cancers were less likely to spread in the first place, while the virulent variety usually proved deadly even *with* treatment.[15]

Even something as mundane as widsom-tooth surgery is based on questionable diagnostic logic. According to a study financed by the federal Agency for Health Care Policy and Research, tens of thousands of operations and at least $150 million would be saved if oral surgeons only removed wisdom teeth that actually caused problems. Their routine removal in teenagers "makes about as much sense as removing everyone's appendix just because some people develop appendicitis."[16]

One medical consumer advocate told me, "Sometimes diagnosticians create an entire class of patients by coming up with a new screening procedure for basically healthy people. If the screening defines you as ill, then you're supposed to go get treated. But sometimes you aren't really a patient at all: your 'disease' is that you're defined as 'being at *risk*' of getting sick."

Broadly, contemporary practice in diagnosis may in many ways be compared with the military's method of assessing an enemy's strength. I was struck by a pronouncement by a Defense Department specialist criticizing the idea of a post–Cold War "build-down" of American forces in Europe. "Military strategy has to be geared to the enemy's maximum capabilities, not his perceived intentions." But his diagnostic view of the "Evil Empire" (which turned out to be rotting from within and poised for change) has not been borne out by history.

A DIAGNOSIS OF EVIL?

> *Between good and evil*
> *How great is the distance?*

> —LAO TZU

The treatment of disease does often seem to be nothing less than a crusade against evil. Armed with such an outlook, the doctor can only be a "hawk" in the war, for evil is an eternal, inimical force we must engage in mortal struggle wherever we find it. Even if treatment side-effects severely damage the quality of life or are arguably worse than the original disease—even if, as the popular jibe goes, "The operation was a success, but the patient died"—these are acceptable casualties in the battle to exorcise the Devil.

Certainly, diseases are often demonic forces that can turn the body into a chamber of horrors. Even the weakest mites on earth—viruses, bacteria, errant genes—can fell us with one blow. It sometimes becomes easy to believe, as did the ancient Persians, that the god they called the Evil Craftsman just walked off the job of creation, leaving us to be minced in the gearworks of some substandard if not downright malevolent piece of cosmic machinery.

We would seemingly be fools not to err on the side of prudence. Every horror-movie buff knows that the character who begs the troops to muzzle their flamethrowers and try to communicate with the monster will be first to sail bloodily down its gullet. We fear if we turn anything but the most opaque "classificatory gaze" upon the Medusa, we will be turned to stone.

But if we diagnosed a disease as an imbalance of forces or, say, as a blocked flow of *chi* energy, we might respond to it quite differently. Ted Kaptchuk notes, "To Western medicine, understanding an illness means uncovering a distinct entity that is separate from the patient's being." By contrast, as we have seen, the Chinese doctor regards illness as a "pattern of disharmony" that cannot be isolated from the person in whom it occurs.[17]

Deena Metzger notes that the Huichol Indians have no word for evil. "Instead, they have an expression: 'In this world, no one goes lacking for something with which to get stuck in the eye.' Evil is only density. I didn't feel my disease was Satan against God." In a similar vein, Debby Ogg told me,

> The one thing that always excited me about Judaism was a rabbi telling me there was no term for sin in Hebrew. The only word was *chrait*, which is an archer's term. It means not evil, but 'missing the mark.' I didn't feel my tumor was evil. I felt it was a signal that something was wrong which I had to attend to. It was terrifying, horrible—I didn't welcome it—but I felt it had happened partly because I had neglected myself. It was the insistent tapping on my arm, "Try to avoid this now."

INNER DIAGNOSIS

In the Grimm Brothers fairytale *Rumpelstilzkin,* a young peasant woman enlists the supernatural aid of a dwarf to convince a king she can weave straw into gold. But the insistent little man exacts a terrible promise in exchange: After she marries, she will be obliged to give him the first child from the union.

This story of romance between a king and a peasant contains interesting echoes of the disease-prone paradigm: The young woman's childhood apparently has been dominated by a father who, like narcissistic parents everywhere, can see her only in terms of his own needs—in this case, how her good looks might better his social status. It is he, a poor miller who wishes to seem important, who tells the king that his daughter is a prettier version of the goose that lays golden eggs. His lie fires the greed of the king, who imprisons the girl in a cell where she will be left to perish unless she can live up to her father's impossible ideal.

Her royal dungeon is the very predicament of the wounded personality: If she does not pretend to be other than she is, she will be abandoned. Only if she weaves her straw into gold will she be loved. She must devalue her earthy "straw" self—for surely her real self is worthless—in favor of a grandiose "gold" outer one. But this impossible persona can only be produced through deception and terrible self-sacrifice. The trap of an inflated persona is that more and more energy is required to maintain it. Thus with each success, the king only demands more and moves her into ever bigger rooms with ever taller heaps of straw to weave. The "first-born child" with whom she has agreed to pay Rumpelstilzkin symbolizes her own potential for authentic growth.

The young woman marries the king, who, like her father, loves her more for the gold she spins than for who she really is. ("If a simple miller's daughter can spin such riches," thinks the monarch, "then she will be a worthy wife indeed.") Still, her new royal life seems a pond without ripples until a small but impossibly heavy stone roils its surface. At the birth of her child the dwarf arrives, clutching the malign claim-stub of a forgotten promise, triggering her postponed but inevitable crisis.

He is in fact her unacknowledged shadow, an irrefutable reminder of her life of hapless falsity. In a strange way, this "little man" is the only character in the story who values vitality over outward appearance. When the princess offers to pay him instead all the riches in the kingdom, he responds, "I would rather have a living thing than all the treasures in the world." He is, as a symptom may sometimes be, both the thief of life and its unrecognized spokesperson.

We know how the story ends: The dwarf gives the heroine three days to guess his name. The "diagnosis" is accomplished through the agency of a wandering hunter, the fairytale epitome of that honest, free, self-directed spirit that bows down to no one. It is he who overhears the "funny little man" dancing and singing his name to himself deep in the forest.

The act of finding the "hidden name" of disease, the one not located in a diagnostic manual (or in this case, book of demonology), is something many patients told me they found invaluable in their quest for healing. They would by and large have agreed with Arnold Mindell's statement: "I'm not so much interested in the name of the disease, but the way it develops, what it does and says to the person."

When Brian Schultz told me he had been diagnosed with "ankylosing spondylitis," I immediately remarked, "Oh, yes, Norman Cousins's disease . . ."

"No," he replied with some vehemence. "*Brian's* disease." For Brian, redefining his disease in personal terms had been the key to his healing. In his view, no two people could possibly have the same experience of illness. Brian's rejection of a medical label, his trademarking of his own disease, helped him find his own path of healing.

DREAM DIAGNOSIS

Sometimes the bodymind presents us with pictures to accompany the words. Indeed, from the standpoint of PNI, the idea that signals from our bodies can be translated into mental images is not as farfetched as it may seem. The apparent accuracy of such images, however, is sometimes nothing short of astonishing.

Researcher Jeanne Achterberg, studying a group of terminally ill cancer patients, found that the most reliable way of predicting how they would fare against their disease was their mental imagery—more accurate even than immune component levels in the blood (which, since they reflect physiological events that have already taken place, are more like "looking in a rearview mirror").

In one of her studies, she used an imagery-based test of her own devising to measure patients' attitudes about the disease, its treatment, and the body's own powers of recovery. She and her colleagues were able to predict with 100 percent certainty who would die or show significant deterioration, and with 93 percent accuracy who would go into remission.

Achterberg's results are corroborated by a study carried out by researcher Dr. Robert Trestman that examined such factors as white blood cell imagery, the imagined color of the cancer, and various metaphorical qualities the disease held for Stage IV patients. The results were persuasive: "[T]hirteen of the fourteen people with 'good' status described their cancer as red or black, while eight out of the eleven with relatively poorer status described their cancers as lighter colors."[18]

As we have seen, a dream may offer startlingly accurate symbolic information about the clinical nature of an illness. But symbols also often speak eloquently of the psychological significance of the disease. Arnold Mindell, for example, asserts that out of the hundreds of physically ill people he has worked with, he has not seen a single case in which the illness did not represent itself in the patient's dream life. Dreams often provide a missing context, a "hidden name" that unlocks the door to understanding.

The striking aspect of my own case, and the one I have puzzled over most diligently for years, was the way in which my illness was "diagnosed" in a series of extremely vivid dreams; dreams that seemed to conflict so directly with my medical diagnoses—even with my own conscious beliefs—that they became sources of some confusion.

I had put off getting an official diagnosis for several months after my tumor was discovered. Finally, I made an appointment for a needle biopsy with a specialist at the hospital. As I lay on the table, I recalled a dream from several months past, in which a circle of "medicine men" had stuck needles into my "neck brain" and withdrawn dollops of blood. Now, holding very still as the pathologist plunged the long needles into my thyroid, I felt I was undergoing this same courage-ritual. When I received the cancer diagnosis, I had felt weirdly triumphant: My dreams had not lied.

Around this time, however, the dreams had become more complex, more ambiguous, like stage whispers in a strange but maddeningly familiar language. From the time my lump was first discovered, they had begun to address relentlessly the problem of "getting a clear picture" of the disease. Here, for example, are only three of the dreams that crowded for my attention:

I. Magazine photographers are taking a picture of a chestnut horse, but they're confused about whether it's a mare or a gelded stallion. They decide they will have to either "reshoot" the animal, or relabel the photographs. The editor tells the photographer, "It's your choice."

II. I am looking through a camera lens and see what I take to be a "UFO." Then I realize it is some sort of fantastical flying creature with a live bird's head and a mechanical body consisting of a metal box decorated with butterfly-wing swirls. It moves with a whirring sound, like an eighteenth-century automaton. It strikes me as slightly comical, its protruding birdlike tongue spluttering cartoonishly. I am "told" this chimera is a "turkey-buzzard." I also discover that, although I thought I was looking at it through a long-range telephoto, I am actually using a 50-millimeter lens, the type portrait photographers use to get undistorted images.

III. Crabs and beetles made of brightly colored molded plastic are scuttling around ominously on the floor. When I kick one over, it turns out that they are really only tiny ants that have had these disguises welded to their backs. I am revulsed by this discovery.

Each of these dreams, I now see, illuminated the exact nature of my disease, and also reflected aspects of my life and my personality that could have contributed to it.

The "chestnut horse" dream contains a fairly obvious symbol: According to Jung, a horse usually represents the body and its animal vitality, which we "ride" through life. At the time, an ultrasound "photograph" had just been taken of my tumor and I had been told it was almost certainly benign. But in the dream, the photographers are baffled as to whether the horse is a mare (that is, able to reproduce others like itself, like cancer cells) or a gelding. They will either have to take another picture (i.e., another diagnostic test), or give the photos they already have a different diagnostic label, but the choice is disconcertingly arbitrary, a case of "six of one, half a dozen of the other." As it was to turn out months later, my cancer was a "borderline" cancer somewhere between benign and malignant, its classification, from one viewpoint, up for grabs.

Another dimension of this dream was revealed the following day, when a free sample magazine arrived unexpectedly in the mail with a painting of a chestnut horse on the cover identical to the one in my dream. According to the accompanying story, it was an eighteenth-century portrait of a famous racehorse that had died shortly after it had been immortalized on canvas. Apparently the animal, whose body was lathered in sweat and cruelly scored by whip-cuts, belonged to a nobleman who had wagered an enormous sum on it. The horse had been urged on so viciously to its victory that it shortly thereafter died of exhaustion. Magazine horse, magazine editor: I, too, had allowed myself to be ridden mercilessly for someone else's purse.

The second dream involves yet another attempt to get an accurate picture, this time of an "unidentified flying object." It turns out to be, like the horse, another "both/and" creature. I could not tell if it was a quaint mechanism or a living animal; a turkey or a buzzard ("turkey-buzzard," I was to discover in the dictionary, is a synonym for "vulture"); threatening or almost harmless. The dream emphasized that this was an "undistorted" picture, but of *what*?

In retrospect, the odd, griffinlike creature seems to have been a representation of both my actual disease and the modern science of diagnosis itself, which, as Dr. Oliver Sacks remarked, has since its eighteenth-century origins tended to reduce people to "machines, automata, puppets." I was to learn only after my surgery that my disease was a cancer more from a "mechanistic" diagnostic perspective. A malignant cell-type with (in men of my age) usually nonaggressive behavior, it was a paradox, a chimera. Its name, "papillary" cancer, itself comes from the word for butterfly; perhaps the meaning of the cast-metallic (that is, manufactured rather than biological) butterfly designs on my dream-creature's body. The dream seems to have been saying that the label of deadly cancer was as much a technicality as an actual living description.

A vulture is usually a symbol of impending death, but the dream's use of an alternate term to "diagnose" the creature—"turkey-buzzard"—gave it both a pathetic and indeterminate ring. These birds, contrary to their fearsome reputations, *are* a somewhat pathetic species: "They have weak beaks and lack the strength of other birds of prey," I read in the encyclopedia, and "rarely attack other than helpless animals." In symbolic language, the abnormal cells would usually be too weak to attack a body with a competent immune system. (Dr. George Crile has written of papillary thyroid cancer, "There is so much resistance to this type of cell that occurrence of distant metastasis is rare.") The encyclopedia adds that American vultures have no syrinx (a bird's version of a larynx), and thus are "voiceless." Again, psychological meaning merges with physiology in the alchemical crucible of the unconscious.

The third dream depicts an alarming horde of outsized crabs and beetles. The word *cancer*, I was later to learn, is the Latin word for

crab. Both crabs and beetles belong to the phylum *Arthropoda,* creatures with external skeletons. These animals periodically outgrow
their shells; the molting process, according to the encyclopedia,
"permits rapid growth in size and significant change in bodily form."
Such creatures would be apt metaphors for cancer, but in the language of the psyche, also for the process of transformation, metamorphosis. In the dream, the "beetles" turn out to be only artificial
costumes that the poor ants must carry laboriously on their backs.
Like the turkey-buzzard, these cancer-"beetles" are creatures that
initially seem daunting but turn out instead to be relatively weak—
indeed, another species entirely.

In subsequent dreams, various creatures with exoskeletons would
go through a kind of evolution, becoming ever less menacing. In
one dream I was offered some "raw lobster meat" bulging from a
partially cracked, molting shell, but it nauseated me too much to
eat it. In another dream a month later, I was offered half-cooked
crab rolled into sushi as part of a sort of a samurai initiation.

Finally, in a third dream, I had walked into a restaurant and
ordered "crab sticks" (pre-cooked *fake* crabmeat) served in a pita
pocket. When I was told that the dish "wasn't on the menu," I
marched back to the kitchen saying, "I'll fix it myself." Interestingly, my surgeon told me after my operation that the tumor had
been "perfectly contained, like it was in a pocket." In my dream, I
was able to "eat" it, perhaps even suggesting, though this is wildly
speculative, that my immune system could have rallied to "fix it
myself."

It is not surprising that I was unable to interpret these bizarre
symbols with enough confidence to affect my treatment decisions.
Jung, who on several occasions provided startlingly accurate diagnoses based on the dreams of patients whom he had sometimes
never met, said of such images: "It looks as if it were a poet who
had been at work rather than a rational doctor who would speak of
infections, fever, toxins, et cetera." Nor was I able to recognize the
"spiritual diagnosis" they contained—hints of the disease's significance to the psyche, or how the "inner disease" might be remedied.
For it now seems to me it was I who had lived as a "neither/nor"
creature, never quite claiming my authentic being; I who drove
myself like a flailed racehorse toward the finish line; I who had
disguised myself in a garish outer shell, hiding the victimized, workaholic ant beneath; I who had no voicebox; and perhaps even I
who had been molting, transforming, cracking open to reveal at last
the rawness within.

FINDING YOUR OWN NAME

Certainly, it is important to have our symptoms translated into medically comprehensible terminology. For all its unadmitted uncertainties, scientific nomenclature demystifies, replacing our nightmares with dispassionate data. But it also tends to preempt the quest for whatever, in the language of my dreams, might not be "on the menu." It purports to tell us "what we have," and enjoins us to look no further. It is almost as if we are receiving a description of an adversary from a scout perched high on a ridgetop—*covered with hair, tall as a house, a huge bloodshot eye*—when in fact our opponent is right in front of us, available to our own inspection, grappling, and perhaps even talent for negotiation.

"Call out your disease, set it in front of you," urged Jeanne Achterberg to a group of patients at a seminar I attended. "Acknowledge it, give it a story, a metaphor, a sound, a smell, a covering. Then get a picture of internal processes that can heal you, the strengths that come to you from the ancestral human heritage." Achterberg is a medical scientist, but she knew that not all the names for our symptoms can be spelled out with the high-tech alphabet blocks of the pathology lab.

The word *pathology* derives from the Greek words *logos,* or "discourse," and *pathos,* "the quality in something experienced or observed which arouses feelings of pity, sorrow, sympathy, or compassion." The very term implies a dialogue with what is wounded. In shamanic societies, every diagnosis is a story of relationship. "The Gimi people," writes medical anthropologist Leonard Glick, "do not respond to illness as a phenomenon independent of the personal identity of its victim. An illness has meaning for a community, not just for an individual, and this is what is expressed each time a man or woman's kinsmen operate in a treatment procedure."[19]

Tribal medicine, like its modern counterpart, reveals causes and suggests remedies. But tribal medical diagnoses also provide a context. If a disease is diagnosed as the outcome of breaking a compact with nature, an insult to a spirit ancestor, or the magical aspersions of a jealous neighbor, the cure requires the repair of the broken links, a harmonizing of the patient's wider life. The diagnosis by its very name suggests the healing story.

The psychologist Elida Evans proposed that a cancer patient's diagnostic case history must always include things "pertaining to the mind": "[W]hat knock-out blows had been dealt to him in the destruction of his affections, his theories, aims, and ambitions, his hopes? what mental and physical habits? what were his anxieties, his longings, his happiest memories?"[20]

In the early modern medical era, diagnosticians were taught to emulate portrait painters, filling in the details of a static scene, capturing the essence of an individual at a moment in time. But as medicine is just beginning to acknowledge, it is the individual, not her portrait, who becomes sick or gets well. Despite the benefits of technology and the marvelous pictures it can paint, it is up to the journeyer to step out of the frame and claim the still-unknown potential of a three-dimensional life.

7

THE MEETING WITH
THE DOCTOR

The relationship between physician and patient,
if it were literally followed, would give us a world
of extraordinary fertility of the imagination,
which we can hardly afford.

—WILLIAM CARLOS WILLIAMS,
poet and physician

ONCE WHILE leafing through a book on ancient Sumer I came
across the earliest known image of a healing deity. Carved on
a ceremonial beaker of dark-green soapstone during the reign of
King Gudea, the god, named Nin-gish-zi-da, is a chimera: a snake's
head wearing a crown topped by two bull-horns; a neck ruffed with
a lion's mane; the claws and wings of an eagle; the body of a spotted
leopard; and the tail of a scorpion. I was startled to see, clutched
in his talons, a staff and a pair of entwined, ascending snakes—a
caduceus, the symbol, from the days of the messenger-god Hermes
to today's A.M.A., of the healing guild. The figure was suggestive
of the tangled powers that all physicians must address and contain—
the dangerous and liberating paradoxes of transformation (the
snake was venerated for its power to shed the skin of the outgrown
self); the forces of nature; and the noble monsters of the psyche.

The earliest doctors knew that the relationship between patient
and healer is charged psychic space. Illness is a forced descent not
only into the body, but into the self. The founders of Western medicine, the physician-priests of the Asklepian temples at Epidaurus
and Kos, made the transformation of both psyche and soma the
very basis of their art. Healers in traditional cultures were not only
physicians but psychologists, masters of ritual, social mediators, spiritual mentors, and often survivors of illness themselves—were doc-

tors of both body and soul. The Healing Buddha, the Asian equivalent of Asklepius as the progenitor of physicians, is said to have devoted himself to "aiding beings to change their negative patterns. He is especially concerned with prompting beings to a great awakening, a momentous turning point."

Our contemporary healing god, personified by the M.D. ("for 'Medical Deity,'" as one doctor wryly remarked), may seem more straightforward. My own doctors by and large communicated their belief that the psyche did not count; that it was at best an irrelevancy, perhaps even an impediment to their task. Their message was: "Your machine has broken down. Leave it with us for a week, and we will perform the necessary repairs."

But though we may inure ourselves to expect little more than a professional body repairman, the M.D. stands in the stead of the eternal physician. We inevitably see him through the camera obscura of the psyche—as comforter or judge, parent-surrogate or confessor, savior or clay-footed god. As one doctor confided to me musingly, "The patient creates an aura around us that sometimes seems quasi-mystical, divine. The fee transaction tends to cloud this, but it's there. It always will be." For the patient who enters his consulting room in search of healing, the doctor reflects the chimerical hopes and fears not only of the moment, but of a life that now hangs in the balance.

"I wanted my kind medical pastor with his scalpel to also be an expansive human being," said lawyer John Studholme. "Someone I could imagine reading the Kama Sutra, meeting strange women in afternoon hotels." Significantly, during the period before his illness, John had begun to mourn the "loss of passion" in his life. His sinecured "trade-off between aliveness and respectability" suddenly felt like an intolerable cheat. Having been diagnosed with terminal lymphoma, he now longed for a passionate doctor, one who could not only conquer the forces of death, but somehow embody the vitality, even the Eros, of his own unlived life.

John was calling upon the most fundamental archetype of the healer: one who administers the curative medicine, but who also, like Hermes, whose caduceus guided souls through the underworld, acts as ferryman across the waters of renewal. He wanted his doctor to cure his body *and* rekindle the fire in his heart. He was seeking not just a physician, but a wizard.

THE DOCTOR AS WIZARD

When we think of the Wizard of Oz, we think of a fraud, a vaude-villian mountebank who could no more perform the Tin Woodman's wished-for heart transplant than cure a bad case of heartburn. But seen in another light, the Wizard is a typical shamanic healer whose goal is to rouse his patients' dormant self-healing powers.

The Tin Woodman's meeting with the Wizard is a classic en-counter. He and his fellow patients arrive in the waiting-room of the imposing Emerald Palace, awestruck supplicants to the world's greatest heart surgeon (or so the Tin Woodman hopes; the Scare-crow is praying for the world's greatest *brain* surgeon).

The healer's authority and the patient's trust, according to the psychologist E. Fuller Torrey, derive in nearly every culture from certain common elements.[1] These include the patient's expectations, usually intensified by a trip or pilgrimage; the impressiveness of the healer's building, dubbed the "edifice complex"[2]; the healer's special regalia and paraphernalia, whether stethoscope or sacred gourd; his exalted social stature; and the aura of power, mystery, and even fear that surrounds him.

One physician remarked to me that "patients in crisis often come to us in a near trance, with all its openness to hypnotic suggestion and psychological change." The Wizard uses the Tin Woodman's awed susceptibility to goad him toward a quest that will lead beyond physical well-being to psychospiritual growth. The Wizard does fur-nish "real" medicine—a patch of fabric for the Tin Woodman's heart (silk, though most heart surgeons prefer Dacron) and a green phar-maceutical vial for the Lion. But his most lasting effect is to reveal to each character his or her own innate potential for wholeness. To get well, the Tin Woodman and his companions must do more than conquer demonic forces or receive new organs (common symbolic features of shamanic initiatory rituals); they must awaken the healer within.

The idea that doctors should treat the whole person rather than just the broken parts still remains, despite recent progress, somewhat foreign to the Western outlook. Former *New England Journal of Med-icine* editor Franz J. Inglefinger has written flatly: "The doctor should not be expected to play a major role in changing whatever lifestyle may be seriously detrimental. He has enough to do . . ."[3]

It is an irony for physician and patient alike that the whole-person approach may also be more clinically effective than the strictly medical model. Maverick cardiologist Dr. Dean Ornish, as noted earlier, has astonished his peers by reversing coronary artery disease in hopeless cases with a "life-style" treatment of diet, exercise, and meditation. Ornish is adamant in his conviction that the healing profession must cast a wider spiritual net than is currently the norm:

> I originally wanted to call my book *Opening Your Heart*. Not only in the literal sense of clearing your arteries, but in the metaphorical sense of "opening up." I'm interested in more than curing heart disease. I want to see how it can be a catalyst for changing how patients perceive the world, their self-worth, their values.
>
> If you can get patients to work toward personal transformation, you win on several levels: When their lives become richer and more joyful, they'll *want* to live longer. And that gives them the motivation to make the changes that could make them well.

What might be called a new mind-body-spirit approach is not without its critics: In a blistering column in a women's magazine, one doctor decried "quasi-religious" stances and "heady, wildly optimistic transcendentalism" that prefers "belief rather than evidence."[4] But it is precisely recent evidence of linkages among the brain, the organs, and the immune system that Ornish and others use to justify their stance. These findings, they argue, imply that psychological medicine is physical medicine, and vice versa—and that not to acknowledge this in practice is to put one's head in the scientific sand.

THE POWERS OF THE HEALER

Ornish is part of a small but influential group of doctors, many of whom practice yoga or meditation, whose approach harks back to the craft's most ancient precepts. The doctor's job, in their view, is not just making repairs but pointing the way toward spiritual regeneration.

Dr. Mark Nichter, a clinician with a degree in anthropology, has wrestled with the implications of this point of view for doctors' own lives: "Like it or not, you're part of your patients' pilgrimage. But in order for it to work, they have to associate you with the power of the hand, with having something special, being a healer, a teacher—and that's a responsibility. You're left with this issue of power which is difficult to morally and ethically come to terms with."[5]

Conventional medicine would suggest the question is largely irrelevant. Precisely because it has dispensed with the "power of the hand," modern treatment claims to be a purely objective enterprise, its results replicable no matter how and by whom its medicines are administered. But physicians always have speculated that the doctor-patient relationship contains its own healing power. The Renaissance physician Agrippa wrote, "It is verified amongst physicians that a strong belief and an undoubted hope and love towards the physician and medicine, conduce much to health; yea, more, sometimes, than the medicine itself."

Researchers have noted repeatedly that psychosocial factors, including the physician's bedside manner and the "ritual" aspects of modern medicine procedures, are themselves powerful healing modalities. Dr. Bernie Siegel relates an illustrative story about the chemotherapeutic agent cis-platinum. When it first was used it was greeted with enormous enthusiasm, with doctors reporting its rates of effectiveness against cancer as high as 75 percent. But over time, the new drug's success rate dropped to 25 or 30 percent. Why?

Siegel suggests that the atmosphere of positive expectation created by confident, gung-ho doctors who believed they had a magic bullet mobilized the patients' own healing response. When the agent was later administered by bored technicians minus the "miracle drug" fanfare, its effects may have been diminished.[6] Siegel's admittedly speculative assessment calls to mind the only partly tongue-in-cheek advice offered in 1833 by the French physician Armand Trousseau: "You should treat as many patients as possible with new drugs while they still have the power to heal."

The possibility that the doctor might hold this sort of power elicits profound ambivalence, particularly among holistically oriented physicians trying to dispel medical mystification and to empower the patient.

"We have for too many decades fostered a decline in the independence of the individual," one doctor explained. "We have portrayed ourselves as being able to perform all rescues, fight all terminal battles, even resuscitate the dead if only we have the opportunity and the funding for our incredibly powerful technology. We have to come down from the pedestal."

A doctor friend once exclaimed to me in near despair, "I just want to be the patient's 'partner in health,' not some all-knowing demigod." But the insistent tug of her patients' expectations, she says, sometimes made her feel as if she should "play the game, put on the magical mantle, create a little atmosphere—maybe make lightning strike!" This doctor eventually took a hiatus from her practice of internal medicine and spent several years studying Jungian psychology, slowly incorporating it into her practice of physical medicine.

She is typical of doctors who are currently struggling to find a place for the psyche within the context of scientific medicine. At the 1991 meeting of the American Holistic Medical Association in a Colorado ski lodge, doctors exploring the potential for a new medicine compared the situation to the Soviet Union before *glasnost* and *perestroika:* "The present system is about to collapse," ventured one endocrinologist. "Everybody senses it. The old paradigm is crumbling, the new paradigm is here, but most of my colleagues still refuse to acknowledge it." The task such doctors confront is how to practice a medicine congruent with startling new theoretical benchmarks. If healing *can* be enhanced by attending to the psychological dimensions of the doctor-patient relationship, what form should that relationship now take?

At one workshop, a small group of self-proclaimed "physicians-in-transition" struggled to describe how their patients saw them, and how they as doctors wished to be seen. Sitting in a circle, they called out in breathless profusion: "enabler . . . listener . . . magician . . . consoler . . . confidant . . . problem-solver . . . loan officer . . . possessor of undeserved wealth . . . clergyman . . . teacher . . . marriage counselor . . . role model . . . fixer . . . a divinity . . . guide . . . motivator . . . pointer-outer . . . facilitator . . ."

Judging by patients' reports, however, doctors engaged in such earnest questioning of their roles remain a rarity. Medical schools, hospitals, and pharmaceutical and insurance companies by and large continue to promote a model in which considerations of the "whole person" are viewed at best as luxuries next to the necessities of standardized treatment.

As a result, when the healing path inevitably leads to the doorstep of one reputed to have the power of deliverance, the ill may find their emotional needs largely ignored, and the psychospiritual dimensions of the healing relationship unacknowledged. The average physician may accept that the patient's mind should be the central focus of psychotherapy, but behaves as if the treating of disease depends on the body's near complete severance from the psyche. But acknowledged or not, a psychic "subtext," one which may affect the outcome of the treatment, is inevitably created by patient and doctor—even if both are unconscious of the roles they are playing.

THE DOCTOR AS PARENT

One common role patients ascribe to doctors is that of "parent-surrogate." In our hour of great helplessness, we may find ourselves seized by an inarticulate hope that the all-powerful parents of dim memory might magically appear, scoop us up in their arms, and make it all better. If not they, then perhaps the doctor will stand in their place, heir to unresolved issues of autonomy, authority, and nurturance.

"The *only* times Mom and Dad were there for me were when I got sick," says former melanoma patient Samantha Coles. "I think I was hoping that when the Real Big Number came up, they'd show me they really did love me. But they didn't come through. So I transferred all my unmet needs for love to the doctors." She grimaces. "*Wrong.*"

For their part, doctors may almost deliberately play upon the parent-child dynamic. Dr. Wang, faced with my reluctance to have surgery, made a plea I found well-nigh irresistible: "If you were my own son, I would beg you to have this operation. I promise it will make you well. I would not risk harming you any more than I would my own child. I only want to take care of you."

What might have left me skeptical under normal circumstances—here was a man who, for all his good intent, was avidly promoting his own professional agenda—instead moved me to tears. Maybe, like a parent, he knew better than I did what was good for me. In an echo of the dysfunctional family dynamic, he was holding out the prospect of love—but only if I permitted him to change me unutterably.

I don't know how he would have behaved had I insisted on challenging his authority, modulating or even refusing outright the treatment he offered. Authority has two faces: seduction and coercion. The latter often appears when the patient exhibits too much independence ("After twelve years of expensive training," one doctor told me, "I don't like the patient telling me my business"), or when the doctor fears that a remedy he believes to be necessary and proven might be rejected.

This coercive stance can be seen in the story of Winnie Scott [not her real name], an early leader in the environmental movement.

When she developed a suspicious spot on her lung, she resisted exploratory surgery. "I immediately got a label: 'Noncompliant Patient.' My doctor told me, 'Come in by Monday and let us "crack your chest," or else you will get a registered letter disowning you as my patient.' What he was telling me was, 'Do what we say, or you'll die.' "

Over the objections of her husband, a former medical journal editor, she decided to work with an unconventional "energy healer" who specialized in a practice called polarity therapy. The shadow on her X-ray, presumed to be but never diagnosed as cancer, disappeared within three months.

When another patient told her doctor that she was dubious about an experimental chemotherapy treatment, the man "threw a tantrum. He told me, 'If you don't want to do this, if you want to die, just go somewhere else.' " Such medical ultimata, even when only implicit, recreate a common childhood anxiety. According to one author, "Studies of chronically ill people have shown how intense the fear of abandonment is. It is feared more than death itself."

The same writer adds that a patient's sense of isolation may be intensified by the doctor's "inability to accept the emergent emotions."[7] Given what we are beginning to suspect about the role of emotion in the healing process, this is truly a prescription for disaster. For if illness is an inner crisis as well as a sheerly physical one—if emotional states may sometimes even *affect* the course of the illness—then the patient's rebelliousness, childishness, or other "inappropriate" responses, so often viewed as obstructions to treatment, may be critical factors in his or her healing. For example, numerous studies have suggested that the willingness to express negative feelings is a trait associated with an enhanced immune profile. (Bernie Siegel reports an account by a Dr. Charles A. Janeway of a lupus patient who, in Janeway's words, "cured herself [by spending a year] unloading all her deep-seated and concealed hostility toward her father"—on *him*. "All the stories I've heard about recovery from lupus," writes Dr. Siegel a bit expansively, "involve confronting authority.")

But it is not only the climate more typically fostered by the doctor that may inhibit "healing feeling"; the patient, too, may find the upswelling of emotion threatening. Alice Miller notes that when patients in psychotherapy begin to gain access to long-buried grief or anger, the tendency is to stuff it back, "to deny, pacify, and control the child within." When the upheaval of disease brings up similarly unresolved emotional issues, patients who once controlled their feelings to win a parent's conditional love may find themselves in the same pathogenic bind with their caregiver.

An odd collusion can develop between doctor and patient which reinforces the same psychic deformations at the root of the "disease-prone personality." As described earlier, psychologist Lawrence LeShan has observed that cancer patients often suffer from a sense, traceable to early disturbances in the parent-child relationship, that their lives are governed by an uncaring, implacable Fate. If this is so, what is the effect upon the patient of entering the domain of oncology, where prognoses of doom are so common? One medical historian told me, "Most oncologists are therapeutic nihilists. Given the poor results of most of their interventions, they are often demoralized men in a demoralized profession." Many of the patients I spoke with complained that their doctors sometimes reflected them in a dark glass; they seemed dismissive or even fearful at a time when journeyers desperately needed inspiration.

Consider this in light of a recent University of Pittsburgh study which demonstrated that therapy aimed at reducing cancer patients' pessimism also improved their immune systems.[8] The influence upon immunity of a pessimistic doctor is suggested by a poem the eighteenth-century poet John Donne wrote from his sickbed: "I observe the Physician, with the same diligence, as hee the disease/ I see he feares, and I feare with him."

A physician's attitudes also may augment the patient's sense of helplessness, another immunosuppressive emotion often carried over from childhood. Particularly within the confines of institution-alized medicine, the doctor's stance may come to resemble "poison-ous pedagogy," a term coined by Alice Miller to describe child-rearing methods that radically undermine personal autonomy. Many patients described being treated by their doctors much as the eighteenth- and nineteenth-century pedagogical manuals Miller quotes from advised teachers to treat their pupils:

> [O]ne should never allow the impression to arise that an adult might be wrong or make a mistake . . . but that the adult should, on the contrary, conceal his or her weaknesses from the child and pretend to divine authority. . . . The greatest problems are presented by surgical operations. If only one is necessary, say not a word about it to young children ahead of time, but conceal all preparations, perform the operation in silence, and then say, My child, now you are cured; the pain will soon be gone.

THE DOCTOR AS TEACHER

This style of "pedagogy" is particularly ironic in light of the very root of the word doctor, the Latin *docere,* "to teach." But to teach what? Much of conventional medicine still subscribes to the same sick-making dividedness—body from mind, inner from outer, emotion from intellect, individual from social context—the patient needs to reconcile to become well. Our health-care methods, quick, external, and fragmentary, travel the same cultural mazeways as our diseases. What the shaman might call loss of soul—an ebbing of self, a loss of capacity for vivid experience, a tearing of connection with the Whole—is not antithetical to the conventional definition of health; in some sense, it is required.

We might imagine a more radical, affirmative, and in a strict sense countercultural role for the doctor: as an encourager of the patient's uniqueness; an ombudsman for long-deferred and often unsuspected needs; a facilitator of self-discovery; a change agent helping to pry the patient loose from pathological life patterns; a helper urging him away from mere "normalcy" toward authentic being. The educator-doctor might furnish her clients with a practical map to the bodymind, teaching them to reawaken what the Taoist sage Lao Tzu called "profound intelligence . . . that penetrating and pervading power to restore all things to their original harmony."

Some "physicians-in-transition" are already bringing this attitude into their practice. One described giving her patients what she calls "a personalized course of study. I'll see them for two-hour sessions each month, and in between, I'll give them 'homework assignments' of various health practices and ways of looking into their lives. They have to complete them before I'll see them next."

Dr. James Gordon, a clinical professor at the Georgetown School of Medicine and cochairman of the National Institutes of Health's "Panel on Mind/Body Interventions," described his unusual medical practice:

> My office is in Washington, D.C., so my patients are mainly hardnosed political organizer types. They come to me to get fixed, not to search their souls. I'll routinely ask them why they think they got sick. After they get over their "what the hell are you asking me for, that's why I'm paying you" response, I've found that ninety-five percent of them will come forth with

deep, powerful reasons that it happened to them at this particular time and in this part of their bodies.

I'll almost always "prescribe" some form of meditation to them along with any medicine I might give them. *Meditation* and *medicine* come from the same root: "to care," and "to cure." Sometimes I'll even try to trick them into looking at themselves in a new way. I'll tell one to try dancing naked in front of a mirror, or hum into their diseased organ, or jump up and down yelling nonsense syllables just to shake things loose.

I told one patient, a very serious computer analyst, that he had to look into the mirror every day and laugh. He came back complaining he couldn't, until one day he realized he'd been telling me he'd do *anything* to get well, but wasn't even willing to have a sense of humor about himself. *That* made him burst out laughing. I think that's when he started to really improve.[9]

According to Ruth Inge-Heinze, a scholar of Asian shamanism, this sort of induced cognitive shift is at the core of the tribal medicine man's approach: "The healer," Ruth told me, "creates a ritual space for the patient that is outside the ordinary. He transposes him or her into a realm of possibility where their habitual limitations can be cut through. He restores the patient's contact with the universal energy, mends the broken wires, plugs them back into the socket.

"But in the West, the whole affair becomes mechanistic, anonymous. The patient is excluded from the healing process, treated as a robot, a piece of matter, a lung, an appendix. It's a travesty."

THE DOCTOR AS WOUNDED HEALER

Some physicians are becoming painfully aware of this debasement of the healer's craft, which the critic Ivan Illich calls "the transformation of the doctor from an artisan exercising a skill on personally known individuals into a technician applying scientific rules to classes of patient."[10]

When I first met Dr. Adan Rios, he was a highly regarded immunologist at Houston's M. D. Anderson Hospital. His wife had been one of my sister's nurses, and I'd been struck by the deep empathy of this soft-spoken man with probing brown eyes. Ten years later, I ran into him unexpectedly at a conference on AIDS.

His professional involvement in the epidemic had changed him, he told me in his lilting accent. He wanted to talk about it. "Maybe it's because I was raised a Catholic," he began with a faint smile. "We are trained in self-confession.

"In the past, I could apply a protocol almost for its own sake, and stay galaxies away from the patient. If things went badly, I might feel temporarily sorry. But I felt I needed the distance to guard myself against hurt. It was an instinct of self-preservation. I think my biggest transformation has been in realizing that the doctor must have not only the desire to treat but the *intent to heal*. If I want to heal someone, I must be intimately connected. I must as a human being identify with the one who is sick and whom I wish to see cured."

Japanese shamanic healer Ikuko Osumi makes a similar distinction between the "dualistic" approach to treatment and what she calls "one-being therapy." In the former, the patient is acted on as a passive object, with the intention of

> restoring the status quo, without any change or learning on any meaningful level. It is a way of treating illness which is designed not to upset or inconvenience the ego (the conditioned self) any more than inevitably happens when one is ill. Such therapy too often denies the patient responsibility for, and knowledge of, his or her own condition and the treatment he or she is receiving.[11]

In the second type, by contrast, patient, healer, and healing process are one. The patient becomes an active participant, bringing discipline, self-inquiry, and a willingness to reorient his or her life. Perhaps the shaman is more at home with this approach than Western doctors because the shaman is almost by definition a "wounded healer," someone whose own initiatory descent permits a depth of fellow-feeling for the patient's suffering, and a profound faith in the healing powers of the bodymind.

"One thing missing from my medical education," muses Dr. James Gordon, "was anything that would lead to insight into my *own* woundedness, into the things inside *me* that needed healing. There was no equivalent to the psychiatric training analysis, to the idea that you have to attend to your own pathology. There's a real germ of wisdom in the idea that you cannot do for anyone else what you have not done for yourself."

As is the case with many tribal medicine people, Dr. Gordon can trace his understanding to his own struggle with affliction, in this case a serious back ailment. "All the old healing traditions," he observes, "say the physician has to go through not only technical education, but a process of refinement, an alchemical transformation. In the Orient, in Africa, in Native American cultures, probably for twenty-five thousand years of medical history, you couldn't become a healer of any kind until this was accomplished. It's only very recently we've forgotten."

The medical training that has produced most of today's doctors has hardly been geared to fostering sensitivity. According to *The New York Times,* a recent study of twelve American medical schools revealed that "abuse and mistreatment of medical students are widespread and often leave long-lasting emotional scars that may affect their care of patients as physicians."

An astonishing *80 percent* of fourth-year students at one school reported experiencing "repeated verbal insults, harassment and denigration by arrogant teachers," and many reported physical attacks and sexual abuse. Medical residents are subjected to long sleepless shifts that cause high levels of stress; to disruption of their key relationships (a high percentage of marriages don't survive med school); and to unrelenting criticism—all, interestingly, techniques used in brainwashing and cultic indoctrination.[12]

Several doctors remarked to me that it wasn't until they began to attune themselves to their patients' inner lives that they were able to recover parts of themselves that had been stifled in their professional tutelage. As one put it, "The more I'm myself, the more room I allow for my inner life, my intuition and feelings—all stuff that got cut off in my early training—the more my patient and I seem to heal *each other*." Another quoted Dr. Albert Schweitzer's observation: "Medicine is not only a science, but letting our own individuality interact with the individuality of the patient."

Ken Rothenberg, coauthor of *The Second Medical Revolution,* notes that while the conventional doctor "exercises control: The patient comes with a problem, the doctor addresses it," the evolving new style of practice is "dominated by mutual feedback, so that both patient and doctor are participants in the healing process. The doctor isn't just a spectator."

Many cultures have long considered the doctor's own inner life to be an important healing modality in itself, part of his or her power to make sick or make well. "In the Tibetan view," writes Terry Clifford in *The Diamond Healing,* "the healer's state of mind is not just a moral question which has no effect on the patient. It is held to be a vitally important influence on his condition. . . . Whatever kind of medicine is being practiced, the Tibetan healer will also be practicing internally various mystic healing exercises, visualizations, mantras, etc."

The healing thoughts of the doctor may have effects on the patient beyond the obvious psychological benefits of being treated by a physician who radiates inner peace. Prayer may be a palpable force with scientifically measurable effects upon biological systems. One double-blind laboratory experiment showed that prayer can promote the germination rates of rye seeds. Interestingly, the greatest positive effects were seen in seeds which had been exposed to severe stress (salt water, which would normally inhibit growth), perhaps indicating the "openness" to healing forces of an organism in crisis.

In other laboratory studies, prayer has been shown to detectably slow the growth rates of leukemic white blood cells, increase the healing rates of wounds, and shrink the size of goiters and tumors in rats. Well-designed human experiments—where individuals were not told they were being prayed for—have reported positive clinical outcomes in cases of asthma and heart attacks. Dr. Larry Dossey notes that several studies suggest that a "simple attitude of prayer-ful*ness*—a feeling of empathy, caring and compassion—seemed to set the stage for healing."[13]

Although he estimates that prayer does not seem to affect more than 20 percent of cases, Dossey states in his fascinating book *Healing Words,* "I gradually decided that *not* to employ prayer with my patients was the equivalent of deliberately withholding a potent drug or surgical procedure from them. I simply could not ignore the evidence for prayer's effectiveness without feeling like a traitor to the scientific tradition."[14]

In ancient traditions, the healer joined in the patient's struggle for health in every region of human experience, the metaphysical and the physical. Healers sometimes undertook metaphorical journeys on behalf of their patients, paddling their spirit-canoes to the fortresses of disease-spirits to battle for the souls of the afflicted— even at risk to themselves. In a sense, the medicine man's job was the constant reenactment of his *own* story of sickness and healing.

How much a doctor is also a healer may be precisely the extent to which she is able to meet a patient in the realm of body, mind, and spirit—a realm fraught with peril and potential. Such healers form a living bridge between the world of the psyche and the world of matter. They know the way out of illness because they have learned, often firsthand, the way in. Dr. Rios told me, "I now feel that what happens to my patient will in a sense also happen to me.

If he is hurt by something, I will be hurt too. It's almost like we're traveling the same road together."

Similarly, the Wizard—who, it should not be forgotten, was a fellow sojourner rather than a native of the land of Oz—is personally affected by the journeys of his "patients." It is through his interaction with Dorothy and her friends that he removes his mask, rediscovers his own humanity, and finally makes his own way homeward. The battle with the Witch is his as well. His fate is tethered to theirs: The same wound, and the same healing, affects them all.

❧ 8 ❧

BIG GUNS, MAGIC BULLETS: THE CITADEL OF MEDICINE

*I have the conviction that when physiology will be
far enough advanced the poet, the philosopher, and
the physiologist will all understand each other.*

—CLAUDE BERNARD, founder of
modern physiology

First, do no harm.

—HIPPOCRATES

TODAY THE archetype of the "wounded healer" is split: All powers of healing seem to reside with the doctor and all pathology with the patient.[1] This dualism may account for the peculiar cast of Western medical practice. When the doctor is "no longer in touch" with his own wound, suggests Dr. Oliver Sacks, he tends to see diseases as "not parts of ourselves, and parts of the world" but "purely alien and bad."

This veritable demonizing of disease has serious implications for patients, sometimes leading to a style of medicine in which a doctor may "attack the disease with all the weapons one has . . . with total impunity, without a thought for the person who is ill." Sacks states bluntly that, though progress is being made, such notions still "dominate the landscape of medicine."[2]

THE WAR AGAINST DISEASE

The more resistant a disease is to rapid cure, or the more diabolical its depredations appear, the more powerful—and potentially destructive—are the big guns and magic bullets arrayed against it.

Particularly in the case of "big diseases," our physicians too often become dichotomizers, wagers of war, tacticians of what philosopher Michel Foucault has called "the healthy-morbid opposition." In such cases the patient—already a conscript awaiting doctor's orders—too often risks winding up an incidental casualty on the battleground of his own body.

I have often wondered how I, a supposed skeptic and resister of standardization, wound up a medical draftee in a small war so relentlessly prosecuted that even thyroid glands with *benign* tumors are taken out with stunning regularity. (According to studies of groups of patients "operated on by the more aggressive surgeons, ninety-six percent had operations that were neither necessary nor useful," writes noted expert Dr. George Crile, himself a thyroid surgeon.) Perhaps the answer was that I *believed* in the Enemy; I *asked* to be classified 1-A, convinced that Death, in the form of ravening hordes of faceless cancer cells, was storming my own beachhead. My younger brother's careless rebuke at the time, that I was a "coward" for trying to avoid surgery, stung me as a public slap would have an able-bodied man too craven to enlist in the Good War.

Dr. Jacob Zieghelboim, a former cancer patient and an associate professor of medicine and immunology at the UCLA School of Medicine, observes, "Since the beginning, cancer has been likened to diseases caused by foreign invaders such as bacteria and germs. What we perceive to be foreign threats to our existence are almost always handled in militaristic ways. . . . We want to kill the cancer, to destroy the enemy and take over."

The war on cancer was formally declared in 1971 when President Richard Nixon signed into law the sort of campaign-unto-victory that was elsewhere eluding him. But after billions of dollars and countless deaths, another technological war of attrition has been pronounced largely a stalemate. In a 1986 landmark article in the *New England Journal of Medicine*, Harvard epidemiologist John C. Bailar declared:

> We are losing the war against cancer, notwithstanding progress against several uncommon forms of the disease, improvements in palliation, and extension of the productive years of life. [There is] no evidence that some 35 years of intense and growing efforts to improve the treatment of cancer have had much overall effect on the most fundamental measure of clinical outcome—death.[3]

The apparent progress trumpeted by the National Cancer Institutes, Bailar stated, was largely "spurious"—filled with statistical flukes, some innocent, others bordering on meretricious, that made any jingoistic dispatches from the front suspect. In a 1987 *Los Angeles Times* article entitled "Chemotherapy: Snake-Oil Remedy?" UCLA internist Martin F. Shapiro writes that for four of the most common cancers (colon and rectum, pancreas, stomach, and lung), there is "no convincing evidence that chemotherapy offers any benefit whatsoever." Chemo is highly effective on several cancers occurring in younger people, but only 2 percent of the patients who die of cancer are under thirty in the first place. Despite its questionable benefits, a *fourth* of cancer patients in all age groups and categories receive chemo during their initial stay in the hospital.[4]

"For a dangerous and technologically exacting form of treatment," says Harvard epidemiologist John Cairns, "these are disturbing figures." Even more disturbing, Cairns points out that in many instances "there may be no way of determining whether any particular patient's survival was predestined or should be attributed to the treatment."[5]

All this is not to suggest that doctors are ill-intentioned, uncaring, or conspiratorial. Like the public, they operate (literally) on the assumption that medicine's foundations—long-standing, undergirded by common practice and "common sense"—must be solid. In point of fact, however, according to an Office of Technology Assessment report, "It has been estimated that only 10 to 20 percent of all procedures currently used in medical practice have been shown to be efficacious by controlled trial. . . . Evidence indicates that many technologies are not adequately assessed before they enjoy widespread use."[6]

And history tells us that institutional practices in which costs outweigh real benefits, from Aztec ritual sacrifice to Pentagon procurement budgets, have great powers of persistence—bolstered by the fear that there are no viable alternatives; by suasions of economics; by the belief that to relinquish these practices would be to risk catastrophe; by a perception that the shortcomings of the system are anomalous rather than paradigmatic.

Big Medicine's prosecution of the war on Big Disease has become something of a national jihad. We tend to view the complications, dubious procedures, and outright failures of medicine as flukes, the unavoidable detritus left in the wheel-ruts of the victorious legions of science. It seems small-minded to cavil over a few inevitable casualties when the campaign goes so gloriously.

But a number of dreams I had during the maddening time I was trying to decide on treatment in retrospect seem stark reminders that there is an underbelly to medicine's Gilded Age. Just weeks before I discovered I was ill I dreamed:

> *I am being taken down to the basement of a building in a freight elevator by a "maniac." He holds a bloodstained executioner's ax with two notches on it, signifying he has already claimed two victims. I know that when we reach the bottom, he will add a third notch by chopping off my head.*

I believed at the time that this terrifying figure represented Death, some dream-variant on the Grim Reaper and his harvester's scythe. The notches had surely stood for my sister and my grandmother, his significant victims in my life, whom I feared—somewhat unreasonably, as it turned out—I might soon join on his final threshing floor.

I only realized years later that the deaths of my sister and grandmother had something very specific in common: Both had occurred in a hospital following a dubious "heroic" medical procedure. After experimental leukemia treatments had left her comatose, my sister was taken down to the hospital basement in a large elevator and didn't come back. We were told she had exhaled gently in the midst of a lung-function test and never taken another breath. A few years later, my grandmother succumbed in her hospital room to a blood clot, a few days after an operation to install a pacemaker in her frail, eighty-one-year-old body. Both procedures had seemed to me products of an almost mad hubris.

Hubris, I was later to learn, seems to be at the mythological root of Western "heroic medicine": After Asklepius, the physician-deity, had perfected the surgeon's art, he dared to use the Gorgon's blood given him by Athena to bring two dead men back to life, and was slain by Zeus. My sister's treatment had been more gleamingly high-tech. First she was placed in a humming, shielded radiation torus that killed off her bone marrow in what amounted to a personalized Hiroshima. Then she received an injection of my brother's inexactly matching but healthy marrow cells, but they failed to "take." In her last fluttering struggle for life, sealed in her germ-free laminar flow room, she had reminded me of a yellow monarch butterfly feebly beating its wings against a camphor jar.

This image, it goes without saying, was terribly unfair to the sincere ministrations of the hospital. The doctors and nurses who had so selflessly cared for her—indeed, had loved her—wept bitterly when she died. Nonetheless, I had from the start doubted the experiment; the manner in which it ended—as it had for each of the previous dozen subjects—seemed to me an obscenity. Such thoughts seemed a little less churlish when, a few years later, I happened on a newspaper article reporting the reprimand of one of my sister's enthusiastic young doctors for having on a previous occasion used an unauthorized experimental procedure on a human subject.

I was later to discover that, given the then-high mortality rates for bone marrow transplants, "there is heated dispute whether the hopelessness of the cases justifies this extreme intervention," as one book of the time put it. It is only now, fifteen years later, that bone marrow transplants have moved, as Dr. Peter H. Wiernik was recently quoted by *The New York Times*, "from the world of evangelical religion to the world of science. We are just now at the point where we can look people in the eye and say this is the treatment for your disease."[7]

But perhaps it just boils down to *You pays your money and you takes your chances*. You can't blame the doctor for failing to produce a medical miracle first crack out of the box. When the Reaper is at the door, isn't it prudent to shoot first and ask questions later, even if the gun is a blunderbuss that could blow up in your face?

My experience with my own disease has left me skeptical that the picture is usually that simple. Thyroid cancer in people of my age group has been shown to be almost invariably *caused* by medical hubris: As I was later to learn, back in the techno–Stone Age of the fifties, it was fashionable to irradiate infants born with large thymus glands, which were erroneously thought to lead to respiratory problems unless shrunken to "normal." Subsequent research has revealed that there is nothing dangerous about an "enlarged" thymus; on the contrary, the thymus, once dismissed as "vestigial," is now recognized as a factory for the maturation of the lymphocytes (a key immune system component that medical texts until recently labeled "a white blood cell with no known function").[8]

A certain percentage of these irradiated baby boomers—like the Marshall Islanders in the first H-bomb test range or the residents of Chernobyl—eventually wound up with papillary carcinoma of the thyroid. Such cancers have also shown up after overenthusiastic use of childhood chest, dental, and tonsil X-rays, similarly prescribed in the name of disease prevention. Because my early and persistent upper respiratory problems made me a frequent X-ray recipient, this may well have been one of the roots of my own disease.

Despite its triumphs, it sometimes appears that our medicine has become so credulous about technological quick-fixes, so inattentive to the cultural deformities that spawn both the human problems they treat and the weapons used to combat them, that it seems to function—like its oddly kindred institution, military defense—outside individual human purlieus, in an abstruse realm of strategies, statistics, and sometimes Pyrrhic victories.

In surgical jargon, to call a doctor "aggressive" is a compliment, even though, as the British medical journal *The Lancet* noted, "Aggressiveness is often a sign of desperation, and surgical aggression is no exception." It takes a Big Gun, the logic seems to go, to take out a Big Disease. When life is at stake, the doctor receives a virtual carte blanche to prosecute the battle. In this regard, Ivan Illich observes, "He who successfully claims power in an emergency suspends and can destroy rational evaluation. The insistence of the physician on his exclusive capacity to evaluate and solve individual crises moves him symbolically into the neighborhood of the White House."[9]

I have seen even the most confirmed, flag-burning iconoclast moved to pledge allegiance to medicine's business-as-usual when faced with what looks like the phalanxed armies of death. I once met a longtime Berkeley activist (call him Walker) who had undergone the same operation as I. When he was diagnosed with cancer, Walker, a founding member of the Free Speech Movement in the sixties and a self-professed anarchist, spent a year and a half trying to cure himself through diet, yoga, herbs, and meditation.

Finally, he told me, "I just got sick of everyone worrying about me, of the uncertainty and the constant conflicting advice. Anyway, I felt I'd 'learned' whatever I was going to learn from my disease." He packed it all in and showed up for surgery. Like me, he had become so convinced of the futility of his self-healing efforts that he hadn't even bothered to get a new sonogram to see if his condition might have changed. A short time after he came out of anesthesia, his doctor walked in and asked him with a certain amount of agitation, "What happened to your tumor?"

It turned out they had removed the gland only to discover that Walker's tumor had disappeared. His doctor's subsequent reassurance—"Your thyroid was still riddled with microscopic focci, so it was a good thing we got rid of it"—mollified him. But in fact, microscopic focci of thyroid cancer do not readily progress to life-threatening malignancy; indeed, they are present in a surprisingly high percentage of the population (in tens of millions of Americans, by some estimates) without causing measurable harm. Had Walker in effect healed himself without knowing it?

RITES OF PURIFICATION

Walker was nonetheless happy to be rid of his "contaminated" organ. I, too, had found the idea of somehow ridding my body of all trace of cancer to have a powerful appeal. The kind of totalizing language sometimes used by physicians can evoke in us the potent promise of bodily purity, a concept we might find absurd under less harrowing circumstances.

To have a disease is to feel unclean, contaminated, defective. For some patients, illness may be a confirmation of an underlying sense of unworthiness. When I found out I had cancer, it was as if a wrongness I had felt simmering inside me all my life suddenly came to a rolling boil. In such a state, it is all too easy to be swayed by an offer to surgically excise a "rotten" part of the self, or chemically cleanse a body that already cloisters shameful, unacceptable feelings. Our bodies and our sense of self are inextricable.

According to Dr. Mark Nichter, a physician and medical anthropologist, "People with diseases are trying to find themselves in reference to their body-state and the life-story it carries. A doctor should help them negotiate an 'illness-identity' that is not pejorative or moralistic. He is in a position to substitute more adaptive metaphors, to help patients experience disease in a way that leads to greater wholeness." Unfortunately, Dr. Nichter adds, "For many doctors, the patient's personal story is heard as subjective noise that obscures the objective signals used for diagnosis and treatment."[10]

But how objective is the signal, and how much diagnosis and treatment is shaped by personal (and cultural) "noise"? In the U.S., hysterectomy is still often performed (by largely male doctors) for fibroid tumors, even though less aggressive treatments like myemectomy have proved equally effective. Furthermore, according to the *Journal of Women's Health*, "Women who undergo hysterectomies for the removal of benign ovarian cysts experience five times the number of complications as women who have the same diagnosis but no hysterectomy." Though the operation's benefits are still unproved, hysterectomy has been the second most performed surgery in the U.S. after Cesarean section.

What can explain such a state of affairs? Leaving aside for a

moment issues of institutional politics, could the fact that an estimated one out of every five American women has suffered childhood sexual abuse, with its legacy of sexual shame and self-hatred,
be one reason women acquiesce to such radical procedures? From
the medical side, justifications like the following, by a Dr. Ralph C.
Wright, are less suggestive of science than gender prejudice: "After
the last planned pregnancy, the uterus becomes a useless, bleeding,
symptom-producing, potentially cancer-bearing organ and therefore should be removed." Although Wright's viewpoint is not widely
shared, it may be, terrible as it is to contemplate, that the attitudes
of a still largely male-dominated profession can have a hand in
shaping treatment strategies.

Nor are women the only recipients of questionable procedures.
"Surgery for prostate cancer in men has little or no benefit," read
a 1993 headline in *The Washington Post*. The article, based on findings
published in the *Journal of the American Medical Association* (*JAMA*),
noted that the practice has nonetheless increased nearly sixfold in
a mere six years. Dr. John Wasson, the report's coauthor and a
physician at Dartmouth Medical School, told a press conference:
"We're doing a lot in this country, yet it's unclear that we know what
we're doing."[11]

Dr. Ed Gilbert is a consummate insider-turned-outsider: Once he
served as a program director for the National Cancer Institute
(N.C.I.); a few months before our interview, he had been testifying
before Congress against the N.C.I.'s new breast-cancer drug trials—
which, he said, were being "ramrodded through" despite questions
of safety. "I've seen how decision-making happens behind the
scenes," he said tersely. "Dogmas get laid down and then become
massively perpetuated as 'standard treatment.' Once a treatment's
up and running, individual doctors can't do anything but recommend it, or risk a major lawsuit.

"It's one thing to talk about a disease like Hodgkins' lymphoma,
where ninety percent of the people used to die, and now ninety
percent can be cured. But what about diseases where only a few
percent are in danger? Or where treatment risks may not justify
benefits? Somehow in the mind of science it becomes imperative to
completely 'wipe out' a disease by treating everyone you can, because
no one, not one in a thousand, dare get sick outside your auspices."

Lynn Payer writes in her incisive work *Medicine and Culture*:

American medicine is aggressive. From birth—which is more
likely to be by Cesarean than anywhere in Europe—to death

in the hospital, from invasive examination to prophylactic surgery, American doctors want to *do* something, preferably as much as possible . . . They often eschew drug treatment in favor of more aggressive surgery, but if they do use drugs they are likely to use higher doses and more aggressive drugs. . . . Surgery, too, besides being performed more often, is likely to be more aggressive when it is performed.[12]

BEHIND MEDICINE'S FRONT LINES

Before my tumor was even diagnosed as cancerous, I timidly asked my doctor about a few clinicians I had heard about who recommended only taking suppressant doses of thyroid hormone instead of surgery.

"Pill doctors!" he snorted contemptuously. "They don't kow what they're talking about."

It was, I now realize, a rare glimpse into the medical palace intrigue between more and less aggressive approaches to illness, part of a competition for hierarchy and turf that has been brewing for centuries. In the 1600s, the physician was a rigorously educated humanist whose principal duty was to diagnose internal disease and prescribe internal remedies. Although he was legally qualified to perform surgery, he depended on lower-status professionals—surgeons and apothecaries—to carry out most physical treatment. But when the nineteenth-century inventions of antisepsis and anesthesia created the preconditions for heroic medicine, the hierarchy was reversed and the surgeon was elevated to princely stature.

In the near future, new biotechnologies and advances in preventive medicine (as well as a growing national sentiment for cost containment) may cause the pendulum once again to swing back toward less aggressive practice. But for the moment, the professionals who wield the most expensive and invasive tools receive the most influential fiefdoms. And though trends in health care reform could alter the picture, studies of nonsurgical or drugless remedies are rarely funded by the drug companies and third-party insurers who are the prime sources of needed research dollars.

Socioeconomic incentives may even affect what kind of person the patient will encounter on her healing path. A British medical student who spent time at Massachusetts General Hospital notes:

There seemed to be an overwhelming number of so-called "Type A" personalities around—and the only explanation I could offer for this was that American medicine selects and is being selected by a different type of student than in England. "Big" money and a position of enormous social and academic prestige are conferred on successful American doctors—perhaps it therefore attracts "business men" who react to it as they would to private enterprise.[13]

But beneath the structural scaffolding of "big medicine" is a foundation of philosophical beliefs that remain largely uninspected—by either those who live in the citadel or those who enter its gates. The worldview of a culture, its working models and metaphors, its ideologies of good and evil, tend to impinge on all aspects of its institutional and private life. How we conceive of a pathology, be it social or biological, determines what avenues we will take in our attempt to cure it.

During the signing of peace accords in the war-torn country of El Salvador a few years ago, an assistant U.S. secretary of state, Bernard W. Aronson, remarked, "If we had vigorously defended the democratic election there in 1972, perhaps we could have avoided the polarization that drove decent people to become guerrillas."[14] Tragically, the war against what President Reagan diagnosed as "the cancer south of the border" cost tens of thousands of lives and hundreds of millions of dollars—monies and lives that could well have healed the social ailments that caused the "disease" to break out in the first place.

Was El Salvador's ravaged body politic a problem for the internist/statesman or the surgeon/warrior? Which would have been more effective—building up the health of a democratic "immune system," or attacking the communist "disease" with an aggressive "medicine" that included excision by death squad? Like the civilian in a war zone, the patient in the medical arena is sometimes an unwitting victim of both policy decisions from on high and the crossfire on the ground.

In fairness, medical policymakers are faced with bedeviling tactical questions. As science philosopher Richard Grossinger points out:

> There are two different types of disease: those that occur from external forces, injuries, poisons, germs, malnutrition, etc.; and those that arise from the organism's being in battle with its own mind/body. . . . It is when that technology attempts to cure a

disorder of the second type as if it were a disease of the first category that it is overmatched and disruptive—for the forces which caused the disease will continue to erupt as long as they are untended and unresolved. It is not always possible to distinguish functionally between the two categories, and they overlap in any organism.[15]

In one of the dreams I described earlier, my tumor cells seemed to be symbolized by a group of grizzled old cowpokes brawling in a bar. A paddywagon pulled up, and they were herded, sheepish and blinking, off to the drunk-tank—but not before they were made to sign "forgiveness clauses" ceding back some property to its original owners.

I was puzzled by the mildness of this image. Were these woozy old-timers the marauding, demonic forces of cancer? As it would turn out, my disease was, in the words of one clinician, a "slow-pokey" borderline malignancy in which aggressive metastasis was relatively rare. The dream seemed to imply that my cells were more disorderly than murderous, senescent rather than malevolent; that having in a sense already outlived their time, they might be induced to give up their fleshy property.

This dream came to mind as I read a recent article describing a national trend in the U.S. penal system toward alternative forms of punishment. The article gave as an example three white adolescents who had vandalized an African-American church. As their sentence, they were required to stand before the congregation to ask forgiveness before being accepted back into the community. Despite their antisocial actions, the court decided to treat them not as evil criminals but as dysfunctional people who needed to be reabsorbed back into the body of society. The article quoted a New York federal judge: "Sentences for nonviolent criminals should help them get back on their feet, not knock them to the ground. What you want to do is work with the healthy part, so that the person isn't utterly destroyed."[16]

This unique legal remedy implies a different model of pathology and its treatment. Of course, our task here concerns deadly diseases, not petty criminals; real bodies, not the body politic. But Dr. Zieghelboim, for one, believes that a new scientific medicine will arise from a philosophical reconceptualization of the nature of disease itself—a medicine that regards cancer, for example, less as a demonic aggressor than as a case of "arrested development. Cancer cells are permanently immature. Because of this, they don't die off.

We may actually find drugs which will make cells mature and normalize their function. I also foresee that surgery, radiation, and chemotherapy may become archaic in the near future. We won't be using them, or we'll be using them much less. . . . Psychospiritual and psychosocial points of view will play greater roles. We'll see movement away from the aggressive therapies towards less militaristic immunological approaches."

MAKING PEACE WITH THE BODYMIND

Whether in the realm of international affairs or interpersonal relations, of psychological or medical treatment, polarized, unyielding propositions of good and evil often are not conducive to long-term wellness and vitality. Plato declared that the doctor "ought to be able to bring about love and reconciliation between the most antithetic elements in the body."[17] In almost identical language, psychologist Alfred Ribi writes that the psyche "integrates a complex by including it in the framework of the personality in such a way that it is no longer antithetical."[18] These two comments suggest a possible theoretical meeting ground between the often competing logic of mind healing and body medicine.

Indeed, older medical systems insisted that the laws of the psyche were, broadly speaking, the same ones that ruled the body. As the early Arabic physician Ali Pul expressed it, "The medicine of the body is the image of the medicine of the soul."

Today, diseases and cures in which the mind is suspected to play an indeterminate but significant role may be bringing the "soft" practice of psychology and the "hard" one of medical science closer together. Holistic medicine, with its openness to the mind-body model and its use of biofeedback, hypnosis, diet, and life-style counseling, has been deemed particularly suitable for a variety of chronic ailments: skin disease, allergy, warts, chronic pain, angina pectoris, atopic eczema, migraine, and asthma. By and large, an invisible class system is enforced in medicine, whereby diseases diagnosed as "psychosomatic" are exiled to the outlying "alternative" provinces, while the Killer Diseases—objective, isolable, quantifiable, presumably wholly material—are attended to in the glittering capitals, the great institutions built on government research grants, biotechnology investment, and insurance industry support.

But the territory claimed by mind-body medicine has been steadily (and, for those who believe in a strictly materialistic explanation of the body, disconcertingly) expanding. Theorists like cardiologist Dr. Herbert Benson, author of *The Relaxation Response*, have already suggested that "75 percent of the illnesses that bring patients into the doctors' offices are in the mind-body category." Similarly, Dr. Deepak Chopra maintained in a recent interview that "maybe ninety percent of procedures that are now done, and of drugs that are now used, will become obsolete. Most illness will be treated by changing the way people behave, or think, or eat, or live their lives. For the remaining ten percent or twenty percent, we will have much more effective technology."

To explore such questions—and to give patients access to some of the putative answers—departments of "behavioral medicine" in major hospitals have become outposts for "biopsychosocial medicine" and have begun, through what Dr. Benson described to me as a "Trojan horse strategy," to subtly export the mind-body approach to adjacent bailiwicks. Biologist and Buddhist meditator Jon Kabat-Zinn has guided over five thousand patients through a stress-reduction program, based on contemplative practices, that focuses in part on the participants' achievement of spiritual wholeness.

I once had occasion to watch Dr. Kabat-Zinn work with a group of chronic pain patients at the University of Massachusetts Medical School. One hand stuck in the pocket of his chinos, the other emphasizing his points, he genially exhorted his group on the need to "develop transparency to the things that drive you up a wall."

His patients, some sitting on molded plastic chairs, others on Japanese meditation cushions colored powder-blue, daffodil, and strawberry, listened avidly. One back-injury patient in a Chicago Bears shirt, his belly spilling from his jeans, his grizzled brushcut upswept in a pompadour, raised an arm etched with a tattoo of a dripping faucet to ask for advice on "how to stay centered."

"Put out a welcome mat for the pain," counsels Kabat-Zinn. "Don't tense against it, don't resist it. You're developing inroads into your own body. Establish a beachhead, a perimeter, in the place of the pain. Befriend it. Work constantly at your limits. There's nothing a human being does that you can't bring awareness to."

He writes "centered" in large block letters on the blackboard. Only his folksy manner keeps his talk on meditation from becoming a caricatured homily on the Wisdom of the East. He tings two small Tibetan bells together, and their silvery, wavering chime oscillates almost visibly in the air. "Live in the moment. What else is there to do? Why go through your life half-awake? The only time you've got is right now."

Later, after the patients slowly filter out, trailing an aroma of sandalwood incense down the neon-flooded institutional hallways, Kabat-Zinn tells me, "We are mobilizing our inner resources for coming to peace with ourselves. We're not magically trying to meditate our tumor away. I tell my patients the point is to be as true to themselves as possible. To authenticate their own experience."

Dr. Kabat-Zinn also cautions against approaches that "exploit psychoneuroimmunology more than the evidence warrants. How is someone supposed to face AIDS or death," he demands with an uncharacteristic flash of irritation, "when they're hearing irresponsible promises and wishful thinking? That's *horse*shit!"

Indeed, the mind-body approach can open the door to a good deal of seductive quackery, and worse. I was surprised a few years ago to read that a well-known doctor I had once met, a wry, fatherly man who ran a high-profile holistic education center and a cancer counseling clinic, had been forced to surrender his medical license for sexually abusing his patients. He had apparently told one woman that sexual relations with him—including a procedure he dubbed "vaginal Rolfing"—were required to cure her cancer. Another woman, herself a professional health care worker, described the premise of her similarly sexualized "treatment" to newspaper reporters: "He said cancer was about fear, and that if I ran away from him, I was running away from my own fear. The implication was that if I left, the cancer might come back."

THE MAGIC BULLET

Such egregious cases seem to be the exception. But the relevance of soul-work to body-medicine remains a controversial line of inquiry. Psychoneuroimmunology (PNI) and associated research, at least for doctors who take time to ponder its implications, have added an imprecise and unpredictable X-factor to the medical equation: As long as the mind rolls through the body like a loose cannon on the quarterdeck, how can we demarcate between purely physical and purely mental disease—or between "pure" scientific treatment and the effects of attitude, imagination, and emotion? One part of the puzzle is that some diseases seem to hopscotch back and forth, one minute psychological complexes in the purview of the mind-workers, the next minute adamantly physical. Consider the case of obsessive compulsive disorder (OCD), a psychiatric syndrome that causes sufferers to, for example, spend sixteen hours a day ritualistically washing their hands in order to eliminate all possible traces of "germs." The disease was originally diagnosed as purely psychological, an expression of hidden guilt, unexpressed aggression, or forbidden desire, a logical candidate for the psychoanalyst's couch. But standard psychotherapy relieved few patients of their symptoms.

Then PET (positron emission tomography) scans revealed that OCD sufferers had curious abnormalities in the brain's basal ganglia, as well as an abnormal flow of neurotransmitters like dopamine, serotonin, and noradrenaline. To top off the evidence for a physical disease-basis, a drug, Clomipramine, has been shown to cure many OCD patients of their symptoms, as have Anafranil and the antidepressant Prozac. The seeming proof that OCD was a result of faulty biology showed, in the words of one research psychiatrist, that "these people are not kooky,"[19] no small boon in a society that often judges people for their existential conditions.

Nevertheless, although OCD has been found to be a condition *associated* with biological anomaly, it cannot as yet be *reduced* to it. One reason is the parallel success of a form of psychotherapy based on behavior modification. The technique consists of forcing OCD patients to face an obsessive fear of, say, germ contamination by making them wear the same dirty clothes for five days. Unsettling to the "pure biology" thesis, this form of therapy—in effect, an artificially induced emotional crisis—has proven roughly as effective as drugs.[20]

What is going on here? From the perspective of institutionalized medicine, either OCD can be cured psychologically, showing its origins must be in the mind, or it can be cured physically, thus proving its cause is biological.

A breakthrough answer did not come until the spring of 1993, when researchers at UCLA discovered, using PET scans, that the brains of patients cured by behavioral therapy exhibited the same kind of physical changes as those treated by drugs. As one article stated, for the first time it had been unequivocally proven that "words can be just as powerful as drugs in correcting errant brain pathways." Said UCLA psychiatrist Lewis Baxter, "Any time you have a change in behavior, you have a change in the brain."[21] He might have added that we may also have the beginning of a new branch of science, one which might properly be called the biology of meaning.

Dr. James Gordon of the NIH's Panel on Mind-Body Interventions recalls the moment he first glimpsed common ground between mind and body healing. Suffering from a painful back injury that had finally driven him to the odd prescriptions of an alternative healer, he had reached a point where his symptoms seemed to be taking an excruciating turn for the worse. The healer, undismayed, suggested that he was undergoing a "healing crisis."

"All of a sudden," says Dr. Gordon, "this light went on. As a psychiatrist I learned that you have to work through resistance and defenses to get to a crisis. It's at that point that the complex, the stuckness, can begin to move. The light that went on was not only hope for my own condition, but joy that the principles of emotional healing might also apply to healing the body. The common thread they shared was the need for *transformation*."

Crisis is transformation's crucible. As some theorists, notably psychobiologist Ernest Rossi, have long claimed, emotional crisis itself may cause lasting physical alterations in the brain. In the case of OCD, for example, a deliberately induced crisis—the forced "contamination" with germ-laden clothing—also changed a pattern of neural connections.

The brain/mind already has been proven capable of delivering its own powerful drug therapy from its "medicine cabinet." The author of a recent medical journal article marveled that "the average effectiveness of a placebo accounts for over half of what can be accomplished by even a potent agent like morphine." On the basis of a variety of studies, Dr. Rossi suggests, "there may be a fifty-five percent placebo response in many, if not all, healing procedures."[22]

The placebo is one of the benchmark concepts of mind-body medicine, a by-now well-marked intersection between psyche and soma. But what exactly do we *mean* by the term? Is it enough to say, as I heard the host of a radio call-in show remark somewhat dismissively, "A placebo is when a person gets better only because he thinks he's going to get better"? Why *only*?

A recent study of pain reduction accomplished by using only sugar pills[23] concluded that "the placebo effect is based on the release of endorphins." But mind-body proponents shot back a challenging question: Wouldn't it be as accurate to say that the "endorphin effect" is based on the "release of *expectations*?"[24] Why, they were asking, do we assume that events in the mind—and the diseases and cures to which they may contribute—are somehow less medically "real" than those in the body? Why are we so reluctant to acknowledge the *physical* therapeutic power of the biology of meaning?

Dr. Adan Rios musingly recounted to me the story of a cancer patient and friend who, after undergoing radical neck surgery and radiotherapy treatment, developed multiple lesions of malignant melanoma. Rios started treating him with an experimental protocol: "It was a product which has since proven to be ineffective in treating cancer, yet he went into a complete remission! I struggled for months trying to figure it out, and have yet to come up with an answer, except that he is still alive and doing well. I am convinced the drug didn't do it. So what did? I just cannot help wondering what unraveled inside this man, and whether we will ever learn to reproduce it."

Dr. Rose Papac, an oncologist at the Yale University School of Medicine, described a similar rare case to me. A man in the terminal phases of acute myelogenous leukemia, my sister's disease, had been treated with a standard but rarely effective drug. Compounding the unlikelihood of a cure, Dr. Papac told me, was the fact that the dosage order had been incorrectly written, so that the man received "what might as well have been a homeopathic dose, one-quarter of normal, too low to possibly have any effect."[25] Nonetheless, the man had, according to her report, "developed a complete hematological and clinical remission, and this has now been sustained for twenty-two years."[26]

Could cures such as these be the product of the unpredictable healing powers of the bodymind? If so, we are forced to ask an even more difficult question: To what extent might the so-called "placebo effect" be a factor in the success of even *proven* treatments? How much "real" medicine owes a still unknown portion of its curative power to mind-body factors?

Jeanne Achterberg inserts herself as a radical gadfly in this still-marginal but highly significant debate. She writes challengingly in her book *Imagery in Healing: Shamanism and Modern Medicine:*

> Apparently, anything can work if you believe in it enough, including wheat grass, Navaho sand paintings, healing waters, and chemotherapy. . . . There is no logical reason to believe that the people who recover after having major poisons assault their systems, such as in chemotherapy, are not also instances of spontaneous remission; they, too, can be regarded as having gotten well because of their attitude and in spite of treatment.[27]

Few in the mind-body field would go so far out on a theoretical limb. But the work of Dr. Dean Ornish and others has shown that even "big diseases" like heart disease must now be considered bio-psychosocial conditions amenable to mind-body treatment. It is becoming increasingly difficult to dispute doctor-theorists like Larry

Dossey, who, along with James Gordon and Jeanne Achterberg, chaired the 1993 N.I.H. Panel on Mind-Body Interventions, part of the recently formed office of Alternative Medicine. Dr. Dossey exclaimed at a recent lecture, "We are talking about mind-body techniques that impact life-and-death issues, but the scientific literature is still virtually unknown even to specialists in the field! How much more evidence do we need before we admit that so-called 'psychosomatic medicine' should no longer be limited to the domain of tension headaches?"

Some might argue that the question may soon be entirely moot. With stunning breakthroughs being reported almost daily in genetic mapping, with laser surgery, real-time body scans, and organ transplants (and someday, perhaps, even organ cloning), we are witnessing an incandescent moment, an apogee, in the history of pure physical medicine. When cures for currently intractable diseases are discovered—soon, surely, given the lightning pace of gene research—won't all the stargazing claptrap about "healing journeys," attitude-change, and "mind-body consciousness" become, like the colorful shields of the Plains Indian ghost dancers or chunks of the Berlin Wall, mere historical curios, their function superseded by progress?

From the perspective of the new mind-body healers, the answer is clear: Any treatment that dismisses feeling and fantasy, that fails to honor the quest for meaning, that disdains the intelligence of the body, cannot make the patient whole. Even when it comes to the newest classes of genetically engineered magic bullets, some suggest that the effects of consciousness cannot be ruled out. Ernest Rossi, a member of an informal movable feast-cum-roundtable of international mind-body pioneers, told me,

> We still haven't learned the lesson from endorphins. Remember, everyone went, "Aha!" at last we've got the ultimate silver bullet, and it's going to solve the pain problem of mankind, because the endorphins are neurotransmitters specific for pain. The drug companies spent millions and millions of dollars just nailing down the patents, but it hasn't panned out. For one thing, endorphins often have terrible side effects. And their potency for pain reduction is kind of weak.
>
>   Why? My speculation is it's because *endorphins are specific to the mind-body interaction.* Maybe they don't even work in a purely molecular way. The drug companies may waste billions more,

trying to hang on to the old mechanistic model. This approach *will* yield results with substances like insulin, a more purely physical process modulated by stress. But I think it may always fall short when the molecule you're trying to synthesize has any link with the limbic/hypothalamic area of the brain. *There* you're inevitably dealing with the mind, emotion, and learning.

Similarly, endocrinologist Deepak Chopra notes that treatments using "magic bullets," synthesized versions of natural immune system anticancer agents called interleukins, have been successful with only 5 to 10 percent of patients. Chopra maintains that this is because science has yet adequately to explore "the whole issue of how intelligence and matter are paired":

> If interleukins "know" when and where to fight cancer, then it is not their molecules that should interest us, but something invisible—the cell's ability to recognize that a cancerous [genetic cell-] memory is present and needs to be eradicated. This cannot be injected into the body. The body's war against cancer pits intelligence against intelligence. . . .
>
> When our emotions join up with molecules, like riders on a horse, the mounts they choose are almost identical to interleukin. For all intents and purposes, to feel happy and to fight cancer are much the same thing at the molecular level. We could call both of them healing messages.
>
> We desperately need a medicine without bullets.[28]

SOLVING THE ALGORITHM

Jungian analyst James Hillman once proposed that if Asklepius is the god of healers, then Hermaphroditus must be the archetype of the *process* of healing. Hermaphroditus is a symbol of nonduality, of gathering into the same sphere "oppositions between conscious and unconscious, masculine and feminine, positive and negative, private soul and public world."[29] Hillman might have added oppositions of physical and psychological, body and mind, material and spiritual, all ancient conundrums medicine must now struggle to resolve.

When I was trying to decide on a direction for my own treatment, I went with my daughter to a movie in which a child was called upon to solve a complex mathematical logarithm. That night, I had a dream in which I was being "forced to solve the *algorithm*." I awoke puzzled. I vaguely recalled that *loga*rithms had something to do with "powers of ten." But what was an *algo*rithm?

Looking the term up, I discovered that it describes a mathematical procedure involving "direct manipulation of figures without regard for the underlying principles of the operation." The dictionary gave as examples division and subtraction. My first thought was that the algorithm symbolized *my* operation, the surgery proposing to divide me and subtract something from my body, certainly a "math problem" I had to solve.

But it also struck me that "to solve the algorithm" was, at least in mathematical terms, a meaningless statement. If an algorithm is a rule of computation, a *method* of problem-solving, then "to solve the algorithm" meant little unless the methodology itself was the problem.

I had left the dream aside until a few years ago when a doctor friend happened to mention that algorithms are fundamental tools in the practice of modern medicine. Doctors are taught from first-year med school on to use algorithms to determine, through a series of choices based on Aristotelian logic, the correct diagnosis and treatment of a patient's symptoms.

Later, I had occasion to mention my dream to Dr. Dean Ornish. He smiled, then explained with some passion, "So much of medicine has evolved—or *de*volved, depending on your point of view!—into algorithms: step one, step two, step three." In a fast, singsong litany, he recited an example to me: "Do they have chest pain? Yes? No? If yes, what do EKG findings show? ST depression, yes, no? If less than one millimeter do this, if greater, do that. Go to thallium lab. Thallium lab shows reverse profusion defect? If yes, go to Cath Lab . . ." He trailed off with a curt laugh. "Algorithms show how uncreative medical training really is."

Dr. Larry Dossey writes, "The most elaborate treatment algorithms—the flow diagrams in medical textbooks that show the next step in the treatment of an illness—never contain a box that says 'LOVE!' or 'CARE!' And that is why the algorithms fail, although they appear to be foolproof and take every eventuality into consideration."[30]

Algorithms may fail for another reason: They exclude the wild card of consciousness from their calculations. I was intrigued to learn that although some cybernetic theorists believe software algorithms may yet be designed that would enable computers to become truly "conscious," others, like the Oxford mathematician Roger Penrose (*The Emperor's New Mind*), believe that such logic has

THE HEALING PATH

a fatal flaw: The human mind, unlike a computer, has a unique
property: what Penrose calls the "strange and wonderful feature"
of being able to perform operations that are *not based on algorithms*
at all.[31]

To some extent, consciousness itself is the "underlying principle
of the operation," the intervening variable at home equally under
the rubric of "PNI," or "soul," or a "biology of meaning." Minus
this understanding, conventional medicine can be sometimes inadequate for or even hazardous to the task of promoting wholeness.
Many patients found at some point on their path that they could
no longer passively depend on big guns and magic bullets to prosecute the struggle for health on their behalf. They could not find
sufficient shelter in the impressively buttressed citadel of medicine,
but had to search for healing in the many mansions of the self.

9

TAKING BACK CONTROL: FINDING NEW FOOTING

*None will improve your lot
If you yourselves do not.*

—BERTOLT BRECHT

IF WE ARE to walk the path of healing, we must first gain some measure of control over our direction. But illness is a fundamental *loss* of control, a form of possession by bodily forces we cannot contain, and by social forces—doctors, hospitals, even family and well-meaning friends—that threaten to contain *us*. Gears whose existence we never suspected whir into motion, oiled by decades of cultural consensus. Suddenly, ordinary coping mechanisms are rendered null and void, our identity is subsumed under the badge "patient." We are dispossessed of ourselves.

Too often, as patients we are deemed not only medically naive but non compos mentis—too emotionally involved in our own case to be trusted with decision-making. Weakened by illness, fear, and uncertainty, patients are immediately placed under strong pressure to conform to a variety of imposed schemas. Great resources—respected specialists, crisp-uniformed nurses, sophisticated equipment—are typically marshaled on the sufferer's behalf. Most patients do not wish to appear ungrateful, to disappoint the clinicians and relatives now busying themselves in preparation, to risk refusing, while it is still being offered, a last best chance for rescue.

Officially, medical authorities urge patients to seek second opinions and to research other treatment options. But in reality, writes Michael Lerner, director of Commonweal, a cancer retreat center in Bolinas, California, "patients are often rushed into treatment immediately following diagnosis. . . . The presumption, sometimes made explicitly, is that any delay will have grave consequences. . . . This compromises the therapeutically valuable feeling of patients that they have made an informed personal choice after consultation with their physician and others, and that therefore they have some real control."

One patient, a college professor who always prided herself on her forcefulness and mastery of logical thinking, told me how she quickly found herself reduced to a helpless observer of her own fate after her diagnosis of thyroid cancer:

> Things happened so fast. Biopsies, blood tests, second opinions, and suddenly I found myself lying in stiff hospital sheets, with bars on either side of the bed, waiting for surgery. I wasn't quite sure why I was there. The doctors were making decisions about me based on information I wasn't allowed to have. Who knows what they were deciding, or how accurate their information was? When I asked to see the doctor, the nurse told me she could answer all my questions, and that a consultation with the doc would cost another three hundred dollars. I thought about just throwing on my clothes and running out. But I figured they knew better than I did, so I stayed.

Patients on the healing path have a double burden: They face the challenge of affirming their own individuality precisely at a time when everything—their disease, their clinicians, the world at large—seems intent upon eroding it. Shortly after my first meeting with my doctor, I had a dream that in retrospect spoke volumes about the task of self-empowerment:

> *I am trying to escape on a child's sled from a man with a rifle that does not have an accurate gunsight. I yell over my shoulder at him, "I guess one size doesn't fit all!" Then I see some Indians who are angry because someone has stolen their "power bundle."*

The sled in this dream was a Flexible Flyer, an icon of suburban childhoods in the fifties, prized for its nimble steering. I loved the feeling of freedom it gave me as I whizzed down hills, master of my destiny. It had been a Christmas gift, and I regarded it as supernatural transport, a varnished and gleaming wooden talisman. A "power bundle," too, is a fetish: I was later to read that shamans in many Native American cultures carry "medicine bundles" which contain artifacts representing the supernatural protectors they have encountered in their dreams. Such objects hold their owners' unique psychic history and talents, acting as guardians of authentic being. Both the "power bundle" and the "flexible" sled symbolized the opposite of the one-size-fits-all approach of most modern medicine, with its invariant protocols, "acceptable" side effects, and normative definitions of health and illness.

Many other images of the theft of something unique and precious appeared in my dreams of this period. In one, a barber—the surgeon's medieval predecessor—was chopping off my sister's cascading blonde hair, trademark waist-length tresses that had taken her half her life to grow. In another nightmare, "hoodlums" were stealing my antique baby carriage. (The dictionary says the term *hoodlum* originally referred to toughs hired to beat up Chinese immigrants—intriguing in light of the fact that I was then considering the "immigrant" Chinese tradition of acupuncture.) Months later, medical treatment did finally "steal" a biological heirloom, one that could well be said to be the "power bundle" of my body. But even before that, it had subtly made off with my power to determine my own course of healing.

THE SURRENDER OF CONTROL

When we first enter the physician's domain, he seems to be in a position to know us better than we know ourselves. He reaches in through the open spaces in our bodies, or makes openings where there are none; probes us with shining metal; plumbs our inmost secrets with occultly precise instrumentation. And because the doctor promises that in exchange we will receive succor, deliverance from pain and fear and infirmity, we willingly comply.

Disease is the one occasion in life when, as one doctor put it, "You willingly hand over your most precious possession, your body, to the control of someone you may scarcely know." It occurred to me only after my operation that my doctors could scarcely have had a clue who I really was. I had spoken briefly with an endocrinologist and seen my surgeon for twenty minutes. My hopes, fears, dreams, loves—anything that made me other than an anonymous customer at the service counter of a smooth-running franchise—were not on the charts. Beyond sonograms, X-rays, blood tests, and a cursory medical history, I was simply another faceless candidate for a routine protocol.

But with the same naïveté that leads a child to believe his parents to be omniscient, I irrationally felt that my doctors *knew* me, and could wisely divine what was best. Awash in illness's moony tidepools, I imagined they would titrate the elixir of wholeness, and so relinquished myself. Jungian analyst James Hillman observes that illness is a state of "momentarily abject helplessness. In this condition one too easily hears the collective voice in oneself that does not understand or believe, and so turns the matter of oneself over with suicidal relief to the professional."[1]

We are, after all, under doctors' care from the moment we are born. We are trained as children to be "good" patients, to accept treatment that may seem to us bizarre, painful, or humiliating. I am old enough to have had a pediatrician who made house calls, who would materialize in my sickroom like a doting, seldom-visiting uncle with his black bag and red lollipops. I can remember how proud I was that I coughed so well on command; that I didn't gag on his tongue depressor, flinch when he kneaded my aching abdomen, cry at his hypodermic, or betray any fear when he took me for a ride on a wheeled gurney down a long hall into the room where he would pluck out my tonsils.

Now, facing another throat operation, I wanted to be reasonable, even complaisant toward those who held my fate in their hands. It is ordinarily difficult enough to find the courage to, in Walt Whitman's words, "Resist what insults your own soul." It is all the more so when the price of intransigence seemingly could be life itself. This paradigm is nowhere more implicitly enforced than in the hospital. In my mind (consciously at least, for my dreams dissented nightly), it was a place of anchorage and enclosure, of access to the highest powers of healing. Like that Greek proto-hospital, the Asklepian dream-temple, where ailing pilgrims threw themselves on the mercies of the Divine, it was the place to go when ordinary methods had failed—the focus of a simple hope (that I would be made well) and an equally simple fear (that I would not). For the hospital is an institution like no other: It is our birthing ground, our first nursery, and the likely place we will go to die. It is at once hard-nosed business and mission of mercy; laboratory, school, secular temple, house of quarantine.

Lifted out of ordinary life, patients float through a neon-lit limbo in white gowns (like angels, like spirits of the dead), garments slit up the back to enable easy access to their bodies. They are shepherded on a disorienting journey that oddly mimes the shamanic descent into the underworld—an (anesthesia-induced) near-death experience, a ritual dismemberment, and a return, transfigured, to the world of the living. They become, in effect, what the anthropologist of tribal life Victor Turner calls "liminal entities":

> Liminal entities, such as neophytes in initiation or puberty rites, may . . . wear only a strip of clothing, or even go naked, to demonstrate that as liminal beings they have no status, property, insignia, secular clothing indicating rank or role or position. . . . Their behavior is normally passive or humble; they must obey their instructors implicitly, and accept arbitrary punishment without complaint. . . . It is as though they are being reduced or ground down to a uniform condition to be fashioned anew and endowed with additional powers. . . . Among themselves, neophytes tend to develop an intense comradeship and egalitarianism. Secular distinctions of rank and status disappear or are homogenized . . . in a symbolic milieu that represents both a grave and a womb.[2]

In tribal societies, this loss of control and ordinary identity was a prelude—indeed, a catalyst—for psychophysical transformation. But for the hospital patient, who also surrenders to a portentous rite of passage, suspended between a familiar self and one yet unknown, the soul-making dimensions of the journey remain unacknowledged. The journeyer passes before the doctors like an auto chassis before an assembly-line riveter. Each day, I was told by way of reassurance, my surgeon performed the momentous act of removing the thyroid glands of two people he had barely met.

The rituals of official medicine are slowly changing, driven by both new science and a new generation of doctors. Increasing numbers of hospitals teach patients relaxation, biofeedback, meditation, even humor: Now that it is surmised that laughter can increase secretions of pain-reducing endorphins, such institutions as Atlanta's DeKalb Hospital train personnel to don Groucho Marx funny noses, deliver shtick, and trundle "laugh wagons" bearing comedy videos down the halls. However superficial some of these attempts to humanize the hospital may seem, it is not far-fetched to imagine that the slow triumph of a more thoroughgoing medical *perestroika* will put the human being back at the center of the healing drama. But for now, treatment of the whole person remains an anomaly, existing side by side with techniques that may weaken natural mind-body healing mechanisms or even violate the Hippocratic maxim, "First, do no harm."

From patients' points of view, modern medicine may represent an invasion not just of the body but of the renascent sense of self, of the long-neglected interiority they are struggling to reclaim. The predominant style of medicine too often runs counter to the patients' own healing requirements: They need to develop autonomy, but are instead infantalized, kept in the dark; they need to actively affirm their uniqueness, but are reduced to passive recipients of normative "protocols"; they need time, but are rushed onto a virtual conveyer belt; they need to build up their immune system, but are given therapies that may debilitate it; they may crave life's messy vitality, but are instead sequestered in a sterile ward; they need a hopeful vision of the future, and are instead provided with often pessimistic ("realistic") prognoses; they may need to reacquaint themselves with their bodies (particularly the diseased parts, where emotional issues may be "somaticized"), but instead receive drugs that block function and sensation, or surgeries which may remove these parts altogether.

Upon being diagnosed, lymphoma patient Arline Erdrich had to struggle with a sudden and shocking loss of autonomy:

> The medical people told me this was what had to be done, they knew exactly what they were doing, and if I didn't cooperate I would certainly die. I was just swept along.
>
> First they gave me a laparotomy, where they open you from under your breastbone all the way down the pelvic area. Then they take biopsies of all your organs: A little slice of your liver, a little slice of your kidney. They even stick little tags in there, like your body's a delicatessen display case.
>
> One time, a doctor felt around in my neck and insisted I had cancerous nodes. I asked him how he could tell without a biopsy.
>
> He told me, "I can tell just by the way they move around."
>
> So I let him put me under general anesthesia, I let him take them out, and then it turns out the nodes were normal, benign! Another time, they took one out on the wrong side of my body!
>
> I began to feel like a slab of meat. I was infuriated. I did a cartoon of a woman with a doctor sticking his hand in through her back and the hand coming out of her mouth, with the caption, "We're going to keep doing it until we get it right." The sketch, my little revolt, circulated through the hospital, and believe me, there were reverberations.

Arline showed me an assortment of other drawings she made during her stay in the hospital: A woman in a negligee under a robotlike machine that brandishes a multitude of probing tentacles.

A woman behind an X-ray screen, her body sectioned off by dotted lines into portions labeled "prime" and "choice."

"When I say to people I used to be a very shy person, they say, 'Who are you kidding?' But I was. I was *forced* to find my power. I started to find my real voice in that place, and that voice has made me healthy."

CONTROL AND HEALING

Arline's belief that she owes her life in part to her gradual assertion of control may have some basis in science. In one experiment, tumors implanted in rats given some measure of control over random shocks grew more slowly than those of their helpless fellow lab animals. In another study, healthy rats were placed in cages wired to deliver electric shocks. One cage was designed so that the shocks could be modulated if the rat pushed a lever, while the second was rigged so the shocks were uncontrollable. Researchers discovered that the immune system of the rat with the control-lever was only slightly impaired, while that of the rat which had no control rapidly became extremely suppressed. In a human study suggestive of a similar principle, terminal breast cancer patients who had received behavioral therapy that included self-assertion exercises and "autonomy training" lived longer than patients who had only undergone chemotherapy.[3]

Other studies have shown that uncooperative patients, those who refuse to fit obligingly into their medical slot, often have the highest survival rates. It has been suggested that such an "empowering" attitude may somehow stimulate the immune system, giving the patient fighting strength, enhancing the will to triumph. Whatever the mechanism at work, a UCLA study revealed that longer-term AIDS survivors shared a number of common characteristics: a refusal to accept the fatality of their diagnosis (this has been referred to as "positive denial"); a stubborn, even ornery insistence on not following doctors' orders until they could make sense of them; and the direct expression of emotions like anger. Similar results have been noted with longer-surviving cancer patients, who displayed traits like "poorer adjustment to the illness" and "poorer attitude toward the physician." These findings tallied with my impressions of many of the patients I interviewed.

We must wonder if this feistiness might not also be a stage in the healing of the "disease-prone personality," the abreaction process Alice Miller describes as "reliving earlier traumas with intense feelings of anger, rage, impotence, despair, helplessness, and—eventually—grief." Surprisingly, many patients whose life history would seemingly have primed them for passive submission told me that their illness had liberated them to stand up for themselves when everything around them seemed to call for acquiescence.

REGAINING AUTONOMY

When, in the course of a single office visit, Samantha Coles's doctor told her that she had malignant melanoma, that it was "very likely" she would be dead in six months, and that she would have to check into the hospital immediately to be prepped for surgery the next morning, she balked.

> I'd always been this person who looked rebellious, but underneath believed I should do as I'm told because everybody knew better than me, and whatever I was feeling or thinking had to be wrong. But as much of a mess as I was, especially by this point, I amazed myself by telling the doctor, "No, I *won't*." I think it was the first time in my *life* I really stood up for myself. I said, "I'll see you in the morning," and then spent the night out on the beach with a bottle, looking up at the stars.

Samantha thinks of her tiny act of rebellion as the first step on an idiosyncratic course that led not only to her healing, but to an overturning of ingrained, lifelong psychological patterns. She is an example of the paradox that Jungian analyst Elida Evans puzzledly observed in more than one hundred cancer patients she studied in the early part of this century. Although they were typically emotionally damaged as children (as was Samantha, an incest victim) and prone to seek outer approval to compensate for inward self-contempt, Evans was surprised to note that her patients had found in the midst of illness a source of stubborn, resistant self-affirmation.[4]

Examining these patients' life histories further, Evans found that they had often displayed an unusually "strong individuality" in their youth which had either been suppressed or become dormant. "When I was a kid," says former arthritis patient Joy Ballas-Beeson, "I was very stubborn and independent. Mom once told me, 'You weren't nasty. You'd listen politely to what I said, and then just go do what you wanted anyway.' But I lost that as I grew up, particularly during my marriage." The crisis of health somehow allowed these lost strengths to be retrieved. One former patient told me: "I got back in touch with that part of me I'd given up, the part that doesn't care what anyone else says. I knew I'd always had it, but I'd kind of thrown it away. Cancer was the signpost that told me I'd been living ass-backwards. It made me start to find my own way again."

A normally equable Colorado postman's prickly attitude during treatment became a matter of pride to him. "I told my oncologist straight out," John Geuther said, " 'It's my body, I'm in charge, I'm a powerful person, I just want your expertise.' " Coming in for a second test after the first had revealed the elevated white cell counts of chronic myelogenous leukemia, Geuther says, "The first thing I told them when I walked in for my bone marrow test was, 'I want another blood test *first.* If the counts have gone down, I'm not doing this.' They were taken aback, because they had a courier waiting to go down to Denver with the spinal fluid. When it turned out they *would* have to do the test, I told the doctor, 'I've got strong legs, and if you hurt, I will kick.' "

John's behavior has a childish ring to it, perhaps reflecting Evans's observation that her patients' long-forsaken individuality did not always reemerge intact. The resurgence of lost selfhood, Evans noted, could sometimes be rigid and "unyielding," lacking in what she referred to as the "plurality of personalities" that characterizes well-integrated adulthood.

In that light, lawyer John Studholme's plaintive comments about his doctors—"They didn't listen well; they didn't seem to be with me, but always thinking about their next patient; they made me feel I was keeping them from more important things"—might be heard, at least in part, as an echo of the unmet childhood needs for mirroring and respect common in the "disease-prone personality." If many patients' self-assertion had a raw, reflexive quality, perhaps it was in the service of a cry for identity. Patients often felt they were being pitted against powerful forces which were, in effect, trying to shove things down their throats at the very moment something long-silenced within them was trying to give voice.

One afternoon during my odyssey, I was visiting a friend who received a midday call from the vice principal of the local grade school. "It's about your son," he was told. "He has a serious behavior problem. He just hit another boy for no good reason." Apparently, a child had tried to shove a piece of dessert into Fred's son's mouth during lunch, and his son had reacted by smashing the kid in the face.

"Put my son on the phone," Fred said sternly. I waited for him to light into his son for overreacting to some innocent lunchroom horseplay. Instead I heard him tell his boy tenderly, firmly, "It's okay. You don't ever, *ever* have to let anyone put anything in your mouth that you don't *want* in there." I was moved nearly to tears, struck by how rarely we receive this message as children, let alone as patients. The health professions, notes social critic Ivan Illich, too often "destroy the potential of people to deal with their human weakness, vulnerability, and uniqueness in a personal and autonomous way." Perhaps, then, it should come as no surprise that patients' reclaiming of autonomy often began with small, highly personal instances. Arline Erdrich says, "I wouldn't stay in bed, even in the hospital. If I was able to be ambulatory, then I was. I was absolutely determined to conduct myself as a well person. I wouldn't wear nightgowns or pajamas. They gave me the nickname of 'the hostess' on the ward, because I always wore my own outfits and was always gladhanding new arrivals. They had to *make* me get into bed, even when I was home. For me, bed is a place to sleep, or be sick, not to live and be well."

RECLAIMING MIND AND BODY

Though the search to regain control may begin with any number of idiosyncratic gestures, it typically included a number of stages: Journeyers often began their struggle to reassert autonomy with what was closest at hand—their own bodies and minds. Arline taught herself a form of self-hypnosis to endure the pain of her lymphangiograms, and this soon became a catalyst for other forms of inward reclamation. Many others started with meditation practices which seemed to provide them with an ancillary guidance system, a method of inner listening that counterweighted the daily burden of impositions from without.

Sometimes control began as a subtractive process, a refraining from an accustomed unhealthy pattern and gradually substituting a new one. "When the doctor told me there was no physical cure for AIDS," says George Melton, "I decided that just because he didn't have the right pill didn't mean there was nothing I could do. It became obvious to me that my body had its own strength and intelligence, and there had to be ways I could encourage it. I was still telling my body to die by feeding it junk food, drugs, cigarettes, liquor. When I began to see myself as a living body, I began to put living food in it instead of dead chemicals. I looked into detoxification, fasting, fruit juices. I started going to a chiropractor, starting having massages and other kinds of bodywork done."

SELF-EDUCATION

George's new perspective was the direct result of a reading campaign he began as soon as he was diagnosed. He and his lover, Wil, who had also been diagnosed with AIDS, filled their apartment with stacks of books. George undertook an avid study of metaphysics and religion, while Wil, a former Naval engineer, began soberly wading through denser texts, determined to "develop a computer model of a surviving cancer patient and then applying these same principles to myself. It gave me the feeling," Wil says, "that I could take at least a portion of my fate into my own hands."

Arline Erdrich discovered an intense desire to explore the Old Testament. "I'd never even owned a Bible. But now it seemed filled with sages who had survived all sorts of terrible adversities. It was as if they had created this word puzzle, and if I could somehow get through it, there would be this secret in there just for me. I was constantly trying to piece it together."

Inspired by its teachings of "a time for every season unto Heaven," Arline began painting scenes from Ecclesiastes. Soon she found herself combing the public library stacks for books on other spiritual traditions, omnivorously gobbling tomes on near-death experiences, paging through lush coffee-table books of Renaissance religious frescoes. "I was suddenly interested in things I'd never cared about before. I became fascinated with the life of the painter J. M. W. Turner, and then with the life of Monet. I'd just pile books up around the chair in the family room. My husband was furious—he wanted me to watch TV with him, not sit by myself and read."

This personal engagement with learning was cited by many patients as a turning point in their journeys, a sort of declaration of intellectual independence. Many studied their diseases, treatment options, and alternatives, mastering some of the intimidating jargon spoken by doctors, equipping themselves with tools, however rudimentary, to assess their own healing process. Books also seemed to provide an inviolable private space, where the inner life could not be contested by others, and a new sense of self could germinate between the lines.

Sieving through books, many journeyers described feeling a peculiar sense of receptivity, of resonance, as if for the first time the words on a page were directly addressing them. This is perhaps part of a syndrome of heightened consciousness that often seems to accompany illness: The world suddenly begins to "speak." Ordinary events and objects may seem to fairly pulse with significance. The crisis-activated psyche begins to perceive a world pregnant with unexpected meaning. In this way, books become a way to access sources of wisdom beyond the immediate environment; not only to gain information about the body, healing, and medicine, but to draw from a well of inner sustenance at once personal and collective.

THE HEALING PARTNERSHIP

Many of the patients I spoke with claimed the right to be partners in their own cures, requiring that their sometimes reluctant caregivers take extra time and effort to acknowledge their thoughts and feelings. (One called this strategy, "Neither compliance nor defiance.") "A major part of getting well, I think, is to find a way to center the doctor's attention on your case," says John Studholme. "You have to take the attitude that nothing is more important than you, because most of them sure as hell won't do it for you."

Writes researcher Glenda Hawley, "Some patients feel that if they are to have the full attention of the doctor, they must be a 'good patient,' i.e., non-initiating, obedient, and compliant. These 'good' patients may often actually be in a state of helplessness and depression, which is deleterious to recovery."

She cites a study by Suls and Mullen (1981) showing that health is adversely impacted not only by uncontrollable circumstances, but by how much they are *perceived* as uncontrollable. It follows, she suggests, that patients assuming "appropriate control" could create "a major condition to promote healing. One way to feel a sense of control is to be an active participant in their own health care team."

John Studholme was bolstered by his years of experience forcefully arguing cases in the courtroom. Deena Metzger, too, felt that her lifetime as a "major warrior" who had once taken an academic freedom case all the way to the state supreme court lent her a reserve of strength when she most needed it: "I had read statistics that patients who assert themselves survived the longest. I think at one point I terrorized everybody at the hospital just by asking them questions. I told them I wasn't sure I was going to go along with their usual procedures. I quoted from literature they'd never heard of. I made myself a real pain in the ass! When I walked into the surgeon's office—he's actually a very nice man—and called him by his first name, he seemed to jump back three feet."

Annie Nathan also refused to be intimidated by the medical setting. She had been working as a psychotherapist at Langley Porter Neurological Institute when a breast cancer that had ostensibly been cured by an earlier lumpectomy suddenly recurred.

"It had been a very hopeful time in my life, I was nine months into a wonderful, fabulous marriage," Annie told me as we shared a sandwich on her sun-speckled back porch. Her golden retriever, Flicka, dropped a well-chewed tennis ball at my feet and looked up expectantly. Reaching over to toss it to the far end of the yard and watching the dog scamper after it, Annie paused with a far-off look, as if mentally retracing the distances traversed: "He told me I had terminal cancer, then handed me a book called *Good Grief,* about dying! I said, 'Forget it! Tell me someone you know who has survived. Give me the names of four other doctors.' Most of the doctors seemed very depressed, just gave me a year or two, maybe three to live. But there was one who was really arrogant, too bright for his own good, no bedside manner whatsoever. And he was the one I liked!"

She paused to admonish the dog, who had crept up to slyly tug a shred of my incautiously dangling sandwich. "How rude, my darling, you're *so* unrelenting!" she scolded, then laughed at the dog's abashed look.

"Anyway, I called this guy back and just said, 'Look, what kind of person are you? How are you when the chips are down? Are you a hopeful person, or do you buy into these statistics? I don't expect you to be God, but my death isn't a *fait accompli.* I believe there are things in this world that we don't understand, stuff you never learned in medical school. I'm not going to hold you responsible for what happens to me. But I'm holding try-outs for my healing team and I want to know if you want to be on it.'

"When I went back to see him, I laid it on the line. 'You don't have to love me,' I told him, 'but we have to have a real connection. I need you to search your own heart, because this is the most important decision I'll ever make in my life.' "

The doctor, she says, sat stunned and silent. After a long pause, he quietly nodded assent. "Then come down from your ivory tower,"

Annie responded. "Let's talk like two real people and figure out how to fix this mess."

BARGAINING

Many patients insisted on the right to alter procedures to take into account their unique needs. Connie Zweig, a lifelong partisan of alternative healing, realized to her dismay that conventional surgery seemed to offer the only hope of curing an agonizing herniated disk in her spine. But, she says, "I told the doctors I had some conditions: I wouldn't let them do anything structural—they had to get the nerve out of the way without altering the disk itself. I told them I would take their medicine, but I wouldn't eat their food. Cedars-Sinai Hospital said they wouldn't let me bring my own health food in, so I ditched them, chose a smaller hospital, and arranged to have friends bring me my meals with all my gallons of carrot juice and vitamins. I even had an acupuncturist come in there to treat me."

Others bargained for time with doctors who were otherwise intent on immediately applying standard treatment. Deena Metzger went through an excruciating, convoluted decision-making process before she settled on her medical course. A deeply committed poet who had made a career of self-exploration, she had wondered whether choosing surgery "might be kind of undermining the gods. You know, if I threw myself into the medical model, would I be giving a message to my psyche that I didn't believe in its healing powers?"

She sought advice from a friend who was "a physician and a healer," an M.D. who had left classical medical practice for a career as a spiritually oriented therapist. He advised her that very few people had the capacity to, as he put it, "fight cancer on the cellular level." He suggested instead she concentrate on her own inner work after having the operation. At the end of a "hellish week" during which she wrestled with "the enigmas of surrender and purposiveness," Deena decided to proceed with treatment, but on her own terms. She opted for surgery, but not radiation or chemotherapy.

Ji-on, a female Zen priest at a contemplative center in California, insisted that her treatment take into account her long training as a meditator. A decade before, when tests had revealed precancerous cells in her uterus, she had made "a bargain" with her doctor to be regularly tested for a few months but not rushed into surgery. "He was very skeptical," she says. "But I had been sitting *zazen* for about five years, and knew how to 'hold my spot.' " Meditating on what felt like a "lack of physiological harmony," she began to notice small, subtle changes in the way she felt. "After a month, it felt like the 'atmosphere' of my body was shifting, and these shifts seemed to coincide with different measurements that would show up in the lab tests. In the end, after doing this for five months, I actually tested clean."

Years later, when she was diagnosed with a form of leukemia, Ji-on "shopped around for a doctor who was willing to keep me company" without insisting on immediate chemotherapy. They settled on a six-month observation period, after which time Ji-on would agree to consider standard medical procedures. She was unusually fortunate, for her approach—which involved intensive meditation, dietary changes, and Chinese medicine—led to an apparent cure: At the time I met her, she had been disease-free for six years.

THE LIMITS OF CONTROL

The drive for control can also be counterproductive. Certainly, it is a salient feature of the "disease-prone" personality and a primary coping mechanism in dysfunctional families, where the emotional undertow ever threatens to drag down any but the most hypervigilant water-treader. For people who have survived such backgrounds, surrendering to treatment—any treatment—may feel tantamount to drowning. From this standpoint, resisting may become a way of fortifying a hard-won sense of identity against the threat of change, even if that change could lead to growth and healing.

An emphasis on control (and a certain penchant for denial) seems particularly prevalent in many "new age" circles, where it is sometimes asserted that anyone, furnished with the proper off-the-shelf psychospiritual techniques, can obtain total mastery over all conditions of mind and body. In his book *How Shall I Live?* Richard Moss, M.D., describes the case of a patient named Earl, a handsome, up-and-coming young advertising executive who was scheduled for surgery on a benign tumor that had spread to his middle ear. Earl, who had attended a half-dozen spiritual growth workshops and sieved through a plethora of popular books on metaphysics, concluded he had "given himself" his disease and was therefore responsible for healing it.

But Earl's symptoms—facial paralysis, dizziness, hearing loss—were worsening despite all his efforts. Dr. Moss quickly perceived that his patient was trapped in a self-made dilemma: He had come to equate medical treatment with passivity and lack of self-worth, and saw a natural, more "spiritual" approach as the only way to achieve his idealized path of self-development.

In Earl's case, Moss suggests, resistance to conventional medicine was in fact a refusal to surrender to the healing process itself. The patient had dug in his heels to such an extent that he was unable to move forward. "No one," Moss observes astutely, "can touch the full potential for healing by believing that one treatment is good for the body but in conflict with the soul, or vice versa. . . . The fullest potential exists when the inner consecration and the outer action unify." Over a series of four therapy sessions with Moss, Earl made a "transformative shift" in which he turned his inner purpose toward what was at that point the only appropriate healing choice. He even began to anticipate his surgery as a potentially life-changing experience. Because Earl was able to bring his whole being to his treatment, Moss reports, his operation was a great success: "As he was rolled through the hospital corridors, he felt a joyous rapport with the orderly who was wheeling him. The elevator up to the operating suite made him laugh. He was like a child on an adventure. When he entered the operating room and looked at the people there, he was filled with a sense of loving gratitude."[5]

Earl's surgeon reported a number of unusual phenomena: tissue which stopped bleeding almost as quickly as it was cut, as well as an extremely rapid and pain-free recovery. While recuperating in the hospital, Earl came to the decision to radically change careers, a breakthrough Moss attributes to the "unified state in which he met the profound stress of surgery."

Here the patient established a sense of control by consciously choosing and even empowering an inevitable treatment. Similarly, cancer patients who visualize their chemotherapy as "liquid sunshine" or radiation as "healing rays" have been found to experience less nausea and hair loss, as well as better clinical outcomes. "Reframing" impersonal medical events in highly individual terms may be a way to regain a feeling of autonomy as well as a method to actually enhance healing.

Perhaps "control" is an inappropriate term. To take a "soul-approach" on the path of healing includes whatever brings together our disparate, sometimes warring parts in the service of becoming more alive. "If we approach our life and healing from the depths of ourselves," Dr. Moss writes, "any experience has within it the power to transform and heal."

CROSSROADS

But it is hard to be wholehearted when the way forward is unclear, the atmosphere murky, and each choice part of a clattering roulette wheel of life or death. Each patient I spoke with eventually arrived at a crossroads, a point where it became necessary to commit fully to a plan of treatment. Here the power of autonomy and choice can become an onerous burden that most patients feel ill-equipped to carry. Samantha Coles reports,

> I was taking myself around to all the hospitals, all the little body-garages—"Okay, X-ray me again, take another CAT scan, another blood test, let's do it again, boys."
>
> But when I asked the hospital tumor board, "What's the up-shot, here, ace?" they didn't seem able to make a decision. They *did* tell me chemo and radiation wouldn't work on my melanoma. By now, I'd had three surgeries. It felt like those dreams where something horrible's coming after you, but you can't move, you can't run, you're rooted to the spot.
>
> Part of me still wanted my mommy—"Just tell me what to do, I'll be the good kid, I'll do it right so you'll love me." But finally I took a little bit of control, just told them, "Give me my records," and started searching.

Samantha joined "I Can Cope," a self-help group for cancer patients, and began to ask members for medical referrals. Eventually she was given the names of several top doctors at one of the nation's leading hospitals.

> These guys were the godfathers of cancer. They looked at my slides, but within fifteen minutes, I had three different diagnoses! Everything from, "We think you should take out the lymph nodes in your groin immediately" to "There's really nothing we can do." Finally, I realized I would have to make the decisions myself, even though I felt pretty damn clueless.

The crossroads is difficult to negotiate even for those who are far more knowledgeable about medical options. Dr. Jacob Zieghelboim was diagnosed with the very form of cancer he specialized in. As a leading researcher he was in a position to get the best advice in the world. He flew up to Stanford to consult with two celebrated col-leagues, certain that "we could all discuss the treatment together and decide what would be best."

One of the doctors, a friend of his, was a warm, kind, and fatherly man. The other, a giant in the field of radiation oncology, was a more astringent personality. Jacob was shocked when the two men convened to present their recommendations: "We have fundamen-tally agreed," they told him, "that we cannot agree." His friend was suggesting a relatively less aggressive regimen. The other doctor was pushing for a more protracted treatment, in the course of doing so exclaiming with great fervor, "If we went easier and you had a recurrence, I would rather die!"

Jacob was in a quandary that is agonizingly familiar to all patients, regardless of their degree of sophistication. "How could I make the right choice? Here was a critical moment, when the disease was still restricted to a small area, the best time to do something. But what?"

His means of deciding was, in the end, more intuitive than ob-jective: "Harry, the radiation guy, had a different *feel* about him. Radiation oncologists work underground, don't see the sun, and at the time all of that seemed symbolically relevant, as if it had somehow impregnated him. Also, my friend was willing to tailor my treatment to more than just the structure of the tumor or what stage it was. He was approaching it as I would, from the 'art' side as well as science, blending his treatment with what he knew of me as an individual."

Fortunately, the treatment his friend had recommended fulfilled its healing promise. But many of the patients I spoke with found that conventional medicine held out little hope for a cure of their particular disease; or that when one was offered, the physical costs and risks had seemed too high.

A calligraphied plaque hangs over former cancer patient Ted Lothammer's desk: TO BE UPSET OVER WHAT YOU DON'T HAVE IS TO WASTE WHAT YOU'VE GOT. Ted, a former long-haul trucker, gives the impression of a man who will brook no nonsense. Possessed of an angular, lived-in face that bears a more than passing resemblance to late jazz trumpeter Chet Baker, and a ferocious, bristling vitality for a sixty-two-year-old (he bounds up and down the staircase like a man half his age), Ted's tough-guy looks are belied by a soft lisp and a fairly extensive teddy bear collection. On the wall above his head is a flyswatter whose business end is shaped like a bear seated at a garish purple-and-turquoise piano. A white stuffed bear wear-ing a red spotted hat squats on a snare drum in the corner.

His office at People House, a crisis-counseling center he founded after his illness, is filled with enough curios, clippings, and artifacts to give the effect of a memorabilia collection-cum-shrine to some departed country heartthrob. Ted professes surprise at the cluttered evidence of his rich and varied life. "I wasn't supposed to be around long enough to take up so much room," he grins ironically.

When Ted was admitted to the hospital with abdominal bleeding, he was told it was too late—the cancer had spread throughout his body. "Four or five guys in white came into my room—the head of oncology, the surgeons—and told me, at best, that I'd be dead in four months. They did offer me chemo, but when I asked them, 'Will it cure me?' they said probably not. 'Will it give me a fifty-fifty chance of living?' They said, 'No, you might live a year at best.'

"They'd officially given me up. But an inner voice said, 'That's not right.' So I told them, 'You guys are wrong, I'm going to take care of this myself. I don't know how, but I'll figure it out.' "

Ted's loyalty to his inner voice flew in the face of both logic and convention. His insistence on finding his own way met with frequent resistance. People who struck out on their own path of healing sometimes reported being treated like outcasts, fugitives, or recalcitrant children. "When I refused to play the good little patient," one told me, "it pissed off just about everyone."

But with their lives in the balance, it was a risk they felt obliged to take. Survivors, as the numerous studies touched on earlier suggest, frequently are *not* "good little patients." With stubbornness and surrender, confusion and clarity, a faint ray of hope and cold, clutching fear, some patients, by choice or necessity, set out for parts unknown, searching for a way to bind their wounds.

❧ *10* ❧

THE QUEST FOR MEDICINE: A WORLD OF ALTERNATIVES

*I would like to try the
sea that brings all chances
To what land no matter
So that it heal me of my wound.*

—TRISTAN AND ISEULT

THE QUEST FOR treatment is at once the most hope-filled and most anguishing juncture on the healing path. Which doctor is the wisest, which hospital more advanced, what option the most failsafe? Which approaches can complement each other, and which slam the door on other methods of healing? Many patients I spoke with found themselves caught up in an epic quest for answers even as the clock was balefully ticking. Often they foundered between the seeming aggressiveness of mainstream medicine and the apparent "flakiness" of the available alternatives. For although these two approaches, the conventional and the unconventional, are moving glacially toward each other, the chasm separating them still gapes alarmingly. For patients trying to plant one foot on each side, there is a real and present danger of winding up with no footing at all.

All cultures have footpaths—anthropologists call them "systems of resort"—which an individual can follow to seek resolution of a crisis. Depending on the social mazeways, a marital conflict can wind up with the clan matriarch, the revolutionary block committee, the priest, the shaman, the family therapist, or the divorce attorney. Similarly, in different cultures the same health problem might be defined variously as personal, familial, communal, or spiritual, with correspondingly different remedies applied.

In a Kung Bushman tribe a disease is also a social problem, to be treated through collective ceremony ("If one is sick, all are sick"); while in Western cultures, illness is mostly a private affair ("between you and your doctor" or to be "kept within the family"). And whether the doctor prescribes a dried root or a scalpel, the "whole weight of the tribe's religion, myths, and community spirit," as anthropologist Edwin Ackerknecht writes, "enters into the treatment."[1] From this standpoint, *all* medicine is ethnomedicine.

The full weight of our own culture presses toward rapid aggressive intervention. Visible, instantaneous relief of symptoms is privileged over gentler, slower progress toward health. In recent years, we have witnessed the public ritual of America's First Ladies—Betty Ford, Nancy Reagan, and Barbara Bush—duly reporting, as if to reaffirm the dominant medical paradigm, to Bethesda Naval Hospital for invasive procedures. (Compare this, say, with the well-publicized affinity of the British "royals" for homeopathy and other alternative forms of healing, played out against the backdrop of a more pluralistic English health-care system.)

"Doctors say" is still our society's most powerful imprimatur (consider, by comparison, "lawyers say," "politicians say"). For all the malaise over health care in the opinion polls, we still tend to view medicine as a category unto itself, a guild of bodhisattva-scientists dedicated to the alleviation of human suffering, hovering above the vagaries of commerce, politics, or ideology that taint normal concourse.

But medicine, as we have seen, is not simply a repository of scientific truth. Intramural politics, cultural biases, doctors' personalities, institutional funding and governmental policy—all come to bear upon which treatment a patient has access to and ultimately receives.

It would be foolish to conclude that because the "medical-industrial complex" may be inadequate—or even dangerously wrong-headed—in some areas, alternatives are available to supply the missing pieces. Unconventional techniques are often insufficiently tested and thus of uncertain efficacy. They may be based on erroneous assumptions, inflated claims, the charisma of a single practitioner, or on sometimes perilous procedures. Their application tends to be less predictable for not being beholden to a standardized protocol. Some "alternative" practices may be nearly as disruptive as the conventional remedies they try to circumvent, may subscribe to equally mechanistic models of the bodymind, and may, in the end, be equally dismissive of the psyche. It is possible for a patient to fruitlessly pursue "nontoxic" therapies while losing a chance to treat a curable disease by more conventional means. As Richard Grossinger writes in his book *Planet Medicine:*

> Orthodox medicine has a standard humanitarian argument: If a patient gets bewitched in the maw of alternative and fantastical treatments, he or she may delay getting competent professional help for a condition that then becomes incurable. What makes this kind of situation so confusing is that sometimes the argument is provincial and self-serving, while other times it is an accurate warning.

THE APPEAL OF ALTERNATIVES

Still, nearly all of the people I interviewed opted for some form of alternative, sometimes exclusively but more often in tandem with or following conventional therapies. Many cases had come to me via the new age grapevine, where there is much suspicion of orthodoxy and a marked, sometimes exasperating preference for anything presumptively "natural." But in most cases, the reason for turning to alternative approaches was not so much a knee-jerk subscription to a heretical gospel as a feeling that standard treatment for their disease was too debilitating, inefficacious, or even thwarting of their own search for a deeper, more thorough process of healing.

Carol Boss, a long-surviving breast cancer patient, told me, "Again and again, I'd seen friends have surgery or chemo and be sent back into the world quote-unquote all better. Then six months or two or three years later, it would recur again, and with a vengeance. I could see that just taking away the symptom is not taking away the disease; there is more to this profound change we call healing. It's like a tree growing. It doesn't happen overnight." Carol had been given a weeks-to-months fatal prognosis for her rapidly progressing metastatic breast disease. Like many, she turned to alternatives when mainstream medicine simply threw up its hands.

She is only one of millions of people who seek nonconventional treatment (in her case, a regimen of acupuncture, diet, and meditation). In 1990, Americans spent $10.3 billion out of pocket on alternative health care, rivaling the $12.8 billion they disbursed on conventional hospitalization.[2] Psychologist Barrie Cassileth and her colleagues at the University of Pennsylvania Cancer Center undertook a study of "the sustained and apparently growing appeal of anti-medicine, non-medicinal, lifestyle-oriented alternatives during a period of technological advance in orthodox medical care." Cassileth found, somewhat to her surprise, that patients who made such choices did not fit traditional stereotypes of "poorly educated, terminally ill patients who have exhausted conventional treatment. Similarly, although some unorthodox practitioners may well fit the characteristic portrait of quacks and charlatans, many are well-trained, few charge high fees, and most, on the basis of patients' views and our own observations, sincerely believe in the efficacy and rationality of their work."[3]

Only 8 percent of the patients Cassileth surveyed had refused conventional treatment, and 60 percent continued seeing their doctors even while undergoing unorthodox procedures. Significantly, 30 percent of their doctors supported them in their search. In a 1985 Associated Press opinion poll, more than half of the nearly 1,500 adult Americans surveyed said they would opt for unsanctioned treatment if they were seriously ill; only 36 percent said they would not.[4] Another more recent poll (1992) revealed that nearly one-third of Americans had tried some form of unconventional therapy, half of them within the past year. Alternative medicine has grown into a $27 billion-a-year industry.[5]

In general, most of the journeyers I met saw alternative medical practices—which ranged from acupuncture to herbalism to "bodywork" and "energy medicine"—as a way to address needs they felt were neglected by ordinary medical practice. They reported that alternative practitioners tended to

- Spend more time with them, from the initial intake and history to individual appointments to gentler, more gradual treatment programs.
- Diagnose symptoms as an interaction of many "cofactors," helping the patient bring healing to diverse areas of his or her life.
- View the body as a whole, and concern themselves with possible relationships between what conventional M.D.s might consider disconnected symptoms and systems.
- Build up the body's general tonus of health, on the assumption that "the patient is not sick because she has a symptom, but has a symptom because she is sick."
- Tailor treatment to the needs of individuals rather than standardized protocols. Many alternative healers believe that illness is less a fixed condition than an ever-changing process—that the same disease behaves in different ways in different people

at different times, calling for shifting treatment strategies.

- Favor prescriptions that include changes in personal habits, both mental and physical, and offer self-care regimens that encouraged the patient's autonomous maintenance of health.
- Treat illness within a psychospiritual framework that encouraged both inner development and a fuller, more balanced outer life.

Few cultures, in fact, present the seeker with choices so polarized as our own tend to be: Doctors, partly out of fear of malpractice suits or professional censure, may refuse to treat patients who are using alternative modalities. One medical writer observes that the Western paradigm is exemplified by "the dominance of one medical theory above all," whereas Asian medicine allows several working models to be embraced simultaneously, "depending on which best fits the need of any given case."

Countries vary widely on the degree of medical pluralism they allow. Michael Lerner, co-founder of the Commonweal Cancer Help Program and a former U.S. Office of Technology Assessment consultant, notes there are 120,000 prescription drugs on the market in West Germany, while Iceland only permits 100. In modern Morocco, anthropologist Loring Danforth points out, "There is no single, socially chartered therapeutic system with final authority."[6] Instead, as in late antiquity, individuals have a choice of different systems, and tend to base their decisions on a "support group" of relatives and friends who help gather information about healing.

But for many of the patients I talked with, relatives and friends were not always available, and support for alternatives was often nearly impossible to find. Many journeyers found themselves virtually alone as they confronted the momentous decision whether to leave the well-traversed ways of sanctioned treatment without knowing their new destination. Debby Ogg recounts, "I was looking for second and third opinions, so I went to Sloan-Kettering and Mass General [in Boston]. But they treated me pretty horribly. We'd go five or ten minutes, and then they'd tell me, 'Dead. You're going to be dead.' When I asked them about things like meditation, visualization, diet, exercise, they all said, 'Hogwash, hogwash, hogwash.' My own brother Bobbie, who's a brilliant doctor, told me my cancer was *incurable*. For a while my sister wouldn't speak to me because she thought I was chasing phantoms.

"Luckily, I had friends who came through. They started bringing me books, and I started ploughing through them. I began to see there weren't really any good maps, that I'd somehow have to find my own."

TWO MEDICINES?

Dr. Bernie Siegel once remarked to me that the majority of his patients' dreams concerned decisions between various treatment options. Because they were forced to make crucial choices that carried almost unthinkable consequences, it is hardly surprising that this struggle dominated their nights as well as their days.

Mark Pelgrin, in his book *And a Time to Die*, describes a dream he had following an exploratory surgery that revealed his finally fatal pancreatic cancer. In it, a conventional physician and an odd healer are squabbling over his case:

> I was in a room with two doctors. One was like the surgeon, a modern expert, a true scientist. The other was a crude little guy who kept arguing with the surgeon about the need for what he called "home cures." I was very ill in this dream, and they were talking quietly but intensely over me. Sometimes we were all standing in swamp water. There were crocodiles about but . . . they didn't really terrify me. Indeed, they seemed to be friends of the little ugly doctor with his crazy talk about "home cures."

Pelgrin does not know what to make of his "swamp doctor," who is diminutive, crazy, crude, and makes absurdly simple suggestions. I was shocked when I read his account, because I too had repeatedly encountered such figures in my dreams. In one, it was a strangely impassive little Bushman in a loincloth who, finding me caught in a desert thornbush, proffered a juicy red "healing herb." In another it was a slow, fat, middle-aged "Sherpa guide" who tried to stop me from climbing Mt. Rushmore (*rush more?*). In yet another, a short, plump "Puerto Rican lady" who claimed she knew my grandmother patiently explained how my ancestors would have healed me with "brown rice and soup," while I listened with mounting annoyance.

These figures provoked in me (my dream-self) feelings of the utmost contempt—at their humble status, their primitive appearance, their irritatingly calm demeanor and slow pace, their seeming lack of sophistication. I was outraged at their simple-minded remedies, their lack of urgency about what I was convinced was a mortal condition. Often, as in Pelgrin's dream, they were questioning or fighting with figures who symbolized more conventional medical mores.

Who were these "primitive" little healers? Carl and Stephanie Simonton, authors of *Getting Well Again,* who took note of similar figures in their patients' dreams, wondered, "Is there something in the nature of cancer itself as the 'disease of civilization,' or in the nature of the individuals who get cancer, that makes the unconscious bring up this image of an alternative treatment approach?"

For me, the "little people" seemed to be in part psychological counterweights, shadow-figures who spoke for the rejected, despised aspects of the self, voicing truths I was unwilling to admit consciously. They presented an approach to healing that would put me on a collision course with social norms and the ostensible security of conventional practice. They challenged, with a kind of maddening composure, the hegemony of technological medicine.

The challenge, as I've since learned, is an historic one, along battle lines that have stood for centuries. Medical scholar Lucinda Beier has traced the devaluation of natural medicines at least as far back as seventeenth-century England. Persisting to this day, such attitudes are, she maintains, "self-congratulatory, viewing the adherents and beneficiaries of 'modern' medicine as rational and civilized, while the users of 'traditional' medicines are at best old-fashioned, at worst uncivilized, furry little natives."[7]

Even in first-century Rome, the historian Pliny lamented the disuse into which natural remedies had fallen in an era intoxicated with surgical experimentation. Why, Pliny asks, had the Hippocratic "simples" been abandoned in favor of a new medical art that was "lucrative beyond all the rest?"[8]

A JOURNEY TO THE EAST

While modern medicine still venerates the name of Hippocrates, Western treatment has made a radical break with the largely herbal and noninvasive Greek practices he built upon. One of the few surviving traditions that can justly claim to be heir to the diffusion of Greek medicine (as well as Chinese, Ayur-Vedic, and shamanic healing) is that of Tibet.

Contemporary Tibetan doctors purportedly have had success with some types of cancer using herbal remedies millennias-old. During my own quest for alternatives, I obtained an appointment with Yeshi Dhonden, the Dalai Lama's personal physician, when he happened to be visiting New York. Before seeing him I had called John Avedon, a friend of the Dalai Lama and the author of the gripping *In Exile from the Land of Snows,* for his opinion. "I've seen tumors literally exploded with Tibetan medicine," said Avedon. "I've also seen people Dhonden *thought* he could treat die."

To the modern sensibility, Tibetan medical practice seems a well-preserved (if not mummified) body of archaic doctrines, a quaint museum piece in an age of PET-scans and neuropeptides. Seasons, elements, flavors, and astrological lore factor incomprehensibly into diagnosis and treatment; medicines are compounded to the accompaniment of complex religious liturgies.

However, ancient Tibetan physicians were sophisticated pathologists and anatomists whose texts on embryology predated Western knowledge of prenatal development by over a thousand years. Their surgeons were skilled in anesthesiology and possessed good surgical implements, some texts even claiming that they performed heart and brain surgery. Surgery had been officially banned centuries before, however, when the mother of the thirty-eighth ruler of Tibet died under the knife. Like a person suddenly blinded who develops extraordinarily sensitive hearing or smell to compensate, Tibetan medicine was forced to redirect all its energies toward noninvasive methods of treatment.

Dr. Dhonden already had made several trips to the West and had amazed Western doctors with his powers of observation.

"I went to observe Dr. Dhonden with some healthy skepticism," Yale surgery professor Richard Selzer told Avedon. "I was surprised and elated by what I found. It was as if he was a human electrocardiogram machine, interpreting the component parts of the pulse. We have nothing like it in the West. It's a dimension of medicine we have not yet realized."[9]

During a 1980 visit Dr. Dhonden made to the University of Virginia's Medical Oncology Department, a lab test had been arranged to ascertain the effect of Tibetan drugs on tumor-implanted mice. After only a visual examination of the animals, Dr. Dhonden prescribed a general cancer drug composed of over sixty herbal and mineral ingredients. The first trial extended the animals' lifespans by 50 percent. A second experiment produced the most prolonged survival since work on that particular tumor began in 1967. Dr. Donald Baker, the researcher in charge of the experiment, commented, "There are literally hundreds of kinds of tumors. How often has Dr. Dhonden encountered a KHT anaplastic sarcoma growing in a highly inbred strain of 3CH/HEJ female mice? It would be utterly unreasonable to ask him to decide what would be the best treatment. If he had been familiar with these conditions, he might have effected a complete cure."[10]

I met Dr. Dhonden in a tiny fifth-floor walkup in lower downtown New York. I was ushered in through a kitchen permeated with the smell of simmering Tibetan-style lamb stew. I panicked when I saw that the translator who usually accompanied him on his visits had not shown up. *Fine,* I thought glumly. *I can't even tell the doctor where it hurts.*

Yeshi Dhonden sat cross-legged on a small platform couch, placidly counting a rosary and reciting singsong mantras under his breath. At fifty-five, he looked wise and robust. When he was just thirteen, I had read, he passed a medical college admissions exam by reciting verbatim—in or out of sequence, as requested by his interlocutors—all 156 chapters of the four medical texts of the Tibetan medical canon.

I draped a white silk ceremonial scarf over his outstretched hands, a traditional honorific greeting, and bowed. He seemed delighted, placing the scarf back over my neck as a token of blessing. He gestured expansively for me to sit down next to him, looking at me with eyes crinkled in friendliness as he delicately palpated the pulses on my wrist.

His fingers were as soft as fine calfskin. I felt secure, enveloped in a warm glow. I pointed to the left side of my neck where the tumor was couched. *"Ah."* He smiled, and reached out to feel it, gently pushing until he could seize the lump between his fingers. He smiled reassuringly, then gestured abruptly that I was to pull up my shirt. Reaching underneath with his large hands as I stood before him, he grappled with the flesh under my armpits, apparently searching for other swellings. His directness, curiosity and even outright jollity contrasted pleasantly with the wan diffidence of the M.D.'s I had consulted. He had the buoyancy of one whose entire being is absorbed in his task.

When we called his translator on the phone, Dr. Dhonden said a few short phrases and handed me the receiver. I grabbed it eagerly, excited to hear what secrets this great man had uncovered.

"He wants to know," the translator said, "how long you've had this rheumatism?"

My heart sank. Every prejudice I harbored, that anyone who didn't wear a white coat and stethoscope was a witch doctor rose clamoring to the surface: He'd completely missed the boat.

"It's not rheumatism," I told the translator crossly, though I was to find out much later that in the Tibetan mind this seemingly unrelated ailment was concomitant with my condition. "It's a tumor. I think it's cancer."

I was to find out later that in Dr. Dhonden's system a tumor was merely a symptom of a more general pathology. I was to have a similar experience with a second Tibetan doctor, who gently probed my lower back and informed me I was suffering from "blockages of nerve impulses." *His* translator gave me a complicated explanation that whizzed by me in a cloud of hermetic medical terminology: "Winds" had affected my circulation, bringing phlegm and bile, and I had "shocks in all peripheral nerves."

I was caught in a predicament many patients who approach Asian medical systems must face. Though such traditions often possess an extensive knowledge of anatomy and pharmacology, their central focus is the workings of "energy," of the mysterious life force itself. In Tibetan medical theory, the "precious human body" is conceived of as a treasure trove of hidden awareness, animated by vital forces or humors (*nes-pa*) whose movements coincide with mental events. (Yeshi Dhonden has described, somewhat enigmatically, "a sub-atomic consciousness within the vast landscape of the central inner nervous system."[11]) Some diseases are said to begin with "afflictive" emotions and thought patterns. Tibetan doctors describe a "subtle body" composed of airs and essences, channels and psychic nerves, which correspond to but are not identical with the physical structures of anatomy.

The element of "wind," for example, is considered to "provide the physical basis of the mind."[12] Similar doctrines can be found in the Greek concept of *pneuma*, the Arabic *ruh*, Ayur-Vedic *prana*, and *shen* and *chi* in the Chinese medical system. Ted Kaptchuk, an acupuncturist and scholar of Chinese medicine, writes:

> Chinese medical theory does not have the concept of a nervous system. Nevertheless, it had been demonstrated that Chinese medicine can be used to treat neurological disorders. Similarly, Chinese medicine does not perceive an endocrine system, yet it treats what Western medicine calls endocrine disorders. Nor does traditional Chinese medicine recognize streptococcus pneumoniae as a pathology of pneumonia, yet often it effectively treats the disease.

"Dr. Dhonden says you shouldn't have any operations," the translator told me finally. "This could be harmful to you, because it cuts the energy 'channels' in the neck. He says to take his pills and that in ten months they will dissolve the lump." I was not sure whether to feel relief or incredulity.

Dr. Dhonden and I had sat drinking tea together in silence while his assistant fished out the appropriate pills from a large plastic bag. Some were *rinchen ribus*, or "precious pills." One of the some 2,000 drugs in the Tibetan pharmacopoeia, they are considered a panacea, often containing gold, silver, pearl, ruby, sapphire, and diamond, ground-up holy relics, and powerful herbals. Their manufacture, according to Avedon, sometimes takes up to three months of around-the-clock labor by a team of twenty druggists.

The pills had had a pleasantly bitter taste, like ancient unsweetened baker's chocolate. Still, I thought, I had a terribly serious disease, one which would supposedly take the full armamentarium of Western technology to cure. How could a few herbal confections slay the monster?

THE POWERS OF NATURE

Our usual opinion of such nonpharmaceutical remedies is that they are placebos, either patent medicine or patent nonsense. It is sometimes difficult to determine the active ingredients, if any, since ethnomedicines are so often buffered with magic and ritual. It took Harvard researcher Wade Davis months of exhaustive fieldwork and chemical analysis to discover that Haitian "zombie-making" potions, made with such eye-of-newt ingredients as corpse bones by voodoo apothecaries, also contained roasted pufferfish, a source of tetrodotoxinone, one of the world's most potent nerve poisons.

Dr. Dhonden, during his training in Tibet, had excelled beyond his colleagues in one medical exam by correctly identifying, while blindfolded, the type, species, and medicinal properties of herbs selected randomly from 200 separate samples. Up until a few hundred years ago, Western physicians, too, were rigorously required to study botany, since most prescriptions still derived directly from plants.

Today, modern medicine will recite, sometimes generously and other times only under prodding, the litany of our debt to native pharmacopoeias: Five thousand years ago, Chinese doctors used medicine derived from the plant *Ephedra sinica* to treat asthma. Today we use its derivative, ephedrine, to dilate constricted bronchial tubes. Its history is most often recounted with a benign, condescending twinkle, a story from the days back when medicine was made from weeds. Though remedies derived from plants remain the primary form of medical care for three-quarters of humanity,[13] Cambridge internist Dr. William Bennett spoke for the majority of M.D.'s when he wrote in a 1988 issue of the *Medicine Tribune*, "The use of herbs or nutrition to stimulate or strengthen the immune system is a nonsense claim . . . and to the extent that people wind up believing such claims, we can say that their brains are damaged."[14]

But recent laboratory analysis has demonstrated, for example, that purple coneflower, known to horticulturists as *Echinacea angustifolia* and used by Plains Indians as an infectious disease remedy, contains a wide variety of active substances with antibiotic, anti-inflammatory, and immunostimulatory effects. Milk-thistle, gardeners' bane, and other long-standing staples of European folk medicine have shown powerful therapeutic effects on the cells of the liver, protecting them from toxic damage and stimulating regeneration through RNA-mediated protein synthesis. Doctors at Walter Reed Hospital have confirmed that a Chinese medicine derived from annual wormwood, a common weed, is a powerful antimalarial. Ginseng, dismissed as a superstitious Chinese folk remedy for impotence and aging, is now known to contain bioactive glycosides with marked effects on the pituitary and adrenal glands.[15]

Recently, there has been an upswing of interest in herbally derived pharmaceuticals. The nonprofit Rainforest Alliance has put an improbable stamp of approval on drug giant Merck and Company's "prospecting" for medicinal plants in the Costa Rican rainforests in exchange for royalties to support conservation efforts. A small California company called Shaman Pharmaceuticals, utilizing indigenous informants, has located a rainforest plant that initial clinical trials indicate is active against the flu and the herpes viruses. (They, too, plan to channel a portion of any profits into ecological conservation.) In India, research into 2,500-year-old Sanskrit medical texts led to a cholesterol-lowering medicinal compound derived from the native guggal tree.[16]

Even animal behavior is being studied in the search for "natural cures." Scientists have discovered, to their amazement, that ailing wild chimpanzees will seek out the *Vernonia amygdalina* bush to cure themselves of intestinal parasites, a remedy they share with—or perhaps even "taught" to—the human inhabitants of Tanzania. Chimp behavior also recently led scientists to investigate aspilia, which contains a red oil called thiarubine-A that apparently kills not only parasites, fungi, and viruses, but solid tumor cancer cells in the lab.[17]

THE WORLD OF ALTERNATIVES

These cases from the "animal annals" are reminiscent of the tale told by the late alternative cancer treatment advocate Harry Hoxsey, who claimed he had received a cancer remedy as a family inheritance. His great-grandfather, he said, had watched a horse afflicted with a cancerous growth graze daily on particular grasses and flowering wild plants in the pasture until its tumor disappeared. Hoxsey added ingredients from traditional home remedies to the formula, at first using the mixture to treat similarly afflicted horses and later administering it to people.

From 1924 until the late 1950s Hoxsey's medicine was offered at clinics around the country. The Hoxsey Outpatient Clinic in Dallas became one of the world's largest privately owned cancer centers, with branches in seventeen states treating a reported 10,000 patients at any given time. After a long series of exhausting legal clashes with the Food and Drug Administration, Hoxsey—a flamboyant, obstreperous man who appears to have had a sincere belief in his remedy—was finally forced to shut his doors.

Still, according to a 1990 report on unconventional cancer treatment issued by the U.S. Office of Technology Assessment (O.T.A.), "Many of the herbs used in the Hoxsey internal tonic or the isolated components of these herbs have antitumor activity or cytotoxic effects in animal tests systems."

Today, years after Hoxsey's death, his onetime nurse continues to supply the mixture from a center in Tijuana, Mexico, issuing unsubstantiated (and doubtlessly highly inflated) claims of an 80 percent cure rate. Michael Lerner, a somewhat sympathetic investigator of alternatives, once told me that most cancer treatments, whether conventional or unconventional, seemed to have at best a 10 percent success rate. The O.T.A. report discusses several follow-up studies of patients whose names were furnished by the Hoxsey clinic, which did not reveal any unusual cure rates for internal cancers.[18] Nonetheless, an improbably entertaining documentary, "Quacks Who Cure Cancer?" by New Mexico journalist Kenneth Ausubel, features moving testimony by former terminal patients who convincingly attribute their unpredicted survival to Hoxsey's elixir.

It is not the place of this book to thrust itself into the highly charged imbroglios over alternative cancer care. A 1991 study by

Barrie Cassileth discovered that the outcomes for terminal cancer patients at a San Diego alternative clinic were neither better *nor worse* than for hospital patients.[19] What is striking is the extent to which many of the purported treatments mirror the worldview of ancient theories of disease and healing: seeing the body embedded in the larger body of nature, obeying the same laws of balance and harmony, possessing an inherent capacity for self-healing.

One proponent of alternative cancer therapy, Stanislaw Burzynski, M.D., postulates the existence of an innate biochemical system in the body, distinct from the immune system, capable of "correcting" cancer by means of "special chemicals that reprogram misdirected cells." He is in many ways the polar opposite of the homespun Hoxsey. Burzynski was an assistant professor at the Baylor College of Medicine and received funding from the National Cancer Institute (N.C.I.) to isolate possible cancer-inhibiting peptides. He believes naturally occurring chemicals—which he calls *antineoplastons*—inhibit malignant growth while leaving normal cells unaffected.

There appears to be a paucity of undisputed evidence for the efficacy of his treatments, though clinical trials are underway in Japan, Europe, and at the N.C.I.[20] Here again is a promising therapy based on the ancient notion that the body is capable of fighting serious disease once restored to its natural balance.

The work of Dr. Emmanuel Revici, another unconventional scientist whose view of nature as a balance of opposing forces—the catabolic (breaking down) and the anabolic (building up)—is strikingly in accord with that of Eastern philosophy. In a fascinating dialogue with the Tibetan physician Dr. Trogawa, Revici stressed that, "All manifestations in nature, including disease, are simply part of this movement between destructive and constructive characters." Citing the ancient principles of yin and yang, Dr. Trogawa concurred, describing a medicine based on "two types of energy, growing or declining," then adding, "I have cured some conditions diagnosed as cancer, but not a great number."[21]

Revici, a former chief of oncology at his own New York hospital, claims to have devised what amounts to an alternative chemotherapy based on nontoxic lipid compounds. Some of his substances were tested at the Imperial Cancer Research Fund and Westminster Hospital in London, and the analyses showed at least one compound to be active on several tumor systems. But the O.T.A. report notes that other studies have been inconclusive or have shown no favorable objective responses whatever, citing a typical absence of "prospective controlled clinical trials."

Revici, in fact, was placed on medical probation for a five-year period beginning in October 1988. (The director of the New York State licensing board would only comment it was "a matter of professional attitude.") Still, one year earlier, the U.S. Federal Court of Appeals for New York had set aside a lower court's malpractice conviction against Revici, stating: "We see no reason why a patient should not be allowed to make an informed decision and go outside currently approved medical methods in search of an unconventional treatment. . . . An informed decision to avoid surgery and chemotherapy is within the patient's right to determine what to do with his or her own body."

But making an informed decision can be well-nigh impossible. The patient who seeks alternatives is often buffeted by radically conflicting claims of legitimacy. Whether due to limited funding, the reluctance of mainstream research and regulatory institutions to engage in full-scale testing, or sometimes simple meretriciousness, proponents of alternative therapies often fail to meet the challenge of providing uncontested "hard data." The patient who pursues such remedies may easily get the feeling she is wandering lost on the far fringes rather than exploring the new frontier.

When I was ill I visited Dr. Revici's tiny, street-level office in New York. The front door had a small brass plaque identifying it as an animal research lab. The air seemed to smell of tar. The staff consisted of two or three men whose chortling camaraderie, combined with the petroleumlike odor, made me feel I was hunkered down in the lube pit of an upstate Shell station. Another man dressed in gray-green workpants and a dilapidated plaid hunting jacket hurried in and out, carrying vials of urine samples and beakers with glass stirring rods rattling in them. The next minute, he was bundling up the office garbage in a plastic bag.

When I was escorted in to see Dr. Revici, he was in the middle of a long-distance call from Vienna. On the cluttered desk in front of me were open test-tubes of fluid trailing the colored streamers of chemical reagents. Small, ancient, and oracular-looking, with a mottled bald head and wise sea-turtle eyes magnified to the size of egg yolks by his thick glasses, Revici seemed a creature out of Lewis Carroll. He felt my neck, took my blood pressure, and checked my facial and patellar nerve responses with an air of attentive dignity, then suggested I consider conventional treatment and bid me good day.

Afterward I spoke with a writer and former lymphoma patient

who credited Revici with his remission after surgery, chemo, and radiation had failed. He cautioned me, "Don't accept optimistic assessments. Revici gets the worst inoperable cases and loses many of them. He still does much better than conventional medicine, but no guarantee."

It seemed like sound advice. I mentioned to him that I was considering the Gerson Clinic in Mexico, which bases its treatment on a grueling thirteen-hour-a-day "detoxifying" regimen of fresh vegetable juices, along with a no-fat, low sodium, and high potassium diet, vitamins, mineral supplements, pancreatic enzymes, and frequent coffee enemas. He gave me an ironic salute: "Wherever you go, a wing and a prayer."

The late Dr. Max Gerson believed cancer to be a disease of an "impaired metabolism," claiming that his rigorous treatment reversed the conditions that fostered the growth of malignant cells, as well as other disease conditions. Gerson won the friendship of Dr. Albert Schweitzer after curing his wife, Helena, of tuberculosis after all conventional treatment had failed. Gerson had what he referred to as a "philosophy of totality" that drew on sources as diverse as the medieval physician-mystic Paracelsus and the work of the cyberneticist Norbert Weiner, and aimed to harmonize the "dynamic forces" and "creative potential" intrinsic in the body.

Eventually, I decided that the rigorous discipline of the treatment would be too demanding. It seemed farfetched that daily gallons of fresh carrot juice, a key Gerson component due to its high concentrations of vitamin A, could actually be active against cancer.

Around the time I was considering this alternative, I had a dream that my daughter was dancing happily around me, holding a lettuce leaf over her head like an umbrella. I thundered at her angrily, "Vegetables can't protect you from *cancer!*" But according to a recent *New York Times* article, compounds linked to cancer prevention (though not treatment) can be found in a number of common vegetables.[22] The National Cancer Institute recently earmarked $20.5 million to attempt to identify cancer-fighting phytochemicals in flax, citrus fruits, members of the garlic and parsley families and licorice root extract. There is already extensive epidemiological evidence that members of the mustard family—broccoli, cauliflower, cabbage, and brussels sprouts—strengthen the immune system, and may be effective preventives against cancer of the colon, stomach, lung, prostate, and esophagus.

"The correlation between folk medicine and phytochemicals is astounding," adds researcher Dr. Chris Beecher. "It convinces me that people's tastes are shaped at least in part by a subliminal knowledge of what keeps them alive."

According to Peter Barry Chowka, a journalist who specializes in investigating alternative cancer treatments, orthodox medicine is edging toward a wary acceptance of the possibility that diet might not only be a preventive, but a form of medicine in itself. Of particular interest at a recent American Cancer Society–sponsored science writer's seminar he attended were three studies showing that survival rates for Japanese women with breast cancer were up to 20 percent higher than for their North American counterparts, presumably due to the Japanese's low-fat, mainly vegetarian diet.[23]

For some of those with a terminal prognosis, no dietary regimen seems too rigorous. Several of the patients I spoke with attributed their survival to stays at the Gerson Clinic and their subsequent adherence to the diet. All commented on the difficulty of maintaining it, but felt strongly that their ordeal had been worth it. Many described experiencing bizarre "healing crises," a frequently reported side-effect of the Gerson treatment believed to signal the restoration of the body's own "detoxifying" mechanisms. "I got violently ill," says patient Margaret Green, who spent time at the clinic. "I would hear the guy coming down the hall with the carrot juice and it affected me like people have described with chemotherapy, where just seeing the nurse makes you throw up."

But despite the program's rigors, and the problems with what Margaret felt was not always confidence-inspiring medical backup, she preferred the clinic's hopeful, highly motivated atmosphere to "the hospital oncology ward, where everyone looks like they've given up."

ALTERNATIVES AS A
PSYCHOSPIRITUAL JOURNEY

Margaret, who later became deeply involved in her own "inner work," points out that many alternative practitioners, anxious to have their treatments validated as purely physical medicine, are unexpectedly leery of mind-body approaches. "If you talk to the Gerson people about psychology," she told me, "they're not interested. They just say, 'Do this for eighteen months and you'll be cured.' Most of them see the mind and body as separately as regular doctors."

Nonetheless, I was struck by the deep psychological transformation that often accompanied journeys through the world of alternative treatment. Marilyn Sanders [not her real name] had been an avid partisan of conventional medicine for most of her life, even volunteering as a "pink lady" at a local hospital. But diagnosed with terminal melanoma, given a grueling course of experimental chemotherapy, and finally sent home to die, she was forced back upon her own resources. When she discovered the Gerson method, she experienced the equivalent of a religious conversion. Her fascinating story is worth recounting at length:

The doctors had given me up for dead, so I was just praying all the time. One day, I was in the grocery store and this book was lying in the aisle. I accidentally kicked it and it spun around and I saw it was titled *How I Purged Myself of Melanoma*. It was only half-price. The minute I started reading it—it was all about the Gerson diet—I knew I'd been spiritually given the answer. That it was natural, it was God's way, and the end result would be good.

After I read it, I started the diet on my own and then went down to Mexico. Within a few days of starting the program, I got a very high fever. Then I just went comatose. I don't remember any external things that happened next. I just felt God was in that room with me, so intimate, like a warmth. It was like He was saying, "I'm not through with you yet, you still have more to do."

Then something really strange began to happen. It seemed as if I began reexperiencing every physical injury I'd ever had. I felt the numbing of my arms from an accidental pesticide exposure the docs thought gave me cancer in the first place. I felt these horrible injuries that had happened to me when I was a child, like my eye popping out of its socket when I fell on a bicycle handle. I went back to the worst emotional hurts I'd gotten from Mom and Dad when I was a kid. It was a combination of mental and physical cleansing, a euphoric feeling of uncovering of layers of the past one upon another. I was coaxing them out, saying, "Come on, it's OK, let's just do it." I knew once each thing was behind me, I would never have to go through it again.

I'd had terrible curvature of my spine as a child and osteoporosis as an adult. X-rays had shown the disks in my spine were all compressed, crushed, no flexibility. I'd also broken my

ribcage; it was so brittle that I could hardly breathe. My posture
had been getting progressively stooped, and I was told the vertebrae would eventually collapse. But suddenly my spine just
seemed to straighten out, *pop-pop-pop*. Then the compound
fractures in my back just went *pow-pow-pow* for about two hours,
a slow snapping. And I could stand again! I knew right then
that I was going to be healed.

After that, the five months of chemotherapy came pouring
out in three days. I could smell it in my perspiration. I had
sooty stuff coming out of my pores and under my arms, and
burns on my face from the chemicals. It was scary at first. The
doctor spoke mostly Spanish, but his name was Doctor Dias—
"Doctor God," I thought—so I felt better.

When I came back home from the clinic three weeks later,
my neighbors didn't know who I was. When I'd left, I was gray-
faced, stooped-over, ugly, awful. I looked dead, because I *was*
dying. Now I was tanned, I was up and moving, I was hopping
around like a twenty-year-old girl. I even started menstruating
again.

Marilyn's miraculous-sounding story does not end, however, with
her walking off into the effulgent light of healing glory and resum-
ing a normal life. When she went off the diet for five months,
"Everything started reversing. It was terrible. The weakness, the
respiratory infections, the pneumonia, the lowered immunity all
came back." She also told me that she recently had "a bad Pap smear,"
and resumed hormone treatment "after a lot of agonizing and re-
searching abstracts at the UCLA Biomedical Library." When I met
her, she had been engaged in an incredible—some might say
frantic—therapeutic regimen for more than four years: drinking
copious quantities of carrot juice, taking enemas, stretching her
monthly budget on an array of organic food products required by
the purifying diet she believes continues to keep her alive.

But clearly, Marilyn had been through an extraordinary healing
experience that had seemingly cleansed both her mind and her body.
The central metaphor of her journey, purification, has a venerable
history in the annals of mind-body healing: At the Asklepian temple
(the inscription on which read BONUS INTRA, MELIOR EXI—"Go in
good, come out better"), the first step was a complete cleansing of
the body. This purification was also said to free the soul from contamination. Many holistic treatments include detoxification, which
is said to be capable of "bringing out the underlying pathology"

through a series of healing crises (much as the psyche is thought to be healed through emotional catharsis).

"Things that came out of my insides were just horrendous. Blood, black, vile stuff," Marilyn says. Symptoms often appear to get worse during this process, which is said to involve the expulsion of toxins from deep within the bodily system; extrusions, as it were, of long-festering inner conditions.

In all, it seems clear that alternative treatments—whatever their efficacy—offered journeyers more than simply an alternative prescription: The daily ritual of ingesting special herbs and vitamins, the various practices to focus the mind on purification and healing, the oft-stressed doctrines of self-empowerment and positive expectation, membership in a community of fellow seekers, the primal act of nourishment itself suggest there were as many spiritual as physiological forces at work.

CAN THE TWO MEDICINES BE RECONCILED?

Part of the attraction and the power of alternatives may be summed up in the old Hindu dictum, "A plant in the courtyard isn't medicine, but a plant on the other side of the mountain is." The act of undertaking a journey toward the exotic and unfamiliar has its own healing power.

The Emperors of the Chinese court reportedly preferred Tibetan physicians to their own. When ten years ago the Gyalwa Karmapa, the head of the Kargyu order of Tibetan Buddhism, had stomach cancer against which his own doctors' herbal medicine proved useless, he reported to the American International Hospital in Zion, Illinois, for surgery. A Westerner who has set up a medical research project in China told me, "I was approached by this old Chinese acupuncturist who said, 'We'd like to learn about your alternative medicine.' It turned out he meant antibiotics and surgery!"

The modern West seems to be in the midst of discovering the "plant on the other side of the mountain" with all its objective and subjective potency. When the *New York Times* journalist James Reston was treated with acupuncture for postoperative pain while he was on assignment in China in 1971, his report on the efficacy of the 2,300-year-old tradition caused shockwaves: "I have seen the past," he wrote, "and it works."

Dr. Jacob Zieghelboim observes, "It may very well be that polarization between Eastern and Western systems of thought and medicine has been essential for the developmental process. . . . But perhaps in this generation, we'll bring forward alternatives that blend rather than discount, that integrate rather than substitute, and that encompass rather than exclude. I feel a greater richness when I can draw upon pharmacology, hematology, oncology, psychology, immunology, spirituality."

But many obstacles still stand in the way of the sort of reconciliation Zieghelboim proposes. As Richard Grossinger writes, "The art of healing often views technology as a shallow impostor, and the mainstream of technology views the art of healing as an archaic, uninformed troublemaker." Alternative medicine operates today under the modern equivalent of the middle Renaissance "Quack's Charter" under which people "having knowledge and experience of the nature of Herbs, Roots, and Waters" were permitted to practice, but only when ministering to the poor. Particularly in the United States, alternative practitioners often receive the marginal cases on whom modern medicine has given up; they are the helpers of the last rather than first resort.

Most conventional doctors continue to regard their unconventional counterparts as a prizefighter might regard a practitioner of martial t'ai chi: It is hard to imagine such gentle-looking gestures packing much of a punch. Most alternatives are considered capable of little more than "making the patient feel better" during the course of "real" medical treatment.

A physician recently told me the story of an M.D. who had gone to Greece to learn homeopathy, returned to his hometown in North Carolina, and "started practicing fifty-fifty" between alternative and conventional care. Soon, local physicians were sending him patients with intractable conditions—so-called "garbage" cases—sometimes with unexpectedly favorable results. Encouraged, the doctor switched his practice almost entirely over to homeopathy. His colleague recounts: "Soon patients who used to go to the other docs for their high–blood pressure pills and their heart medicine just stopped—they didn't need it anymore. At that point, the other town doctors *could* have said, 'George, what exactly are you doing, and can you teach it to us?' Instead, they went to the medical board, which sued George not because he was doing bad things to his patients, but on the principle he was practicing an unsanctioned form of medicine."

The medical board, the colleague told me, lost their case at every level up to the state supreme court. But the high court ruled in favor of the board, which it decided had final authority to establish common practice. Similarly, the American Medical Association (A.M.A.) Council, though essentially a trade organization, has vast quasi-legal powers. In an attempt to circumvent the iron grip of what often feels like a de facto (and de jure) monopoly, holistic doctors in several states have established parallel medical boards. One doctor who is trying to organize such a body in his state told me, "I've almost given up on the regular medical community. The major area of change will come through educating the insurance companies. Since insurance companies care about keeping costs down and making higher profits, a bunch of us have designed common forms for our patient data, which we're submitting as evidence of the cost-effectiveness of alternate practice. If you can keep patients healthy, I don't think the insurance companies will care so much what you do. The public will change if the companies will pay. Of course, it may take a generation."

Or sooner. In the first policy of its kind, California's American Western Life Insurance Co. began in 1993 to offer coverage—through a special "wellness health plan"—for alternatives ranging from acupuncture and biofeedback to aromatherapy, herbal medicine, naturopathy, and yoga. Later that same year, Mutual of Omaha, the nation's largest provider of health insurance for individuals (10 million nationwide), announced it would begin reimbursing patients enrolled in cardiologist Dean Ornish's "reversal program"—the first non-surgical, non-pharmaceutical therapy for heart disease to so qualify. Blue Cross and Blue Shield promptly announced they were considering similar measures.

Cost containment may be one of the driving forces: Americans spent $18 billion in 1992 on coronary-bypass surgery, making it the number-one health-care bill in the nation. Dr. Ornish's program costs about one-tenth the price of conventional treatment.

The policy was applauded as "terrific" by Dr. Joseph Jacobs, director of the National Institute of Health's Office of Alternative Medicine, which appeared in 1993 as suddenly as a spring crocus in the courtyard of the nation's firmest bastion of biomedical research. The Office's budget of $2 million out of the $10 billion N.I.H. behemoth—"a flea on an elephant, pen-and-pencil money," said Jacobs, who wryly calls his office "the Starship Enterprise"—is a controversial allotment. Jacobs resigned in 1994, citing political pressures. Even PNI-oriented scientists like Dr. Avram Goldstein, professor emeritus of pharmacology at Stanford University—a man who has studied how music can stimulate the brain to produce endorphins—are skeptical. "What's it going to be under?" he demanded testily of a reporter for *The New York Times*. "The Office of Astrology?"

The Office planned to mollify some of its detractors with some orthodox pharmaceutical testing, likely collaborating with the National Cancer Institute investigating Dr. Burzynski's antineoplastons, which have proven effective enough against childhood brain tumors to warrant clinical trials. But it will also scientifically study the efficacy of everything from hypnosis and biofeedback to "therapeutic touch" and "prayer and spiritual healing."

Other unanticipated forces are accelerating change. The AIDS crisis has led the F.D.A. to approve, in writer Peter Barry Chowka's words, "an unprecedented relaxation of some conventional barriers to less than orthodox research." Much of this new openness has been in response to pressure from AIDS patients, who tend to be "younger, more aggressive, and more organized than cancer patients," as Dr. Adan Rios told me.

Dr. Rios believes that both institutional and alternative practitioners are "starting to drop preconceived notions of each other," particularly as doctors notice that patients they had written off for dead are surviving outside the medical fold. "If we try to force people to abandon some alternate therapy they've found," he says, "they're going to go off and do it anyway, only now we've alienated them and will lose the potentially valuable data they might give us. The protocol ought to be to ask if we could at least follow them, see what happens, and document it."

Rios describes the AIDS patient to whom he attributes his own change in thinking: "I had always considered side effects a minor part of the treatment decision. But one AIDS patient who, over my strenuous objections, decided to stop treatment said, 'No thanks. I'm not into suffering.' He had Kaposi's sarcoma, and I assumed he would go off and die. When he came in to see me five years later, I could only regard him with awe and bewilderment. And, to be honest, with a strange sense of disappointment—I had to admit he was doing well even though I had had nothing to do with it. It hurt my ego. Now I tell people I'll accept healing no matter what the cause."

Accepting the existence of other healing paths remains a difficult hurdle for many physicians. It feels galling to acknowledge the possibility that, in the words of one, "Someone other than ourselves might be more appropriate—the hypnotist, the chiropractor, the spiritual healer, the massage therapist, the nutritionist, clinical ecologist might have a better key to that patient's healing than we do."

Alternative medicine might be seen as a continuation of an ancient "empiricist" tradition that believes in the uniqueness of each symptom and individual, and seeks insight by examining the functions of the living whole rather than its discrete chemical or mechanical parts. By contrast, writes Professor Richard Grossman of New York's Montefiore Medical Center, the scientific rationalist

> seeks to generalize the laws of healing. To achieve this he studies the etiology (the origin and "natural" course) of disease processes, and his intent is especially focused on the application of a quick, mechanical treatment of a dominant single symptom. . . . In modern, organized, consensual medicine—the medicine increasingly paid for, monitored, and managed by governments in an unsettled partnership with corporations—the rationalist view has clearly triumphed.[24]

In many crucial ways, the rationalist view may have earned its currently dominant place. But the fact remains that technological, "heroic" medicine has represented a detour from traditional practices that saw body, mind, and spirit as a unity; believed the body itself was the hero; instinctively understood the role of immunity; and saw the bodymind as a dynamic, energetic system whose contents were not merely biochemical, but sacred.

Only now has the opportunity emerged to bring together what historian Harris Coulter calls medicine's "divided legacy." Despite the often vicious struggles that are waged between different forms of medicine—struggles that not only divide the healing community, but are painfully reflected within the hearts and minds of those who are seeking healing—there is new hope that bridges may be built. I recently saw, sandwiched into the evening news, a human interest story on an arthritis patient and her two doctors. One scene showed her M.D.-rheumatologist sifting diligently through a pile of herbs in the exotic pharmacy-office of her other physician, a wizened Chinese acupuncturist. As the Chinese doctor beamed, it seemed to me a trifle bemusedly, in the background, the M.D. said resolutely to the camera, "I'm sure that there must be an active ingredient in here *some*where."

The quest for the future of medicine may be leading us, on a long looping itinerary, back to the wisdom of the past. A few years ago I attempted to schedule a conference in Boulder, Colorado, with some of the most academically respectable lights of the new medicine. The plan was defeated by scheduling conflicts: One prominent doctor was preparing for a trip to Nepal to measure the physiology of Tibetan Buddhist meditators; another was in China at a conference on the ancient art of *chi-gong;* another, a program director at Boston's Beth Israel Hospital, was studying with a renowned yoga teacher in southern India; and another had embarked on an on-site investigation of Balinese healing rituals.

Still, such practitioners remain the exception in this time of the Great Divide. It is still up to patients to wend their own way through confusing and competing domains of the realm of healing. But they cannot do it alone. Inevitably, each journeyer I spoke with found a guide—the figure I call the Helper.

THE HELPER: THE WAY OF
THE WOUNDED HEALER

What strength have I that I should endure,
And what is my limit that I should be patient?
Have I the strength of stones,
or is my flesh of bronze?
Have I not helper,
and has advice deserted me?

—JOB 6:11–13

These souls turn back at such a time if there is none who
understands them; they abandon the road or lose courage.

—ST. JOHN OF THE CROSS,
Dark Night of the Soul

ONCE THE MYTHIC hero embarks on his own unique odyssey, observed Joseph Campbell, he inevitably encounters a guide or protector. This figure, who often steps out of the mists just when the journeyer becomes discouraged by the obstacles to the quest, is the "unsuspected assistance" vouchsafed to anyone who has "undertaken his proper adventure."

The figure of the Helper appears with some frequency in our own cultural myths: In the film *It's a Wonderful Life* it is Clarence the Angel; in *The Wizard of Oz*, Glenda the Good Witch; in *A Christmas Carol*, the troubling, comforting, relentlessly truthful Spirits. Such Helpers furnish guidance, caution, and encouragement, point the way to change, and confirm the existence of a path through the dark forest.

In mythology, Joseph Campbell writes, such figures are typically "some little fellow of the wood, some wizard, hermit, shepherd, or smith, who appears to supply the amulets and advice the hero will require."[1] When I was searching for help, these figures appeared in my own dreams with almost irksome regularity. Once it was a "tinker," someone who could repair broken things that would otherwise be thrown away. In another dream, it was a "wrestling coach,"who told me that though the opponent who had been chosen for me was "burly," defeating him was not "a task greater than your abilities." Occasionally, these dream figures asked me to perform paradoxical feats that seemed impossible—for example, to grasp the glowing-hot blade of an ancient dagger, which, when I fearfully complied, mysteriously did not burn me.

But the Helper is not merely a mythical figment. Time and again, the journeyers I spoke with described meeting such people at crucial junctures on their path. For some, the Helper turned out to be a doctor; for others, a psychotherapist; for others, a provider of alternative or adjunctive therapies; for still others, a friend of a friend, a relative, a fellow patient or a chance acquaintance. Whether they were located after a deliberate search or through a series of happy accidents, they often were discovered right in the patient's own backyard. Often, the Helper was a kind of externalization of the patient's own "inner healer," as if the psyche had recognized a champion in the outer world who could both provide tangible help and promote the soul's agenda.

Whatever their guise, their function was the same: to guide the patient to the heart of healing, insistent that the resources to proceed could be found within.

Early in my own journey, a friend gave me the name of a Jungian therapist who counselled cancer patients at several Boston hospitals. I was amazed to learn the woman lived five minutes by car from my apartment. Jane (not her real name) was a thin, graying, sharp-featured woman who gave an incongruous impression of ampleness. I felt comforted the instant she opened her door. She exuded an atmosphere of warmth and security, of food on the kitchen stove on a late winter afternoon. We clambered upstairs to the small room she used as an office and sat on floor pillows while I poured out a torrent of dreams and doubts.

"Have you ever seen tumors regress?" I finally asked.

"Sometimes," she answered, with an enigmatic half-smile.

"Have *you* seen anyone get well from cancer?"

"Some do, some don't," she relied cryptically.

"And the ones that don't?" I asked, knowing the answer.

She looked at me sympathetically and nodded. "They die." Her eyes misted. I stared at her silently as tears brimmed at their edges.

"I really shouldn't say this, it's unprofessional," she said musingly, "but I had a sudden intuition perhaps you *could* heal yourself." She brushed her eyes with the back of her hand. "We'll just have to see."

As we got to our feet, she suggested, "Watch the dream you have the night before we next meet. The unconscious will tell us what it thinks about our working together."

The morning before our next visit, I awakened with an unusually simple dream: My daughter had cancer, but was lightheartedly dancing around me, holding a piece of lettuce over her head like a hat while I stood by, infuriated at her naivete. Its meaning seemed clear enough: My ideas of natural healing were childish, silly and ineffectual. But Jane disagreed.

"I think this little ballerina is charming. I love her gaiety. Maybe she's telling you not to panic. Don't be so quick to dismiss her. Her playfulness has power. She's a *good* sign."

Jane looked at me a little sternly. "You must try not to be so literal-minded. The psyche's not some wire service to tear off the news bulletin of the day. Dreams, especially the kind you're having, come in service of a much greater wholeness."

She offered to clear out three days a week in her schedule. "And don't let yourself be pressured into surgery," she added. "You have to feel ready. If you don't, even if it's the last minute, I'd even call the hospital for you and cancel." Here, at last, was shelter from the storm. But I mistrusted myself so deeply at that point, anyone who would trust *me* seemed a little suspect. Jane's advice seemed too simple, too straightforward. ("Don't worry about diet so much," she had told me as we walked back down the stairs in our socks. "Eat a few things that make you happy, spend time with friends, try to relax.")

At our next session together, I told Jane about my plans to fly to California. "I don't like the sound of it," she murmured, her brow knitting. "Why rush off? Let's find out what these dreams are trying to tell you." But I wasn't sure I had time to explore my psyche. Jane could give me neither assurances nor medicine, and I was itching to do something, anything, before sacrificing a piece of my flesh. I could play at psychology later.

But I can see in retrospect that Jane was a classic Helper. A representative of the "low, dark, and small," she made no promises, yet I had intuitively felt safe with her. She respected my dreams more deeply than I did. She not only empathized, but was willing to give both her time and a kind of personal protection. Healing, I now see, may flow from the place we least expect it.

THE HELPER AS TRICKSTER

Psychiatrist James Gordon was working as the director of a National Institute of Mental Health program for runaways when he suffered a serious back injury. He reported to Bethesda Naval Hospital, where he was prescribed muscle relaxants and a week of bedrest. But the condition persisted, forcing him into months of unproductive consultation with orthopedics experts. Trying a few sessions with a chiropractor provided an interlude of drug-free relief, but the effects proved transient.

Eventually, in misery, he sought out a man who had impressed him when they had met some months before as "a cross between a shaman, a madman, and a healer. He scared the hell out of me. But I could sense he knew things I didn't." The man put forth what seemed an absurd remedy—eat three pineapples a day, and nothing else—and supported his "prescription" with what seemed equally thin reasoning. "His justification was something about pineapples containing malic acid," Dr. Gordon recalls, "which he said would affect the colon. Fine: Medically speaking, they do and it does. But he made what seemed to me an absurd set of connections—something about the lung and colon in Chinese medicine being 'mother' of kidney and bladder, and kidney and bladder being connected with the back, and so forth. Still, I was at the end of my rope. I'd try anything."

Starting on this bizarre course of treatment, Dr. Gordon remembers feeling "like a complete idiot." The teenagers he was counseling for drug abuse sniggered at the doctor who made a ritual of devouring raw pineapples. The fruit's acidity caused his lips to blister. And if anything, his condition only worsened. His back began to hurt as much as on the first day he had injured it, and he rapidly developed a 102° fever. "I called the guy up, very disturbed at what was happening to me. But he reassured me that this was all good—that you had to make a chronic disease acute before it could be healed."

"Amazingly," recounts Dr. Gordon, "after another four days, my back was ninety percent better. I went to an osteopath, and this time the adjustment held. I've been on a journey of discovery—of myself, of ways to expand the medical boundaries—that little by little has changed the way I do my own healing work."

Dr. Gordon says he will never know exactly what it was that led to his cure. Though it may have been the arcane physiochemistry of fruit juice, we might speculate that it was in part the sheer illogic of the remedy that finally led to his healing crisis. Many centuries ago, the Greek philosopher Aristides wrote, "Paradox is the highest thing in the god's cures." Jungian scholar C. A. Meier cites records of such "healings by paradox" at the ancient Asklepian temple: a Jew cured by being told to anoint her child with ritually impure pork fat, or a Greek devotee of Adonis directed to eat the forbidden flesh of the god's sacred animal, the wild boar. "[T]he taboo had to be broken," Meier writes, "in order that a cure might be effected. This makes it clear that the primary consideration was the cure of the soul."

The Helper often seems to spark a startling cognitive shift in the way the journeyer relates to disease, as well as to shake up the existing pattern of life. He or she may push the patient toward "shadow-work," helping to uncover rejected aspects of the self that, long sequestered in darkness, contain powers of both sickness and healing. As Campbell remarks, the Helper has "the forces of the unconscious at his side," and may sometimes guide us, for our own good, "to the peril of all our rational ends."[2] Brooke Medicine Eagle, a Native American Helper, writes: "All forms of healing intervention act to disrupt the continuity of the present disorder, the present limiting trance. . . . Anything can be used that, without causing damage or unnecessary distress, creates a radical discontinuity in the way the dis-eased person's reality is assembled. Then the dance toward wholeness can begin."[3]

Dr. Richard Moss, who uses dance and other spiritual-emotional exercises as techniques for wellness, assigns three "assistants" to help those who attend his workshops. In Moss's schema, one assistant is responsible for "creative involvement," suggesting images and feelings that might "break the habitual stimulus/response equation so that a new and unanticipated response emerges." The second is to encourage intensity, "a kind of tension that itself produces attention." This Helper acts as "a throttle": sometimes "urging . . . greater effort, more vigor" to cut through inertia, and at other times, "if the person is trying too hard, decreasing the force." The third Helper is unconditional love. This aide "is asked to merge his or her awareness with the dancer unconditionally . . . to accept the dancer no matter what."[4]

Moss describes a patient at one workshop who appeared "lifeless and self-conscious," barely moving to the music. He urged her to put more of herself into the dance. "She replied that she had cancer.

Before I could even begin to consider this, I heard myself saying, 'Dance! You aren't dead yet!' "

Moss reports the woman later told him his remark had made her "furious, first with me and then with her own apathy. She realized that it was true, she wasn't dead yet, and she tried to dance, although it was not easy and caused her pain." From this point on, her symptoms underwent a marked improvement.[5]

AWAKENING THE HEALER WITHIN

The endocrinologist Dr. Leonard Wisneski observes: "The idea of therapeutic relaxation, which has become such a watchword in holistic medicine, doesn't tell the whole story. It's a little like putting a piece of toast in an unplugged toaster: The toast may relax a little in the darkness of the slot, but it won't change. It has to be plugged in for this mysterious transformation called toast to happen. What provides the power is a powerful motivation: 'I really, really *want* to get better.' Absent this, you'll see *nada* in the way of healing."

From this standpoint, the Helper is less the provider of the cure than an awakener, instigator and even provocateur of the patient's own slumbering inner powers. Neurologist Oliver Sacks, recuperating from the disastrous consequences of a leg injury, relates how he was invited back into the "dance of life" by a friend, who asked him to go to a memorial service being held at Westminster Abbey for one of Sacks's idols, the poet W. H. Auden. Pleading convalescence, he declined. As Sacks describes the episode in his book, *A Leg to Stand On*, he tried to explain to his physiotherapist the day after the service why he was unable to go:

> "I couldn't. I wanted to, but it was unthinkable, not to be thought of."
>
> " 'Unthinkable?' " she exploded. " 'Not to be thought of?' *Of course*, you could have gone. You should have gone. What the hell stopped you? Why shouldn't you go out?"
>
> My God, she was right! Who had stopped me, what had stopped me? What nonsense I had uttered about "not to be thought of." The moment she spoke and said "Why not?" a great barrier disappeared—though I had no thought of it as a barrier, just "not to be thought of." Whatever it was, I was liberated by her words, and said, "Dammit, I am going out right now."
>
> "Good," she replied, "And high time, too."

This urging toward autonomy, toward seizing one's own power, is a common characteristic of the Helper. When Dorothy and her ragged band of supplicants approach the Wizard of Oz, he takes them aback by demanding to know why they think he should simply hand them their cure. The Scarecrow disappointedly complains to his companions that the Wizard "needs a heart as much as the Tin Woodman." But the Wizard is not heartless. Championing the "soul approach," he is spurring them on beyond a mere cure toward more thoroughgoing healing.

"Just giving the person treatment for their disease may not be enough," says cardiologist Dr. Dean Ornish. "Just providing information isn't enough. Most people now know what's good for them and what's not. What may be necessary is a real transformation of how the person lives, of how they feel about themselves."

Dr. Ornish's patients typically follow an extremely low-fat diet, engage in regular exercise, and practice daily stress reduction through yoga and meditation. But their uniquely dynamic relationship with this special care-giver may leave the deepest impression on his patients. "I try to change their belief system as to what's possible, and I think that in itself can be healing," he confides. "It's like when Roger Bannister first broke the four-minute mile, and suddenly the impossible became fairly routine."

THE WAY OF THE HELPER

In *The Wizard of Oz*, Dorothy is not only helped by, but is herself a Helper for, her wounded companions. She first discovers the Tin Woodman by following the sound of his anguished groan, coming upon him alone in the woods, his uplifted ax in mid-swing, "shining in a ray of sunshine" but hopelessly rusted in place.

"I've been groaning for more than a year," he says to Dorothy, "and no one has ever heard me before or come to help me." When Dorothy, moved, asks what she can do, the Tin Woodman directs her to first oil his neck, gently working it loose until "the man could turn it himself." He then directs her to oil his arms (so he can let down his ax) and finally his legs (so he can walk). Dorothy has all the hallmarks of the Helper described by the journeyers I interviewed. She hears and responds to his still inarticulate suffering. She helps to free him from the "rust" of a rigid life-pattern which has frozen him. She restores him to motion.

From journeyers' reports, a composite description of the relationship with the Helper would include:

Empowerment: Helpers refuse to treat the people in their care as passive recipients, insisting that they participate in their own healing. The Wizard tells the Tin Woodman, "If you indeed desire a heart, you must earn it." Helpers also take their cues from the patients. Just as Dorothy accommodates the Woodman's own sense of his healing requirements—it is he who directs her to the oilcan, and indicates where he most needs oiling—Dr. Naomi Remen of the Commonweal Cancer Help Program says, "I find that at the deepest level of the unconscious mind, the client knows what's needed. If I can be present without having any expectations of how he or she is supposed to change in order to be 'better,' what happens is magical. It has a deeper sense of integrity about it, more than any diagnosis I could make on my own, or any therapeutic strategy I might devise."[6]

Challenge: Helpers challenge patients to *change,* sparking a shift in attitude from death toward life, from ignorance toward self-knowledge, from disease toward well-being. "Why should I help you?" the Wizard queries Dorothy sharply. "Because you are strong and I am weak," she answers. "Because you are a great Wizard and I am a little girl." But the Wizard refuses to accept her self-definition. "You were strong enough to kill the Wicked Witch of the East," he says pointedly, ushering her out on her journey. One patient described her Helper as "nurturing, but tenacious as hell."

Acceptance: At the same time, Helpers seem to radiate an acceptance of patients—for who they are, not for how they fit into a preconceived mold. The Helper often performs the function of "mirroring," a particularly vital task for those who carry childhood emotional wounds. Osteopath Dr. Robert Anderson notes, "The art of medicine means giving patients the opportunity to do what they need to do when they are with you." Dr. Anderson remembers an office visit in which he simply sat in sympathetic silence as a woman who had just had a miscarriage wailed in grief for twenty-five minutes. "We can do many things to contribute to healing," he says, "even if it's only to listen, to guide, soothe, encourage, and validate."

Communication: Helpers are typically powerful communicators who appear able to speak patients' "healing language." For Marilyn Sanders, Charlotte Gerson at the Gerson Clinic "seemed like someone I'd known all my life; her *voice* was right." Dr. Jacob Zieghelboim, on the other hand, located a medical doctor who believed in healing as an "energy process, someone who could relate to my inner life but at the same time knew what an electrolyte was." Even when the Helper's language is unfamiliar, what they say somehow rings true.

Empathy: Helpers seem unusually capable of understanding the patient's vulnerability, pain, and potential—often because they, too, have been forced to grapple with serious illnesses and setbacks. Commonweal medical director Dr. Naomi Remen, who underwent seven major surgeries for Crohn's disease, explains, "You may feel lost, frightened, trapped. My woundedness allows me to find you and be with you. . . . We are here together, both capable of suffering, both capable of healing."

Protection: The Helpers provide not only treatment and advice, but sanctuary. Like the Good Witch Glenda in *The Wizard of Oz*, the Helper provides a "kiss of protection" on the journey through a country that, as Glenda unflinchingly tells Dorothy, is "sometimes dark and terrible." Patients have reported that the Helper had an almost uncanny ability to appear when most needed. Like the divine go-between Hermes, the Helper becomes guardian of the dangerously charged spaces Joseph Campbell calls "threshold passages."

Touch: Asklepius learned the art of healing from the centaur Chiron, whose name means "working by hand." Helpers give "hands-on" assistance, often using the ancient balm of touch. One family doctor relates that doing "body-work" on her patients gave her "access to emotional and physical levels of healing the biomechanical model never did." Dr. Oliver Sacks was convinced he was not yet ready to walk. His physiotherapist gave him a long look and then, "seeing the uselessness of words, wordlessly moved my left leg with her leg, pushing it to a new position, so that it made, or was made to make, a sort of step. Once this was done, I saw how to do it. I could not be told, but could be instantly shown."[7] Whether through massage, acupressure, or a simple hug, the Helper speaks to the ailing body in the way it can most tangibly comprehend.

Involvement: The relationship with the Helper often transcends normal professional bounds, becoming something more like a true friendship or sometimes even an apprenticeship. Anthropologist Ruth Inge-Heinze, who made a thirty-year study of medical practices around the world, has observed, "Because what cures a patient is so often not what a practitioner *knows,* but who the practitioner *is,* real and prolonged contact with him or her can be crucial."

Humility: In the hierarchy of the psyche, the Helper is allied less with the high and exalted than with the "low, dark, and small," the undeveloped parts of the self. In that spirit, the Helper rarely promises a cure, but rather tries to help the patient grapple meaningfully with illness at a gut level. "For a while, there was a certain optimism that if only we could get people to visualize or have more positive thoughts and emotions, then they would get better," Dr. Dean Ornish told me. "But now it's more like: Use the illness to get the most out of whatever time you have. Working on emotional and spiritual issues makes your life richer, though you may incidentally find that you live longer than your doctor!"

Individuation: Helpers regard each journeyer as a distinct individual, and tailor their methods accordingly. They seem intuitively able to read what Dr. Bernie Siegel calls "the blueprint that not only turns us into a certain type of physical being, but also maps out the path of our psychological, intellectual, and spiritual development."[8] It is from this unique plan they built an architecture of healing.

Transformation: "Healing is creative, bringing forth patterns and connections that did not exist before," says Janet F. Quinn, R.N. "Rather than a simple returning to some prior level of being, healing involves emergence, and during emergence a midwife is needed. Rather than imposing, a midwife allows the system to move in its own ways; she doesn't force, but facilitates; doesn't push, but receives; doesn't insist, but accepts."[9]

In a traditional Navajo myth, twin warrior gods once set off into the unknown to try to find the house of their father, the Sun. On their way, they met up with a Helper in the person of Spider Woman, who dwells in a subterranean chamber (i.e., in the domain of the psyche) into which they must descend by way of a ladder.

Spider Woman, who though dark and small is the keeper of the web of life, informs them that the way is dangerous, with "many monsters dwelling between here and there." Like other Helpers, she acts as a guide, pointing out particular "places of danger." To help them protect themselves, she teaches them magic formulae to subdue adversaries and gives them eagle-feather charms.

But her greatest gift is the gift of pollen: "Your feet are pollen," she chants, "your hands are pollen, your body is pollen, your mind is pollen, your voice is pollen. The trail is beautiful. Be still."[10] To the Indians of the Southwest, pollen is the symbol of spiritual energy. It represents the energy of birth and the eternal potential for growth. The story contains the essence of the Helpers' role: Though they cannot ensure that the journeyers will reach their destinations, they strive, through word and deed, to make the healing path spiritually fertile.

FINDING THE HELPER

Among the people I spoke with, the Helper ordinarily did not show up until the patient had set foot, however stumblingly, on his or her own unique journey. Only at the point where patients had begun to take responsibility for their own healing process, to follow the promptings of their own feelings and perceptions, did the old maxim apply: "When the student is ready, the teacher appears."

Nevertheless, the search for the Helper was often conducted against the backdrop of daunting odds. Cancer patient Marsha Markels, for example, was determined to find a "holistic oncologist." She was told that "there just ain't no such animal, and I was crazy to waste precious time and energy looking." Uncomfortable in what she perceived as a forbiddingly cold, male-dominated specialty, she at last located a Harvard-educated female oncologist who headed her own clinic, only to be informed by her that "your mind may help your attitude, but it will *never* make a difference in your physical condition."

"The minute I heard that," Marsha told me, "I got up, told her, 'I'm in the wrong place,' and walked out."

She tried another highly recommended specialist, with similar results. Then, on her third try, she found exactly the person she was searching for: an oncologist whom she describes as "tough, the real thing, but also able to work at a deep emotional level. I remember one precious moment during chemotherapy when I lay down and he did a guided meditation with me. I was amazed—it turned out the guy had even studied Zen!"

Art professor Samantha Coles's image of her Helper was not nearly as specific. But setting out alone with her medical records and the unyielding prognosis they contained, she discovered the truth of Goethe's words: "The moment one definitely commits oneself, then Providence moves, too—raising in one's favor all manner of unforeseen incidents and meetings and material assistance."

Looking back, Samantha says, "When you begin searching for your own path, helping hands appear out of nowhere."

When she felt a need for psychotherapy she could not afford, she by coincidence met a therapist who was willing to trade sessions for artwork. When she decided to sit in on a class on the psychological aspects of cancer, she wound up meeting the teacher's husband, an oncologist, who gave her "the first semioptimistic prognosis I'd heard. He told me that if I wasn't dead in the first year, I had an eighty percent chance of staying alive for five years. This was great news, because all the other doctors were telling me I only had six months."

A friend suggested that, seeing as she was going to die anyway, Samantha might as well visit "this crazy lady" who taught "healing sound-and-movement exercises." Samantha's first sessions with the woman were at once soothing and unsettling:

"The first time we met, Elizabeth sat me down, got me comfortable, and then had me pick a single card from a Tarot deck. I got the Death card! But for some reason, it didn't freak me out. In that setting, it seemed almost like a good omen: We were starting out with all the cards on the table, so to speak.

"The truth was, I *was* on a path toward death at that point. I can see it in my artwork from that period. Your mouth says you don't want to die, but slowly and surely, one foot in front of the other, you're walking toward the edge of the cliff."

Samantha began her relationship with Elizabeth with no other goal than to get well. "I thought I was basically just *fine*," she says with a small, ironic smile, "except that I had this little *physical* problem." But her Helper began gently probing into her past, pushing her to explore the other aspects of her life. "One day, we were walking along and she asked if I had any alcoholism in my family. Well, *both* my parents were alcoholics. We started wondering together where that might fit in."

Elizabeth suggested she make one list of the reasons she wanted to live, and another of the reasons she might want to die. Samantha was surprised at how profusely the second list grew, and particularly "how many times Mom and Dad were mentioned." Later, in a session with a hypnotherapist, the long-buried secret story of her childhood was unexpectedly disinterred. "All at once, I remembered the physical and sexual abuse. I'd never dealt with it, but now I began to connect the dots: How in those traumatic situations, I'd left my body 'down there,' put my real feelings off somewhere else. For my own survival, I'd learned to process emotional experience through my analytical left brain instead of with my heart."

Many Helpers are fierce in their conviction that an honest emotional inventory was a crucial stepping-stone on the path of healing. Little by little, Elizabeth helped Samantha reclaim her emotional life. "I was starting to cry for the first time, to be able to say to somebody, 'I'm feeling bad,' and know it was okay. It may not sound like it, but these were *huge* steps to make."

Dr. Emmett Miller, medical director of the Cancer Support and Counseling Center in Menlo Park, California, encourages such brave forays as part of a Helper's credo: "a refusal to settle for less than the whole truth. This means that instead of allowing patients to choke back their tears and forget about the painful thoughts and emotions, I try to create space in which they can explore the sadness in greater depth."[11]

The Helper seeks to jumpstart the ill person's own process of self-insight, to penetrate the morticed bricks of habitual thinking that have walled off healing resources. One osteopath characterizes this aspect of his job as being "an honest yet sensitive mirror. The patient does not have to see the truth all at once, but I do not aid and abet the continuance of an illusion, unless (as happens in rare cases) it seems very important for the patient to maintain this illusion—and then only for the time necessary for adaptation and growth to occur."[12]

Similarly, in *A Christmas Carol* the Spirits prod and cajole the reluctant Scrooge into healing by stripping away his delusions. The Spirit of the past re-opens the still-festering wounds of childhood that they might be cleansed and healed. The Spirit of the present encourages him to shed his encrusted habits and fixed beliefs, to see with fresh eyes his immediate potential for fuller being. And like the Spirit of the future, Helpers try to wrench those they accompany from the straight-laid track of disease prognosis, to instill in them the passion to change what might otherwise be a fast-dimming destiny.

When he was twenty-one , Mitchell May's destiny took a horrifying wrong turn. On his way to a bluegrass festival on a rain-slicked Alabama road, a car struck his van head-on, reducing his vehicle to a twisted wreck, collapsing his lung, and shattering his leg in forty places. A team of several dozen UCLA orthopedic, vascular, and plastic surgeons conferred and decreed the limb unsalvageable. "From just below the knee down to the ankle," remembers orthopedist Dr. Edgar Dawson, "there was just bare bone hanging out with no muscle or skin over it. The leg was grossly infected. It had to come off." But May stubbornly refused amputation.

His mother, desperate for help from any quarter, sought out a healer whose unorthodox methods included laying on of hands, hypnosis, and prayer. Jack Gray was not a healer in the classic image, unless one's imagination ran to old-timers with impasto-thick New York accents and polyester leisure suits. But this odd apparition drove his wheezing Pinto in from the Valley after work each day to stand without sleep by Mitchell's side. "His hands would dance around me," says May. "He managed to take me into very deep trance states, just using his voice." Within three days of these strange ministrations, Mitchell's constant pain was gone. Over a period of months, his bone began to regenerate, the missing nerve and muscle tissue mysteriously filled in, and his never-set fractures began to fuse. Eventually he regained full use of his leg. Dr. Edgar Dawson, his orthopedic surgeon, does not hesitate to use the word "miracle."

Mitchell May's story is nothing if not utterly atypical, a one-in-ten-million ticket stub in a cosmic lottery. Yet it suggests the latent, perhaps vast healing powers the bodymind may sometimes mobilize when the Helper provides the catalyst. Jack Gray threw himself unreservedly into every aspect of Mitchell's life. "He was not only a healer, but a teacher, a magician, and a therapist. He told me unresolved family problems—he called them my 'old umbilicus'—could keep my own healing powers from kicking in, so he would get my whole family into the hospital room to create a sort of transfer of trust. My father, who is ex-military brass, was very impressed this old guy could stand for twelve hours hardly ever moving his feet. For my mother, it was seeing him pouring his whole being into me without even knowing who I was."

Mitchell told me that Jack was also a trickster, performing stunts that "knocked me on my butt, just exploded my frame of reference. Jack had worked in vaudeville, and he'd learned a bag-full of stuff from the Hindu yogis they used to call the Indian Rubber Men. Late at night in my room, he'd persuade some unsuspecting intern to hook him up to the blood pressure machine and amaze us by changing the readings at will. He'd seemingly stop his pulse, or stick a needle in his arm and show how it wouldn't bleed, or hold his hand over a Zippo lighter without any visible pain or burning. He was goading me to totally turn around my thinking about the mind and body."

Over a years-long struggle that took him from a wheelchair to leg-braces to, finally, full mobility, Mitchell became a student of, and finally an apprentice to his healer, spending seven years learning from him until the man died. Now a cheerful forty-two-year-old with a mane of hair that streams off his prominent bald spot like water off a rock, he has gone from patient to Helper. Pressed to describe what the healer had done for him, and what he now tries to do for others, May once explained: "A lot of healing is breaking habits. It's changing the personal story. My story was: 'I'll never walk again, I'll be in pain, I'll be in and out of a wheelchair my whole life.' Then Jack came along. *His* story was that we were created in the image of God and that everything we need is within us. It was his guidance that enabled me to shift."[13] As far as Mitchell can tell, it was this powerful, fundamental change of perspective that was the impetus for his cure.

THE HEALING APPRENTICESHIP

Relationships with Helpers who were health practitioners may also extend considerably beyond office visits or treatment sessions. The Helper becomes an active presence, a mentor, in the person's life. There is an eye-level interaction, as with a senior colleague involved in a common project. Among practitioners who are irresponsible or otherwise deeply troubled, such fluid boundaries may provide the opportunity to engage in manipulative and violative behavior. But much more often, the relationship creates an intensive learning situation in which one person happens to be a student and one the teacher, both bound by a common human predicament.

Marsha Markels's relationship with her oncologist was not always ideal. They sometimes argued: "I had to be willing to be a 'bad' person who didn't always agree with him," she says. "I learned to risk rejection, even though my life depended on him because he had the medicine. I didn't put myself in a position of being less powerful. The important thing," Marsha concluded, "was that it was *a real* relationship, with all the give-and-take."

Ernie Scharhag, who cast off the moorings of conventional therapy while still suffering symptoms of lymphoma, met his Helper in the form of a visiting Tibetan physician. "The minute I saw him," Ernie says, "I felt I had known him for a thousand years. It wasn't even 'Here's this guy who can save me,' but rather, 'Here's a guy who touches my heart.' "

The doctor recommended radical dietary changes, prescribed three types of herbal pills, and taught Ernie special meditation practices to foster healing. To Ernie's surprise, "He never told me, 'I'll cure you.' He did suggest I'd had enough chemotherapy, and any more would be 'poisonous' and could weaken my body's ability to 'transmute energy.' It created this terrible moment of conflict. My first thought was, 'Forget this esoteric crap.' But he was so understated and yet so completely confident, my second thought was just, 'If I'm going to die, I might as well die his way.' "

Ernie was so drawn to the man that he asked if he could assist him in his work. Before he knew it, he was helping to prepare herbs and make other patients comfortable. It was a pattern I noticed in a number of cases: Like the novice samurai who might find himself weeding the master swordsman's garden, preparing tea and sweeping the floors, the relationship between journeyer and Helper became something resembling an apprenticeship.

In traditional societies, apprenticeship accomplishes a variety of purposes. In rendering service, the student becomes more than just an empty, passive vessel, but a person with his or her own resources. Learning becomes grounded in daily experience. By watching the master go about everyday routines, the apprentice learns the details—breathes in the very atmosphere—of the craft. The craft, in this case, is the art of wholeness. In such situations, the Helper places patients in the position of not merely receiving, but offering.

"If you wish me to use my magic power to send you home again," the Wizard tells Dorothy, "you must do something for me first. Help me and I will help you." Such a bargain often proves empowering: Even though journeyers are sick, they discover they still have the energy to give something, no matter how small. They are no longer in a special category, isolated from the rest of humanity, swallowed up by the sheer immensity of their own pressing needs. John Davies [not his real name] believes he contracted the HIV virus from a blood transfusion while stationed with the Air Force in Amsterdam. In the course of his search, he came across a book by a doctor who claimed to have mitigated the disease's symptoms with a natural healing approach. Calling the publisher and finding out that the author coincidentally lived in his hometown, John excitedly looked the man up and "flat-out asked to be his assistant. Amazingly, he took me on, and we became good friends."

A little while after that, John met Clara, a volunteer acupuncturist, at an AIDS patient organization. Clara was a classic "wounded healer," a former medical anthropology student who had fallen ill just before her scheduled departure to study leprosy at a famous Middle Eastern hospital. After being healed with the help of an acupuncturist, Clara had enrolled in a Chinese medical school. When a fellow student came down with symptoms of AIDS, she decided to devote herself to doing what was possible to alleviate his suffering. After she graduated, she dedicated a large portion of her practice to AIDS patients in a loosely organized "healing circle."

John, a member of the same circle, had begun donating Thursday nights to organizing rides for AIDS patients who had no transportation. In the life-during-wartime atmosphere of the epidemic, John became Clara's assistant and later, in his words, "a sort of guinea pig. There *are* no traditional Chinese treatments for AIDS. I was sick, there was no other path of hope, I figured why not? Even the most venerable old acupuncturists have to improvise. So Clara would try different herbs, different protocols, to see if they could affect the virus."

Their collaborative work—one of them patient, one of them healer, each in their own way Helpers—drew them closer.

Eventually, to their mutual surprise, John and Clara became "safe-sex lovers." They moved in together, working as well-known co-therapists among the AIDS community, publishing a newsletter and running an informal network for hundreds of patients.

Debby Ogg's Helper, too, was an acupuncturist, whom she had found after a search through a maze of alternative treatment.

> I was going around trying all sorts of holistic workshops. I started a macrobiotic diet. I did weird breathing exercises that required getting up in the middle of the night. Then, finally, I went to see this Chinese healer I'd heard about on the grapevine.
>
> After Lin [not his real name] checked my pulses, he looked into my eyes, and said, "I can fix this." But then the first story he told me was about a patient of his who *died*. Why did he do that? It seemed very deliberate, sort of laying it on the line so I could make my own choice, eyes open.
>
> Along with treatment, this funny personal relationship evolved. Money hardly ever passed between us. Instead, my

husband and I wound up doing stuff like buying him a new stove, or helping him dig a septic system into his house.

The thing about Lin was, he was always there. Every day, for weeks. He told me that once he took me on as his patient, I would always be his patient, and he would always be my doctor.

Debby says that Lin was true to his word, dedicating himself to her health in ways that were both tangible and emblematic. She recalls one small occasion that convinced her of Lin's commitment to her well-being: It was the time she came to a session with a broken nail, and Lin, over her laughing protestations, insisted on slowly and delicately cutting it off, saying softly, "No hurry-worry, Debby. No hurry-worry."

A CIRCLE OF HELPERS

"I don't want to imply he was a saint," Debby says. "He would sometimes get angry when I would see other healers." But despite Lin's disapproval, Debby, like most of the patients I talked with, arranged to have recourse to an entire network of practitioners. Just as spiritual seekers in India typically collect initiations from a variety of teachers who possess specific "skillful means" of instruction, pilgrims on the healing path often seek out different Helpers for different types of healing. Debby continues:

> For example, Lin wouldn't let me talk about all the feelings of anger that were coming to the surface. It just wasn't his thing. But Harris, who is technically a massage therapist and nutritionist, welcomed it. He's someone who really believes in the power of the mind and spirit to cure the body. He'd help me do dream interpretations. Other times, he would just hold my head and pray. I could feel it go straight through my body, like he was hooking me up with the Force.
>
> I also saw a therapist who I called "The Great Santini." He helped me relive the trauma of my parents' death. I would come into the office and immediately begin to cry, and cry, *and* cry. The well of tears seemed bottomless, but he didn't flinch. He was always present. I knew that one part of my illness was my body trying to resolve physical, emotional, and spiritual questions. Each of these people had part of the answer.

Perhaps this multiplicity of Helpers is needed to once again constitute the archetypal healer whose mantle was a coat of many colors rather than a pair of mechanics' coveralls. The legendary first physician, Asklepius, was described by the fifth-century poet Pindar as treating "those whosoever came suffering by the scores of nature, or with their limbs wounded either by gray bronze or by farhurled stone, or with bodies wasting away with summer heat or winter's cold [to] be loosed and delivered . . . from divers pains, tending some of them with kindly songs, giving to others a soothing potion, or haply swathing their limbs with simples or restoring others by the knife."

As medicine continues its metamorphosis, perhaps more physicians will become, as they were in ancient days, Helpers possessed of wondrously well-stocked kitbags to address ailments of body, and mind, and spirit. But perhaps it is unfair to expect a single practitioner to take on so many roles. Anthropologist Michael Harner notes that the shamanic healer was often only one "specialist" in a "circle of healing," which included other tribal members skilled in plant remedies, bonesetting, massage, or other special rituals.

Physician Dwight McKee describes creating such a healing circle for a patient he calls Lynda. He and other practitioners provided an array of different modalities, including "dream-work" and visualization, family therapy, transactional analysis, psychodrama, radiation, limited chemotherapy, and nutrition. Lynda, his patient, was in the last stages of terminal illness, and eventually died. But, says McKee, "in Lynda's case, the process of stabilizing her physical condition was secondary—a means of buying time for her to explore herself, to understand the meaning of her illness and the shifts she needed to make in order to become psychologically whole. . . . Becoming psychologically whole does not always mean physical recovery."

Like several other Helpers I met, McKee might be said to be working in the spirit of the shaman, for whom, as Jeanne Achterberg puts it, "avoiding death is not necessarily the purpose of their medicine. Healing is a spiritual affair. Disease has origins in and gains its meaning from the spirit world. To lose one's soul is the gravest occurrence of all, since it would eliminate any meaning from life, now and forever. Much shamanic healing is to nurture and preserve the soul."[14]

Dr. McKee is anything but a therapeutic fatalist. He has gone back into residency in oncology to study the latest advances in cancer treatment. He characterizes himself an "integrator," one who is trying to "use modern technology more flexibly while developing ways to approach the psyche. I want to become more familiar with technological innovations and trends so that I can better contribute to the research that tells us how it can all be combined."[15]

But how to know when to apply "soothing potions" or "kindly songs," "simples," or "the knife"—or all of the above? How much meeting ground is possible between "soul-healing" and body medicine?

Anthropologist Ruth Inge-Heinze described an illuminating example of the Helper's flexibility she observed while studying a Southeast Asian shaman. A patient came in who had been diagnosed with a brain tumor. Belying Western caricatures of the medicine man who touts the limitless power of his own magic, the shaman told the patient in no uncertain terms that surgery was unavoidable. "If you had come earlier, I might have done something about it," he informed the man, "but now it is too large for me."

The patient vigorously contested this advice, Inge-Heinze relates, shouting at the shaman that he was too afraid to undergo the operation. "So the shaman, who always tries to find *some* way to help, said, 'Well, I will come right into the operating-room with you and guide the surgeon's hand, and you will recuperate very fast.' Since the patient believed he was being addressed by a supernatural being—a sacred king—who was using the shaman as a mouthpiece, he had no choice but to obey." The shaman accompanied the man to the hospital. The operation went far more smoothly than the surgeon had expected, and the man recovered in an unusually short time.

The late Talcott Parsons, who made vital contributions to medical anthropology, maintained that the relationship between healer and patient is the same in all cultures, based on such principles as "permissiveness, support, scrupulous adherence to professional attitudes [and] bestowal of conditional rewards."[16] But his colleague Edwin Ackerknecht took issue, insisting that, as Ivan Illich has phrased it, "The medicine man and modern physician are antagonists rather than colleagues: both take care of disease, but in all other ways they are different."[17] And so the journeyer who seeks help on the healing path must contend with a fragmented landscape:

The doctor says, "Your machine is broken."

The shaman says, "You have fallen out of relationship with the whole."

The surgeon says, "I can resolve your crisis with biomechanical repairs."

The Helper says, "Your illness is an existential question that ultimately you must answer."

In Mark Pelgrin's dream, he was caught between contending worlds of healing, the dream-witness to an argument between two healing figures. "The surgeon, a modern expert, a true scientist," was alternately disputing and discussing his case with "a crude little guy" surrounded by crocodiles. But strangely, these dangerous animals did not frighten Mark, as they "seemed to be friends of the little ugly doctor with his crazy talk about 'home cures.' " Crocodiles, like other creatures that are amphibious or otherwise indeterminate, are held sacred in many cultures because they inhabit two worlds, water (the psyche) and land (ordinary physical life), without belonging exclusively to either. At the end of this "swamp doctor" dream, Pelgrin found himself "shaping a piece of wood, trying to let a figure buried in it come out. What it was, I didn't know. A crocodile? Or me?" Here the dreamer is already turning his gaze from the outer world of either/or choices, toward the more paradoxical inner realm of his own emergent potential. He is trying to let an unknown, buried self "come out."

This self is an ambiguous figure, full of portent and potency, whose shape he cannot yet discern, but which might contain the shaman's crocodilian powers of transformation. In his dream, his Helpers are awakening something whose existence he has not previously suspected. The faint outlines are beginning to resolve themselves into an imago. Hidden inside him, struggling from dormancy, the mysterious Inner Healer has announced its presence.

12

VISION QUEST: DISCOVERING THE HEALER WITHIN

*So great a power is there of the soul upon the
body, that whichever way the soul imagines and
dreams that it goes, thither doth it lead the body.*

—AGRIPPA, 1510

*Work of the eyes is done, now go and do heart work
on all the images imprisoned within you;
for you overpower them:
but even now you don't know them.*

—RAINER MARIA RILKE, "Turning Point"

WHETHER THERAPIST, doctor, shaman, or friend, the Helper
can only accompany the patient a certain distance along the
path of healing. Inevitably, the journey veers inward, toward a realm
where others may guide but cannot follow. Even as the journeyer
searches for rescuers and companions, it is in the country of the
psyche, writes the Jungian analyst A. Guggenbuhl-Craig, that the
unknown powers of healing are encountered face to face:

> The sick man seeks an external healer, but at the same time
> the intra-psychic healer is activated. . . . The physician is within
> the patient himself, and its healing action is as great as that of
> the doctor who appears on the scene externally. Neither wounds
> nor the diseases can heal without the curative action of the inner
> healer.[1]

Virtually all the patients I spoke with reported direct, vivid, and often startling meetings with this "inner healer." More than an abstraction, it was a living presence that somehow bridged mind and body, conscious and unconscious, emotion and intellect. Sometimes it appeared as a figure in a dream; other times, as a symbol during guided imagery, reverie, or visualization exercises. But even when the invocation of the inner healer began with an artificial technique, the psyche inevitably supervened, producing spontaneous fantasies with all the earmarks of soul-experience: idosyncrasy, complexity, and an unmistakable aura of power.

THE POWER OF IMAGERY

Seated cross-legged on the carpet, Marsha Markels holds up her drawing—a ferocious-looking lion, rendered in a powerful, folk-art style, exploding with primary color. "This is my white cell," she informs the group sitting around her at the Esalen Institute in Big Sur, California. "Frank told me my last image looked tired, so I drew a fresh one." Frank Lawliss, who is helping to lead this weekend seminar on "shamanism, visualization, and healing," nods approvingly. His red flannel shirt hanging over faded jeans on a big-boned frame gives him more the look of a truck driver stopping for a beer on his way to Albuquerque than a nationally respected psychologist. An Indian fetish dangles around his neck, while his belt is festooned with a tiny medicine bag of embroidered deerskin.

"Here are my killer T-cells," Marsha continues as she picks another rendering, this one of multieyed creatures bristling with rocketlike projectiles, each with the word "killer" scrawled like graffiti on its side. "Piranhas," she explains. "The eyes are to spot the cancer cells. And I gave them big brains, so they'd be intelligent."

Then Marsha reaches for another, less fanciful picture which instantly makes clear that this game of show-and-tell is in deadly earnest. It is an X-ray sheet, two feet long, with an ominous-looking dark area marking the spot where her cancer recurred six months ago—a year after she had begun her visualizations.

"I was just devastated when I got this," she says, as the room suddenly falls quiet. Then she triumphantly holds up her latest X-ray. The black area is now mostly white. Against all odds, the cancer, for now, has receded. "I spend two hours every day visualizing," Marsha tells me later. "It's very involved; I'm actually inside my body, making this intimate relationship with it, participating in whatever it's doing." Her conviction that she is helping her body to heal seems unshakable, though most clinicians would say her fantasies could no more turn around her disease than a toddler playing in the front seat with a toy steering wheel could turn around the family station wagon.

The idea that a subjective image could be linked to an objective physiological event is, one skeptical doctor told me, "pure medievalism." It was in some ways an apt comment. Medical theorists through the Middle Ages up to the time of Descartes believed firmly in linkages between mental events and those that took place in the flesh. In 1604, Thomas Wright declared that the mind-body connection was mediated by "Spirits" that "flocke from the brayne, by certaine secret channels to the heart."[2] Nemesius in 1636 asserted that "the Instruments of Imagination are the former[frontal] Panns of the braine; The Vitall Spirits, which are in them; The sinewes proceeding from the braine."

Today physiologists are discovering how close these earlier thinkers came to the truth. We now know, for example, that the brain is directly linked via the "secret channel" of the vagus nerve to the thymus gland above the heart cavity, which governs the production of disease-fighting white cells. It has recently been shown that the "Spirits" of imagery can increase the secretion of thymus hormone. And the brain's "instruments of imagination," the frontal and prefrontal lobes, actually *are* connected via "sinews proceeding from the brain" (nerve fibers) with the seat of emotions—the limbic system.

This connection is in keeping with the doctrines of Aristotle, Western science's first psychosomatic theorist, who observed that strong emotions affect the body, and that these emotions are stimulated by the imagination. His speculations on the intimate connection between imagination and emotion are borne out by physiology: damage to the limbic system, for example, produces individuals who are "not only lacking in emotions, but also unable to . . . hold symbolic images in their heads."

Scientists can now piece together a picture of the "neuroanatomical bridge between image and cells"[3] that runs from the frontal areas of the brain, through the limbic system and hypothalamus, the gland that regulates sleeping, eating, body rhythms, temperature, sexual function, blood chemistry, glandular activity, and immune function. The hypothalamus, in turn, is linked to the pituitary, which by altering hormonal balances affects the ovaries, testes, adrenals, the thyroid and parathyroid, and "conceivably every organ, tissue and cell."[4]

The imagination may be the crucial link between mind and body: According to a study that illustrated this by default, "[I]ndividuals who were unable to fantasize, who seldom remembered their dreams, and who were not regarded as particularly creative had the most difficulty learning the biofeedback response,"[5] In other words, without the imaginative faculty, the bridge between consciousness and flesh is difficult to cross.

What mind-body researchers propose is as revolutionary as it is ancient: If images are the "Spirits" that shuttle between brain and body, might they not carry on their wings the messages of healing?

ANATOMY OF AN IMAGE

Like many other patients, Marsha Markels's images became more elaborate the more deeply she explored the practice of visualization. She imagined her macrophages—the cells often described as the body's "wrecking-and-cleaning crew"—as blue elephants, stamping on cancer cells, sucking up dead carcasses through their trunks and squirting them into her "elimination system." This bustling inner Toontown may not be as pointlessly elaborate as it looks: As we shall see, there is evidence that anatomically accurate images can have startlingly precise effects upon the body.

A number of patients reached this conclusion independently. Lawyer John Studholme, a self-admitted "detail fanatic," took it upon himself to work out a series of scrupulously exact visualizations:

> It was hard to concentrate inwardly on something I could barely see on an X-ray. So I bought an anatomy coloring book. I colored in the locations of my tumors; my spleen and the blood supply that feeds it; my lymphatic system and the nodes that trap and kill the cancer; my mediastinal area where the big mother tumor resided, and all the healthy blood cells available to destroy it; my chemotherapy and how and where it goes after the injections, and how it can work in concert with my white blood cells. I pretended that each time I peed or had a bowel movement, cancer cells, dead ones, were meeting their doom and leaving my body.

Zen priest Ji-on also felt the need to imagine a meticulous visual schema of her body. Ji-on garnishes her Buddhist outlook—equable and ironic—with a twist of American psychologizing. "I come from an alcoholic, dysfunctional family. I'm a textbook case of codependency. I started out at the Center as a secretary, and then moved up," she grimaces wryly, "to one-armed paper-hanger."

Ji-on, found that the more responsibilities she took on, the more she became a lightning rod for conflicts—between austerity and worldly success, private life and community life, secular power and spiritual surrender—that eventually tore the center in two. She considered it a particularly crushing irony that, after years of "bad blood" between herself and the center's abbot she was diagnosed with a form of leukemia, a cancer of the blood.

Ji-on, who with her broad, placid features and wide-spaced gray eyes, calls to mind the writer Gertrude Stein at midlife, had years before discovered the power of visualization. She had been in a car accident that "knocked out all my hairpins," causing injuries to her vertebrae and immobilizing her for the better part of a year. Told by her doctors at the time that there was little they could do, she eventually found her way to a physical therapist she calls "the mad Israeli. He kept trying to get me to visualize rotating my arm, which I could barely move. I was convinced that I had to be able to *physically* do it before I could *imagine* doing it. We battled back and forth about it for weeks: Which comes first, the chicken or the egg? One day, I finally succeeded in visualizing the motion, and was thunderstruck to discover that I could *immediately* do it for real. It was one of those big, penetrating 'Aha's.' "

When Ji-on was diagnosed with leukemia, she ran out and bought a deluxe copy of *Gray's Anatomy*—"one with all those plastic overlays"—and began studying the circulatory system, blood, the immune system, the structure and behavior of blood cells, anything that might yield a clearer picture. She did her visualizations twenty minutes at a time, five times a day, until she felt she could hold an image steadily. "I had learned from my previous back problems that I personally needed to understand things accurately before I could work to change them." Then she diligently pieced together ever more sophisticated mental models.

I used coloring books, I made drawings, I did library research. I wanted to be very particular and precise. I discovered that if I did a certain kind of imaging five or six or seven times a day, it was as if the image was actually there within my body whether I was awake or asleep, active or quiet. And I got very excited about that, so that my whole focus came to be the process of imaging.

I later realized that, blindly feeling my way, I was rediscovering the kinds of psychophysical meditations you find in Eastern and even some Western esoteric traditions. It really became quite consuming, because I was completely *fascinated* with the details. In a way, I almost forgot what I was doing it for! But I could feel a growing sense of well-being.

Various schools of Buddhism, Hinduism, Taoism, and even Judaism and Christianity include spiritual exercises that superimpose an imaginal map upon the human body. As noted earlier, Tibetan medical and spiritual practices in particular include a highly elaborated occult physiology, a mystical body of "nerves," "veins," and white and red "drops," which is visualized with sometimes dramatic results.

The Harvard cardiologist Herbert Benson has documented the ability of Tibetan monks meditating on sacred inner diagrams of the body to raise their skin temperature by seventeen degrees—high enough to dry wet sheets wrapped around them in near-freezing weather. Benson suggests, "We've seen what one set of visualizations can do, in the case of so-called heat-yoga, or *tummo*. Could other visualizations work in other predictable, measurable ways? I think that's where our next studies will carry us—which imaging technique leads to which physical responses?"

Some studies indicate that images can alter not only general processes like the stress response, but specific—sometimes, *highly* specific—bodily functions. One study, carried out in the department of psychiatry at Michigan State University, involved the neutrophil, the most common white cell, which acts in the immune system as a combination beat cop, judge, jailer, and executioner of harmful microorganisms. As it circulates around the body, the neutrophil identifies pathogens, isolates them in a sac called a phagosome, and then kills them by "shooting" them with enzymes, a kamikaze action that destroys the defender as well as the attacker. Experimenters taught a group of college students to visualize the neutrophil and its peculiar, finally self-sacrificing behavior by using relaxation techniques, slides, drawings, readings, and imagery coaching. Blood samples were taken before and after the exercises and analyzed.

The investigators were startled by the results: Total white blood cell count dropped in all sixteen students. But more amazingly, nearly the entire drop was accounted for by *neutrophils*, as opposed to all other white blood cell types. By further refining the students' image-making, experimenters showed that subjects could even change the behavior of their neutrophils—specifically, their degree of adherence to blood vessel walls.[6] The therapeutic potential of imagery has not escaped medical clinicians. Though few doctors will venture a guess at the extent to which images could impact the healing process, interest at several major hospitals is running high.

IMAGERY AS MEDICINE?

The crowd, crammed shoulder-to-shoulder into the small room at Boston's Copley Plaza Hotel, is raptly attentive as the speaker races through topics ranging from healing circles to near-death experiences, a ten-minute bus tour of leading new age attractions. But this is a group with a low flakiness quotient. The lecturer, Dr. Leo Stolbach, is a prominent oncologist at Beth Israel Hospital in Boston, and his listeners are doctors and nurses who have signed up with enthusiasm (or in some cases, uneasiness) for this Harvard Medical School–sponsored conference. The modalities that he describes— positive affirmations, visualization, meditation—are, he insists provocatively, "treatment for medical symptoms and complaints, *not* just psychotherapy. This is a legitimate medical model, and we bill the insurance companies accordingly."

Stolbach orders the lights dimmed, and a film clip of monstrously enlarged immune cells—lymphocytes—fills the video screen. As they writhe toward a cancer cell, their behavior seems cannily strategic. Here are these little . . . animals, each one seemingly operating autonomously, resourcefully, within some group plan of attack, battering themselves against the walls of the looming, Death Star–like cancer. Like guerrillas destroying an enemy supply depot, a few close in and, in a pitiless pincers maneuver, "blow up" a malignant colony. As a dark substance oozes from the stricken enemy, the packed audience of medical professionals erupts into wild victory cheers.

Stolbach blinks happily as the lights come up. Such films, he explains, can be used to help visualize the body's natural defenses. After viewing them, patients are encouraged to imagine their own disease-fighting scenarios and draw them in crayon. Their doctors then evaluate the drawings according to a range of criteria—the size of the image of the tumor; how and where the patient portrays himself in relation to it; the depiction of the white blood cells; the relative strength or weaknesses of their images of treatment and disease, and the character of the interaction between them.

Dr. Stolbach taps his pointer at a slide of a childlike crayon sketch of bluebirds in a cherry tree, drawn by a psychiatrist with breast cancer. "This is a good one," he adjudicates in his cracker-barrel voice. "The bluejays are eating the dried-up, raisinlike cherries she is using to represent her cancer cells. And there are lots more ripe, juicy cherries—good, healthy cells. It's a gentle, life-affirming kind of image."

He moves on to a new slide. "Here's one that's not so good," he says. "The tumor is a hard, green, glasslike object at the bottom of the sea. Even though the 'sharks' of this person's immune system have teeth, they aren't going to be able to do much with a structure like that."

He clicks a button, and another drawing comes into view, this one filled with ants scurrying across the page like a picnicker's nightmare. "Bad," he says, a medical art critic. "The white ants—the immune system cells—are larger and more numerous, but they're not interacting with the black cancer-ants at all. And the difficult thing is," he pauses sadly, "you never get rid of ants."

Finally, Dr. Stolbach comes to a drawing of a group of knights in shining armor mounted on white horses. In this patient's visualization, he explains, the knights' job was to hunt armadillos, each returning from the hunt with their quota of several hundred. But the patient who drew it was being treated for a deadly cancer of the pancreas. His condition began to decline rapidly. As he became clinically depressed, "the ends of his knights' lances became curved," Stolbach says as he clicks to a slide of despondent-looking warriors, their weapons drooping. "His therapist was worried that he was imminently terminal. But then with time, he got over the depression. The lances straightened out again. And then one day, the knights went out and couldn't *find* any armadillos.

"The therapist thought the patient might just be giving up the fight, but there was no clinical evidence of it. They decided to do a CT scan, and lo and behold"—and here the audience lets out a collective, involuntary gasp—"the tumor . . . was . . . gone." The room buzzes—the doctors and nurses are too surprised to clap.

DISCOVERING THE IMAGES WITHIN

The study of imagery is such a new—and unexpected—area of scientific investigation that there is incomplete consensus as to which images, if any, might affect the course of disease.

The late Australian psychiatrist Ainslee Meares reported a patient with advanced breast cancer who had a dramatic remission following weeks of intensive (but nonvisual) meditation. But when she started to use an active vivid visualization—"will[ing] the cancer to go away, so that she could clearly see the lump in her breasts getting smaller . . . bring[ing] herself to visualize the good cells eating away the bad cells"—she had a relapse. The remission returned when she resumed her formless meditation. Meares concluded that the visualization had demanded too much alertness and "active control," which in turn had worked against the kind of "psychological and physiological regression which allows activation of the immune system."[7]

Meares's intriguing paper is, to my knowledge, the only one in this frontier field to take such a position. Jeanne Achterberg, on the other hand, has done interesting preliminary studies to ascertain which *kinds* of images are associated with healing. Her studies reveal that visualizations of archetypal figures who fight for God and country to protect their people presaged good clinical outcomes. Those patients whose disease-fighters were animals with killer instincts—sharks, bears, vicious dogs—fared slightly less well. ("Some people tried to force these images because they thought they were the most likely killers, but at the same time, they got disgusted with the gore.") Vague, weak, or amorphous symbols had poor responses, and those with the worst prognoses could "see" their cancer but could not visualize their immune systems at all.

Former cancer patient Ted Lothammer started out visualizing "big sharks eating little sharks, and white knights killing horrible dragons." But he found the images flat, impersonal, and lifeless. One day, an unexpected picture arose unbidden of "brown-gray mice running all over the place."

> At first I didn't get it at all. Then I realized they must be the cancer. Then a few days later, *white* mice came into my mind. All week I'm wondering why, but then I remembered: When I was twelve, my family moved to a house near some vacant land.

Every winter brown field mice would get into the building. One day, my father came home with two white mice and let them go in the house. Apparently white mice don't like to live with field mice, and they proceeded to chase the brown ones out. I remembered how the white mice would come out of the woodwork all dirty, then lick themselves clean like cats so their fur would be pure white again. They became wonderful pets. They would come up and sit in the chair. In my visualizations, even though there were only a few white mice and hundreds of brown mice, the brown mice just gradually disappeared.

Interestingly, in Ted's visualization, the cancer cells and the white cells are, in effect, the same animal, perhaps reflecting the fact that cancer cells are not alien invaders, but aberrant versions of healthy cells. Though they are killing the patient, they also, in another sense, belong to him.

AIDS patient Wil Garcia also began by using violent imagery in his visualizations. But Wil had decided his healing path would consist of trying to "create as much love as possible," in every circumstance of his life. He soon found himself caught in what became an untenable contradiction. "Every day I would come home, lower the lights, and proceed to visualize a war taking place in my body, with Pac-Men with big teeth eating the virus and spitting it out. In my meditations, the question came up, 'Why am I willing to love everyone, everything, *except* the virus?' I started to think, 'I coexist with the virus—it needs me, my body, in order to live.' It took two or three weeks before I had the courage to visualize—and I know this sounds even crazier—a loving experience between me and the virus."

The symbol that Wil eventually chose was a soap opera-hour staple of TV advertising: Pepto-Bismol. "It was just like in the old commercial, except instead of a pink coating in my stomach, I imagined this pink love-essence coming down and coating my entire body. It made me feel sensations of warmth, gentleness, loving-kindness. I would see it go down to where my lesions were and coat them in a very caressing, nonconfronting way. Then I began to have a conversation with my virus."

Wil, a former Air Force officer who still seems to stand reflexively at attention, had a conversation with his disease that seemed unthinkable, almost traitorous. He felt like a student in Tiananmen Square embracing the tank that would inexorably crush him beneath its treads. Wil's incongruous inner message to his virus was, as he recites: *"You're in a space where you do not need to act up. You're in a body that loves you. You do not need to be fearful. You can rest. You're so safe, you can go to sleep if you want to."*

"And that's what it seemingly began to do," he claims. "My virus began to deactivate itself. The Kaposi's lesions began to get lighter. And as they began to get lighter, my T-cell counts began to go up." Wil's AIDS, for what was to be a period of years, in effect went into remission.

Wil's image was interesting, given some clinicians' view of AIDS as a chronic disease that can be successfully managed by the body for longer periods than previously assumed. Wil believes that the peaceable emotional state created by his revised visualization stimulated his immune system more than an internal "war" ever would have.

His story illustrates a characteristic common to the vision quest: While early efforts often are directed toward devising anatomical metaphors that fit clinical pictures of disease and healing, once the journeyer enters the realm of the imagination, the personal psyche intrudes. Most patients I interviewed reported that mental images quickly became emotionally charged rather than merely technical. Their experiences confirmed Aristotle's observation: The bridge between emotions and imagination is open, unavoidably, to two-way traffic.

THE SECRET LIFE OF IMAGES

The very act of mentally "getting in touch" with their own bodies often tapped unexpectedly deep feelings. Many I spoke with recounted their impression that they had been unconsciously "rerouting" their emotions since childhood, rationalizing them away until illness had forced their rediscovery.

I was reminded of this model in a recent episode with my daughter. Exasperated that she had "blown off" some important math homework after I had spent an hour tutoring her the night before, I barged into her room and cranked up the dreaded Lecture on Responsibility. My tone was caustic, my anger barely suppressed—I had taken time from my workday to help her, and for what? My words clearly shamed her. Leah, head down, her face blank, began doodling unresponsively in the margin of a sheet of blue-lined homework paper.

"Do you have anything to say?" I finally asked, only realizing when she silently shook her head that I had just visited upon her the same crippling sense of inadequacy my parents had frequently placed on me. I suddenly saw in her stubborn, impassive expression not contrariness, but a frozen mask of pain.

Chastened, I knelt beside her and glanced at her marginal sketches. One was of a head that looked as if it had been wrenched off its body. Below was a torso, blood gushing from a crevasse in its chest. Below that was the life-drained face of a Halloween skeleton. What clearer illustration could there be of the "splitting off" of mind from body that occurs in moments of emotional pain, and the psychically grisly consequences? When I asked Leah how she felt, her sullen immobility dissolved into a flood of grief.

"I feel so horrible when you talk to me that way," she told me in between sobs. "I feel myself 'going away,' like I'm leaving my body, because my heart hurts too much. I don't mean to, but my mind just floats off a million miles. Then I get this cold feeling in my chest—empty, like outer space."

This sense of disconnection is commonly recounted by "disease-prone personalities." For some, the simple exercise of visualizing their own bodies is like a poignant reunion with a lost companion. As Marsha Markels described her imagery to the Esalen group, tears began coursing down her cheeks. "These cells were working just for me, they were mine," she said in a small voice that gradually grew stronger. "Nobody else's. We are so *connected* with each other. There's no separation. And the deeper our relationship becomes, the more the cancer seems to shrink. I'm connected to my body, to myself, in a way I've never been.

"I sing to these cells, 'You are so beautiful to me,' and I usually wind up crying. I sing it very loud. Sometimes I don't sing '*You* are so beautiful,' but '*I* am . . . ' We are just melded together."

For Margaret Green, too, imagery became freighted with overwhelming emotion, with a sense that she was not just healing her body but reclaiming a piece of her soul.

When I was in Mexico, I had started having pain in my chest. I went across the border and got an MRI [Magnetic Resonance Imaging] scan, which showed a mass on my thymus connecting to the aorta. I decided just to wait, but a scan six months later showed it was still there.

I decided to spend a week at Carl Simonton's healing center in California, and I imaged "sharks eating cancer cells" as they recommended. But toward the end of the week, I had this extremely vivid, spontaneous vision that wasn't on the program. I saw the mass on my thymus as a piece of ice that just started to melt in these big, amazing drops. I've never in my life had this kind of clear image just come up by itself. And I knew instantly that the drops were really teardrops. My whole life, through all the losses, I'd never been able to cry. Now there was this melting away of the oppression I'd been feeling; the deaths and the abuse in my childhood, the unresolved relationship with my ex-husband. The emotion was suddenly available, and it felt so powerful.

Four months later, I had another MRI, and the mass was gone—there was no sign of it. I hadn't had any new treatment. Whatever this mass had been, they said the only way they could tell it had ever been there was from the previous two tests.

Such experiences may suggest there was a grain of truth in the observation made by the Renaissance philosopher-physician Agrippa: "The passions of the soul which follow the phantasy, when they are most vehement . . . can take away or bring some disease of the mind or body." Perhaps the more emotionally "vehement" the image, the stronger the effect. But such experiences also demonstrate how, once the imagination has awakened, it pursues its own agenda. Entering the realm of the psyche is an open-ended process, and the destination cannot be foreseen. An unknown world awaits the journeyer who, perhaps with the help of a skilled guide, hearkens to the inner voices and discovers a community of neglected selves. Here, images are no longer just toy soldiers waging a cellular proxy war, but figures with their own resources and purposes, enacting their own parts in an unfolding drama. Though the journeyer has ostensibly created them, they may gradually take on a life of their own.

Marsha Markels began to feel that her lion was not just a killer of cancer cells, but "a female lion, symbolizing female power. Having power as a female in my family was *verboten* to me. But my lion goes out into the world, she is strong, she hunts and kills."

Ominously, however, Marsha's image of her cancer started to change as well, eventually taking the form of a fierce black jaguar. Her crayon renderings of it vibrate with the mysterious presence of some forgotten animal-god, a presence that at first terrified her.

But, she says, "I'm connected to this jaguar, too. I'm discovering my dark side, which I've always hidden away. I can't do that anymore," she says, again bursting into sudden tears. "It's been killing me. I've been afraid since I was *born*. I've worked on this issue all my life, now I'm face to face with it. There's so much *fear* trapped in my relationship with my jaguar. I haven't even introduced it into my other visualizations. It seems like evil incarnate, the worst villain imaginable. But every villain has a heart. There's something it wants from me. My dark side, where so much of my power is—it also needs love. When my fear is dissipated, I think that power may be released."

Patients who take the inward journey often find themselves grappling with such terrible ambiguities. The outer world—particularly, the institutionalized world of medicine—presents clear distinctions between evil and good, sickness and health. The inner world is contradictory, inchoate. To what extent is disease outside of us, implacable, irredeemable; and to what extent is it inside, mutable, a wounded part of ourselves which we have never dared approach?

ALICE THROUGH THE LOOKING GLASS

In her remarkable book *Mind, Fantasy, and Healing,* Alice Hopper Epstein describes her confrontation with the seemingly inimical inner forces that she believes led to her eventual triumph over terminal cancer. Her story is worth recounting here in some depth, because it clearly illustrates the power and paradox of the inner experience of illness.

Epstein's personal history provides a textbook example of the disease-prone personality. "On the surface," writes her husband, a psychologist, in the book's introduction, "Alice was cheerful, helpful to others, highly competent, and much loved by many people in and out of the family. The only one who did not love her was herself. She could do things for others, but she could not do things for herself. . . . Her manifest enthusiasm and cheerfulness masked an underlying depression."[8]

Alice's description of her childhood reveals the roots of this divided self. When she was two and a half, her mother's younger brother died suddenly, setting off an emotional domino effect within the family. Alice's grandmother fell into a severe depression, at the end of which "Nana" was discovered to have terminal breast cancer. Alice's mother devoted herself to frantically trying to stave off Nana's death, becoming so distraught that she could not even tell Alice that in the midst of it all, she had become pregnant. Only weeks before the birth of Alice's baby sister was the shocked little girl told of the impending arrival of a new sibling. "After my sister Ruth's birth," Alice writes, "we had two patients in the household: my grandmother, dying of cancer, and my mother, ill and exhausted from childbirth and concern."

And no room for Alice. Any attention her mother did pay her was stained by a deep taint of narcissism: "My mother transferred her ego to *me*." Alice was sent to dancing school she never wanted, entered into contests she could never win, taken for show business auditions that spelled rejection. "I could never be an ordinary person, make mistakes, be myself. There was always this need to be special, to be brilliant."

Even into adulthood, Alice understood that her parents' love for her was conditional on how much she bent herself to their needs and desires. When she announced her impending marriage to a man they disapproved of, her father, "in a voice as cold as ice," told her that no one in her family would ever speak to her again. Estranged from the family for four subsequent years, she was able to return only when her mother was dying of lymphosarcoma.

Alice's experiences limn the classic disease-prone syndrome: the child seen by the mother as an extension of herself; early emotional losses, in this case not just of her grandmother but of her mother's nurturance; a split sense of self—damaged, inferior, and unlovable inside, inflated and "perfect" on the outside—and the futile attempt to win love through inauthentic behavior.

The submerged tension in Alice's outwardly well-adapted personality surfaced two years before the onset of her illness, when she was studying frantically for her Ph.D. exam. She had begun the lengthy program "as if at some level I said to myself, 'Okay, you (meaning my mother) want me to do this? Fine. I'll show you. I'll do it with a vengeance. I'll kill myself in the process, and then you'll see what you have done to me.' "

The exam was fraught with intense symbolic significance. Now it loomed before her as "an event of world-shaking proportions," a "final challenge I knew I could not win," a "last report card." It was in a sense a final attempt to buttress herself against her inner feelings of worthlessness. When her husband tried to reassure her, Alice became infuriated. He didn't understand, she writes, "I had painted myself into a corner." This revelation was accompanied by bitter tears: "I began to realize—to my horror—that there *was* no self inside me, except the self that worked for A's on tests. If I failed, I would know for sure that I was an empty shell. . . . I had to get A's in order to be loved."

She passed the exam, but it was not the brilliant performance her fierce need for approval demanded. She could feel no solace or relief. "I had a degree that I felt was a farce." Like many patients I spoke with, something she had hoped would bring self-love turned out to be meaningless—not because she had failed to obtain a level of success, but because no success could bring her the elusive fullness of being that she really sought.

Not long afterward, Alice was diagnosed with a lemon-sized tumor in her kidney and metastases to one lung. Surgeons removed her left kidney, but within a month, the cancer had spread to the other lung. Her doctors offered only a three-month prognosis. She decided she would spend her remaining time, in her husband's words, "not so much trying to defeat the cancer, but to become the person she wanted to be."

Alice began a daily regimen of what her oncologist disapprovingly called a quack remedy, adopting the Simonton-recommended image of knights on white horses spearing black, slimy cancer cells, in this case in a jousting ring. This latter personal touch is psychologically telling, for her whole life had in a sense been spent in an endless royal contest for wind-blown tokens of approval.

Alice was disappointed that, though she faithfully performed her anticancer imaging at least four times a day for weeks, there was no noticeable effect. She was dying. In the midst of this cul-de-sac, her Helper appeared, a therapist named Dorothy. Among other techniques, Dorothy encouraged Alice to personify various different parts of herself—first creating an image, then letting it "talk," giving it a name, and initiating a "relationship" with it.

The first "subpersonality" to emerge from this new imagery exercise was "Baby Alice," an incessantly fearful two-and-a-half-year-old whose motto was "Mother is always right." Baby Alice hated the clothes she was forced to wear, always lied about how old she was, and sat in a corner weeping continually. Soon an entire gallery of other, more vital inner personalities emerged. Some, like "Amanda the Builder," were strong and stalwartly positive; others were more ambiguous. There was "Little One," a volatile dancer who was "nasty, aggressive, devious, and joyously happy. . . . She pushes, kicks, stabs, claws, spits, bites, strangles, beats with a club, punches, etc., and then runs away. She never gets caught. . . . I hate to admit it, but I liked her from the beginning."

Her most problematic personality was "Mickey," whom Alice referred to as a "manifestation of jealousy," the "skeleton in my closet." In Alice's fantasies, Mickey—a little girl who wants everyone to admire her and is constantly tricking other children out of their possessions—grew from an unpleasant annoyance into a titanic mortal enemy. In one fantasy, Mickey swelled into a towering, earth-shaking "giant chicken" that seemed about to crush Alice.

"In my growing panic there was a terrible new insight: 'This is the part of me that wants me dead! How will I stop her?' I somehow sensed that there was some word that she wanted to hear and that the word was *forgive*. So I turned to her and screamed, 'I forgive you!' To my horror, she did not stop, but instead turned into a huge vampire bat and came straight for me. I had no choice; I wrestled her down and stabbed her to death."

Here was a force that apparently would not be bargained with. But when Alice was asked by her therapist to describe Mickey further, the image of a monster gave way to a young girl wearing "very short dresses that her mother picks out for her," crying because she hates the idea that her new baby sister's crib will be put in her room. Mickey puts on a false front to "the adults," being helpful and making only the most veiled references to the baby's unpleasant smells and cries. Though she was not able to acknowledge it at the time, Alice would come to understand that Mickey—"completely motivated by other people"—was a perfect replica of her painfully distorted childhood self.

Over a period of weeks, Alice continued her fantasy campaign against Mickey, whose impossible standards and punishing self-criticism were squeezing the life from her. At last, she says, "I decided she had to be abandoned." At the moment she made this decision, Alice had a clear image of Mickey all alone in a train station, carrying a little suitcase, sobbing at being left behind. "Suddenly I realized it was she who was in fear of her life and was calling out in pain. . . . I knew that I could not leave her behind, because it was she who contained all my emotions. To live without emotions, even the bad ones, was impossible. I might as well be dead. I turned to her and told her to come, that I was going to take her up the mountain with me once more." Shortly after this pivotal experience, and six weeks after she had begun psychotherapy, the lesion in one of Alice's lungs had, against all odds, disappeared. But the other lung still contained a malignant tumor the size of a large marble. Through another series of physical and emotional setbacks, Alice tenaciously continued her "exorcism" of her cancer and, as she now saw it, her very soul.

As time went on, she allowed her subpersonalities more and more freedom. Her new fantasies seemed to differ from her previous visualizations: "They came freely out of my imagination and then took off into a story line that I did not control." They felt "higher in their authenticity. By following these fantasies wherever they led, I was giving myself the respect that I needed. I was giving myself a form of unconditional love. . . . I intuitively knew that I could trust my subpersonalities to lead me to eventual wholeness."

Her journey, still without benefit of further conventional medical treatment, proceeded through a seemingly unending series of perilous twists and turns. But eventually, X rays showed only a tiny spot remained in her lung. Determined to "sweep away the seeds of some new bloom of self-destruction," Alice continued her inner work, until improbably, there was no trace of the remaining lung tumor. In her visualizations, Mickey—with her flame-red curly hair, her purple eyes, and her green dress—had grown up into an "attractive, mature woman" capable of captaining the imaginary inner "ship" that hunted for cancer. At the time of her book's publication, Alice had been living for more than three years with no detectable recurrence, longer than any of the people in a recent study of more than one hundred kidney-cancer patients.[9]

GUIDES, DREAMS, AND DAIMONS

Alice's "Mickey" had gone from being an evil obstruction to being, in effect, a source of healing energy, a protector and guide. The appearance of such interior Helpers is a commonly reported phenomenon in all forms of inner work. Often they seem to behave less like aspects of the self than independent beings in their own right.

Debby Ogg kept up her meditation and visualization for some years after her illness, even though she had been certified clear of cancer. Her images had changed from impenetrable, thorny brambles of disease to triumphal " 'Mighty Whites,' armies of good cells I imagined from a drawing in the Passover Haggadah, millions of people streaming through the mountains into the Promised Land." One day, she reports, "I was going 'downstairs' in my mind, to this mental space I used to go for healing. I came around the corner and there was . . . *Buck Henry*, the eternal TV guest host! Everyone else gets great, exalted archetypes; I get Buck, with Bermuda shorts and knobby knees and glasses. And I said, 'What are *you* doing here?' And he said with this little laugh, 'Just hanging out.' But he's turned out to be so perfect. He lectures me sometimes, but he's funny. There's something that effervesces about him, just bubbles up."

Jay Simoneaux, a genial, soft-spoken carpenter with sandy brown hair, met his "guide" in his doctor's office:

> One day my doctor had arranged some conference calls to the big East Coast cancer hospitals to ask if I should get my lymph nodes removed. Out of the three experts we called, one said yes, one said maybe, one said no!
>
> I was totally confused. I had decided beforehand I wouldn't just hack at my body if I couldn't see any clear-cut benefit. My doctor, who is very progressive, said, "Why don't we ask your guide?" At this point I wasn't even sure I *had* a guide, though I had been seeing fleeting images during my meditations of this guy who looked like a Kalahari Bushman warrior. So my doctor asked me, right there in the office, to get in touch with this character. To my surprise, this Bushman image immediately appeared.
>
> When I asked, "Should I have this surgery?" the Bushman took his spear and jabbed it underneath my arm where I was supposed to have the surgery, clearly saying, "Cut." My doctor also asked the same question, three times, and each time the same image came, very technical and vivid. I decided to go ahead and have the operation. I don't know whether it really made any difference—the nodes all turned out to be clean—but the fact that I had trusted this inner information seemed like an important step.

But his Bushman, Jay stresses, was "not just an information machine. He was like a real person." What had begun as a contrived exercise in his doctor's office became a process of self-development that grew ever richer as he communed with this inner companion.

> Sometimes I'd check in with him and he'd be completely moody. He wouldn't speak to me, he would be downcast or pissed off if I wasn't doing something I ought to do. But then if I handled the situation on my own, he would come back and be all smiles.
>
> He's also become a sort of inner role model for me, an example of what real manhood is. He's muscular but not muscle-bound. He's sensuous and strong, he moves with grace and ease. He's like the Bushmen I later read about: They laugh easily, play easily; they enjoy walking on the earth. And they have a very deep connection with intuition and dreams.

Such encounters have been reported by many explorers of human consciousness. Jung, too, was awed to discover that his psyche could produce images which seemed to have their own independent life. He reported a dream in which he met "Philemon," a guide-figure who first appeared as an old man with the horns of a bull and the wings of a kingfisher, clutching keys in his hands. As described in his autobiography, *Memories, Dreams, Reflections,* Philemon "brought home to me the crucial insight that there are things in the psyche which I do not produce, but which produce themselves and have their own life. . . . Psychologically, Philemon represented superior insight [but] at times he seemed to me quite real, as if he were a living personality. I went walking up and down the garden with him."[10]

"BIG DREAMS"

Jung's dream of Philemon proved to be a spiritual turning point in both his personal development and professional work. Much of his later inquiry centered around such experiences, which he referred to as "big dreams," dreams which most often occurred in conjunction with major life passages: puberty, love, self-realization, middle age, disease, death—times when the old self was dying and a new one was yet to be born.

As is clear from my own narrative, such "big dreams" can prove to be powerful and sometimes terrifying sources of healing vision. Whether in illness such dreams are caused by a malfunctioning metabolism, secretions by tumors and other pathogens, side effects of therapeutic drugs, or just the mysterious activation of the psyche under stress, their frequency and intensity are often unprecedented in the dreamer's experience.

One AIDS patient told me, "I've been having the most incredible, lucidly real dreams every night. Sometimes I'll get up, go to the bathroom or get a drink of water, then put my head back on the pillow, and the dreams'll start up right where they left off." John Studholme remembers "dreaming *poems:* deep, plunging poems; raging, sexual poems; dark, brooding poems; painterly poems."

These dreams often have an unusual texture: Patients report that space appears larger (descriptions of immense landscapes and great halls are typical); they speak of intense luminosity and color, of the same vivid images repeated again and again, of symbols of anatomical processes, and of labyrinthine dreams within dreams.

Illness dreams often seem to be filled with strong emotions, by a magnification of feeling-tone. Dreamers experience not familiar anxiety, but terror; not aversion, but horror; not desire, but lust; not surprise, but trembling awe. They may have dreams of joy, laughter, and heart-bursting happiness—dreams for which our culture has no working vocabulary (but which the Bantu people of Africa refer to as *bilita mpatshi*, blissful dreams).

Sometimes journeyers report spontaneous imagery usually associated with mystical experience: powerful animal figures, rituals, sacred food, drink, dancing, "books" containing spiritual or medical instruction, gods and demons, wild animals, even psychic phenomena like clairvoyance and precognition—all the components of the shaman's world that have been banished from modern consciousness.

Among the Zulu, for example, it is said that the person in the midst of the shamanic initiatory crisis becomes a "house of dreams." Michael Harner, author of *The Way of the Shaman*, writes, "Dreams, from a shamanic point of view, are of two types: ordinary dreams, and nonordinary, or 'big' dreams. A big dream is one that is repeated several times in the same basic way on different nights, or it is a one-time dream that is so vivid that is like being awake."[11]

Such dreams, Harner says, "are to be taken as literal messages, not to be analyzed for hidden symbolism." But taking dreams too seriously is notoriously dangerous business. In mystical lore, those who interpret them aright are amply rewarded; those who do not may be destroyed.

Jung once described a mountaineer who came to see him with what seemed to be a dream of religious transcendence:

> *I am climbing a high mountain, over steep snow-covered slopes. I climb higher and higher, and it is marvelous weather. The higher I climb the better I feel. I think, "If only I could go on climbing like this for ever!" When I reach the summit my happiness and elation are so great that I feel I could mount right up into space. And I discover that I can actually do so: I mount upwards on empty air, and awake in sheer ecstasy.*

The patient assumed, as many of us would, that this marvelous, ecstatic dream was propitious. But Jung, highly agitated, implored his patient (who was also a friend and colleague), if not to leave off mountain-climbing altogether, at least to take two guides with him at all times.

Jung writes: "Three months afterward . . . he went on a climb with a younger friend, but without guides. A guide standing below saw him literally step out into the air while descending a rock face. He fell on the head of his friend, who was waiting lower down, and both were dashed to pieces far below. That was ecstasis with a vengeance."[12]

Had the dreams which seemed to beckon me towards healing similarly been leading me off a precipice? How can we know when or even *if* we should listen to our dreams? I can recall being carefully quizzed by a Tibetan lama when, years later, I described my experiences to him. What time of night did I have these dreams? he asked. (Tibetans consider the hours leading up to dawn as the domain of prophetic dreaming.) Did I actually see the figures, or just hear their voices?

After ten minutes of interlocution, the lama gazed at me with what looked almost like pity. "Next time you have this kind of special dream," he said, "you may do what they tell you."

But Tibetans, as were the peoples of the ancient world, are in many ways better equipped to navigate the trickier psychic shoals. Buddhist religious training, for example, has always included repetitive visualizations of deities to prepare the student for a direct encounter with higher wisdom. It is a way of giving the ineffable a comprehensible raiment—a standard uniform, off-the-rack, so to speak, with clear symbolic meaning. Encounters with the psyche could be thus more easily decoded.

Tragically, our civilization has impoverished us of these ancient symbols and practices without providing substitutes. "Big dreams" speak to us in a language we are no longer schooled to translate.

We have lost the sophistication of traditional societies, bred from attention, familiarity, and respect, to distinguish one birdcall from another, to understand why one "weed" is medicine and another poison, to know which dreams are wise. Jung insisted that "big dreams" were often impossible for Westerners to interpret without some understanding of mythology, folklore, comparative religion, or "the psychology of primitives."[13]

I recall in the midst of my own fumbling attempts to part the muslin veil of my ignorance, a dream in which I was confidently lecturing a college seminar. A student raised his hand and asked me what I did when I couldn't understand a book I was reading. "Well," I answered breezily, "I get someone who *does* understand to read it to me." Yet when the ever more complex passages in the "book" of my psyche eluded comprehension, I was unable to take my own glib advice. When a therapist offered to clear her schedule to help me puzzle out my dreams, I brushed her aside: Couldn't she see that I was consumed with more pressing matters than the parsing of dreams?

I would have denied it at the time, but I now suspect that I did not want my dreams "read to me," because I did not want to know what they were telling me: I just wanted them to stop. For these "big dreams" may ruthlessly summon us to confront that which we would much rather avoid.

In *A Christmas Carol*, Scrooge tries to dismiss the forces tugging him into his own Underworld as inconsequential imaginings: "You may be an undigested bit of beef, a blot of mustard, a crumb of cheese, a fragment of an underdone potato. There's more of gravy than of grave about you, whatever you are!" Informed by the Ghost of Christmas Past that he has come solely for his welfare, "Scrooge expressed himself much obliged, but could not help thinking that a night of unbroken rest would have been more conducive to that end."

But the Spirit more forcefully repeats its mission: " 'Your reclamation, then. Take heed!' It put out its strong hand as it spoke. . . . The grasp, though gentle as a woman's hand, was not to be resisted."[14]

THE HEALING VISION

Though such encounters may seem fearsome and peremptory—recall Job's cry, "With dreams and visions upon my bed, Thou affrightest me!"—they more often than not come in the name of healing. During the years of China's Tang dynasty, the Emperor Xuanzong (who ruled 712–756 A.D.) fell ill with a serious fever. In a dream he saw a terrifying deity engaged in subjugating and destroying fiends. When he awoke, the fever had left him. The account is reminiscent of the doctrines of the Asklepian temples of ancient Greece, which prescribed that the afflicted receive a vision of unmistakable meaning, called "the effective or healing dream." The right dream, it was said, brought the patient an immediate cure.

It is interesting to speculate whether vivid mental imagery, whatever its content, might have an activating effect on the body's "healing system." There is evidence that thymic hormone levels increase in patients while they are doing creative visualization.[15] And Augustin de la Pena of the University of Texas Medical School cites a 1954 study of cancer in patients diagnosed as paranoid schizophrenics: "As the psychosis becomes more apparent (presumably hallucinations, delusions, and disorganized thinking increase), the cancer remains quiescent; and as the psychosis is treated and the patient thus returned to his conflict with reality, the malignancy resumes its activity."[16]

In these cases, did some unknown physiology of hallucination itself have an effect on tumor growth? Along a similar line of inquiry, a recent article in *Newsweek* magazine described how the jungle plant brugmansia is used by the Shuar Indians of Ecuador as a poultice to heal bone-fractures. The article notes, "The same plant, they say, lets them see God, which raises the question of how much hallucinations promote healing—and whether a pharmaceutical lab could separate the effects."

In any case, the spontaneous imagery of illness is often well-nigh indelible. The Chinese Emperor deemed his vision so compelling that he ordered the court painter to render the deity, called Shoki, just as it had appeared in his dream. From that time on, Shoki, a truculent-looking warrior god, became a universal personification for a force that "routs demons and malignant spirits and drives away pestilence and plague." Anthropologist Knud Rasmussen reports that the Caribou Eskimo shaman Igjugarjuk informed him how "strange unknown beings came and spoke to him, and when he awoke, he saw all the visions of his dream so distinctly that he could tell his fellows all about them."

Scrooge, too, finds he is unable to erase his dreams. At one point, seeing how the Spirit's light was "burning high and bright; and dimly connecting that with [the Spirit's] influence over him," he tries to press a lamp extinguisher-cap down upon its head. But though Scrooge "pressed it down with all his force, he could not hide the light: which streamed from under it, in an unbroken flood."

The light and power of such experiences, as I and others can attest, is impossible to snuff out. (Jungians refer to such visitations as "numinous," from the Latin *numen,* or "command.") Patients report that the figures that spring from the loam of the inner life may remain with them long after the symptoms of disease have subsided. The encounter with the inner world leaves a living mark upon the soul. Jay Simoneaux says his Bushman guide is still with him (and in one recent visualization even introduced him to *his* guide!) Jay credits the intensification of his inner life with not only helping to cure him of cancer, but creating an active spiritual reorientation, giving him a way to incorporate into his life a different image of being.

Not everyone I have described in this chapter was as fortunate:

I learned recently that Wil Garcia, who was one of the longest-surviving AIDS patients, has died. Marsha Markels's cancer (was it her mysterious black jaguar?) did eventually claim her life. But those closest to them insist that their ardent inner journeying was by no means in vain: By turning illness into an exploration of the furthest reaches of the self, they had perhaps extended their lives and inestimably deepened their understanding of its mysteries.

Jay says of his Bushman-figure, "The main thing he did for me was give me a sense of my own part in the general purpose of things. I had felt, especially after I got cancer, that I was just a biomechanical mistake floating through a random universe. Now I feel like I have a place in a larger Something, a clear sense of being included, connected.

"Occasionally I give talks, and people invariably ask me, 'If I visualize, will it help heal me?' And my most truthful answer is, 'I don't know.' The deeper issue is not whether someone will be cured, but whether they're going to resolve their life, whether they're going to change. To me, that's what healing's all about."

13

INNER WORK:
THE RECOVERY OF FEELING

For nothing hidden will not become manifest,
and nothing covered will remain without being uncovered.

—JESUS CHRIST,
The Gospel of Thomas[1]

I N DICKENS'S *A Christmas Carol,* Ebenezer Scrooge, confronted by
visions of his own desolation, asks only one boon of the Spirits:
to affirm his potential to change. "Why *show* me this," he implores,
"if I am past all hope?"

Healing is in its very essence a process of transformation—from
illness to wellness, from dysfunction to integration, from breakdown
to wholeness. It is propelled by an organismic drive toward health
that never falters; by our own human potential, which continually
strives for fulfillment under even the direst circumstances; and by
the ever-moving flow of life itself, which, like coursing water, seeks
ways around, through, and over any obstacles that impede its progress.

But change, especially when illness has radically disrupted our
lives, can seem a frightening prospect. When researchers in one
study asked a group of seriously ill patients which they would choose
if both were of equal efficacy—an operation or a drastic reorientation of life—fewer than one in five said they would opt for personal
change.

Illness can sometimes be traced, at least in part, to our unconscious
resistance to change—to those times when we neglect "obedience
to awareness," to use Jung's term; when we ignore the shouts and
signals from the bodymind that something is not right; when we

stay mired in self-destructive patterns long after our dreams and our flesh denounce them.

But the change demanded of those who embark on the healing path is less a leap into the void than a fresh discovery of the ground on which they already stand. Just as medieval alchemists professed that within the most inert substance was locked the supreme good, awaiting only the right catalyst to reveal itself, some journeyers, through the catalyst of illness itself, found healing resources unexpectedly close at hand: in the hidden powers of the awakening self.

FINDING THE HEALTHY CORE

This, surely, is the central theme of *The Wizard of Oz:* Each seeker already possesses, albeit unknowingly, the very quality he or she needs to become whole: the Lion, his courage; Dorothy, the power of the magic slippers; the Tin Woodman, his heartfulness. His living flesh turned to scrap metal, the Tin Woodman longs desperately for the lost balm of emotion; yet in the original book, we are shown that he weeps "several tears of sorrow and regret" when he accidentally steps on a tiny beetle. If anything, he possesses precisely the tender "awakened heart" that the late Tibetan Buddhist lama Chogyam Trungpa described as the essential element of human development: "sore and soft . . . [and] completely exposed. There is no skin or tissue covering it. . . . Even if a tiny mosquito lands on it, you feel touched."

But the Tin Woodman, numb to his own inner promptings, experiences himself as a soulless automaton: " 'You people with hearts have something to guide you, but I have no heart, and so I must be very careful.' " The Tin Woodman's tragedy is not that he *has* no heart, but that he can no longer *feel* it.

(His plight calls to mind an intriguing study by psychologist Lydia Temoshok. She had a group of cancer patients watch slides containing disturbing statements like "You've done nothing worthwhile" and "No one loves you," each designed to provoke emotions like anger or sadness. During the slide show, the patients sat hooked up to a machine that measured their levels of nervous system arousal. At the same time, they were asked to assess in writing how bothered they were by the presentation. They reported they did not find the statements on the slides upsetting, but the equipment told a far different story: Their physiological readings, showing "the intensity of each person's *inner* reaction," had "skyrocketed." The discrepancy between their lack of conscious response and their strong, unconscious physical reactions led Dr. Temoshok to conclude that these patients were in some ways unaware of what they actually were feeling.)

I have suggested that the Tin Woodman is a classic "disease-prone personality." He has suffered the suppression of a capacity for feeling that in his case seems abnormally vital. His situation calls to mind Dr. Lawrence LeShan's impression that cancer patients often seemed to have "a special 'spark,' a strong potential for being alive . . . with the highest level of emotional force." This is the paradox around which Alice Miller constructed her classic work, *The Drama of the Gifted Child:* Children who are the most "intelligent, alert, attentive, extremely sensitive"—the ones who are "especially capable of differentiated feelings"—have the most acute receptivity to the needs of the dysfunctional parent, and are thus in greatest danger of losing themselves:

> This person develops in such a way that he reveals only what is expected of him, and fuses so completely with what he reveals that . . . one could scarcely have guessed how much more there is to him. . . . He cannot develop his "true self," because he is unable to live it. It remains in a "state of noncommunication." . . . He cannot rely on his own emotions . . . has no sense of his own real needs, and is alienated from himself. . . . Understandably, these patients complain of a sense of emptiness.[2]

How suggestive of the "empty" Tin Woodman's predicament is Miller's conclusion: "We often first cut off the living root, and then try to replace its natural functions by artificial means."

The living root of our human potential, according to the psychologist Abraham Maslow, is our "essential biologically based inner nature." In his landmark book, *Towards a Psychology of Being,* Maslow wrote, "If this essential core of the person is denied or suppressed, he gets sick sometimes in obvious ways, sometimes in subtle ways, sometimes immediately, sometimes later. . . . Even though denied, it persists underground forever, pressing for actualization."[3] Here Maslow is referring to psychology, but the laws of the psyche and those of the body, as we have seen, sometimes have overlapping jurisdictions. Time and again, patients described to me how acutely they had felt the pressing from within of forgotten emotions and longings even as they struggled against the juggernaut of disease.

For if illness is in part a process of progressive desensitization—

a loss of contact with our vital energies—then the task of healing is the opposite: to strip away layers of physical and emotional numbness; to bring movement to what has become stuck; to respond to cues from the bodymind; to reclaim the riches of the feeling world; to find our deepest level of integrity, a word rooted in the Latin *integer:* "untouched, unbroken, entire, whole."

Many patients reported that, after facing their initial terror, they sometimes found themselves filled with an indefinable sense of potential, as if healing powers independent of their conscious will suddenly had appeared unbidden. As we have seen, crisis may engage the innate healing system, stimulating an unusual "orchestration" of body and mind, producing trancelike states or psychophysical "hyper-arousal."[4] These intense states can act as gateways, thresholds to a process of transformation.

In his book *Bone Games,* mountain climber Rob Schultheiss describes the alterations in consciousness that he experienced after a shattering fall during a solo ascent of Mt. Neva. With broken bones, in shock, struggling to make his way back to safety, he was surprised to find himself in a strange "state of grace," his physical prowess and mental faculties heightened: "I crossed disintegrating chutes of rock, holds vanishing from under my hands and feet as I moved, a dance in which a single missed beat would have been fatal. . . . *What I am doing is absolutely impossible,* I thought. . . . One small part of me trembled with fear and fatigue, cried out to be rescued. . . . The rest, confident, full of an unsane joy, reveled in the animal dance of survival. . . . The person I became on Neva was the best possible version of myself, the person I should have been throughout my life. . . . I believed it, down in my very cells."

He reported powerful psychological after-effects to this striking bodymind experience. After climbing down, Schultheiss found his trail home, feeling curiously renewed: "It all lay before me. I felt I could pick it up, the whole world, like a golden apple. My old life, everything before that moment I had let go of the rock and fallen, was gone. It had been a dry, cramped husk anyway; I watched it blow away."[5]

Schultheiss's account calls to mind St. Paul's Letter to the Philippians (3:13) on the subject of *metanoia* (literally, "change of mind"): "But this one thing I do: forgetting those things which are behind, and reaching forth unto those things which are before." In the same spirit, Greek medicine held that healing called for a relinquishment of the habitual self. Patients at the Asklepian shrine at Trophonius were first led to two springs, Lethe and Mnemosyne. The first allowed them to leave behind the patterns of their previous life, and the other gave them the power to recall—and integrate—the new insights they would receive.

The previous lives of many patients I spoke with had been a jittery round of activity binding together divided psyches, conflicting agendas, and fragmented selves. John Studholme says, "One minute I would be gardening, the next minute practicing law, the next running, then playing the piano, then having a drink, doing yoga, reading, worrying, paying bills, buttoning a shirt or taking a shower. But if you had asked me the color of the walls in a room I had been in last night, or the color of my wife's dress, or the title of the book I was reading, or the look of my own face in the shaving mirror, I could not have given you a description."

Actually, many journeyers approached the problem of curing themselves with the same full-bore momentum that had characterized their lives before their illness. Arlene Erdrich reports, "I was going to be one hundred and ten percent. I was going to do five times more than any other lymphoma patient in history. I was going to run the house, take care of the kids, do things for the community, *and* get well. I wasn't really changing, I was just trying to be more of the same."

ENTERING THE MAGIC CIRCLE

For many of us, the initial response to disease may be to grasp frantically at a life that seems to be slipping away. Terminal patients in particular, says Dr. Larry Dossey, may feel that "time is running down, it is being played out. The time sense becomes heightened. Moments, heretofore unnoticed, are savored—but usually with a dread: soon they will be gone, and I with it."

Dossey speculates that there is a direct relationship between the quality of time perception and a patient's length of survival: "One can almost see patients living out their belief that 'since my time is running out, I must turn my body off.' " This constriction of time sense, which Dossey calls "a malignant path for the afflicted," is clearly expressed by one of Job's laments (7:6–7): "My days are swifter than a weaver's shuttle; they come to an end without hope. Remember that life is like the wind; I shall not see happiness again."

Dr. Dossey recommends using visualization, imagery, relaxation, biofeedback, and other techniques known to modify the sense of time. In fact, many of the patients I interviewed reported a sort of natural time-dilation, as if ordinary events, rather than speeding by, seemed to occur in what Jung called the "existence outside time which runs parallel with existence inside time."[6]

My interviewees and I avidly compared notes, puzzled that even as we had hurtled into the black hole of illness, uncertain where or if we might reemerge, we had experienced such an incongruous sense of possibility. Debby Ogg says that her state of mind reminded her of the strange interlude that she had experienced while giving birth to her daughter, Jenny. "It was interminably long and very short at the same time. It reminded me of when I was a child, when the sign for the town of Worcester was only ten minutes from our house, but getting there seemed to me like a day-trip."

Cancer patient Mark Pelgrin wrote in his book, *And a Time to Die*, that he felt himself increasingly plunged into the radical experience of an endless present: "Meaning, or so I discovered yesterday, can be found when a child puts Daddy's hat on her head and laughs. . . . I was always ambitious and so frequently, in years past, I had an uneasy sense of marching somewhere to a wall I must get over, only I didn't know what it was. Now I can say, 'There are no walls any more, no anxiety walls, and to hell with it if they change the doors on me.' So I can do the thing I enjoy for itself, not for what I get out of it. . . . [H]ow could I keep the magic circle working?"

John Studholme, too, found that a new experience of time began to steal upon him. "I began to delight in my own 'hereness,' " he says. "When I watched my boys playing Little League, I wondered about the mental mechanism of the disease. At times I was so slowed down that I could focus on each event intensely, on the arc of the ball as it left the bat, on the motions of the pitcher."

I, too, can recall bouts of feeling suspended in time, of an uncharacteristic simplicity of being. Pelgrin's "magic circle" called to mind a dream I had early in my journey:

> A white worm is slowly, circularly, turning inwards upon itself. When its head reaches the center of its self-made spiral, brilliant "avenues of light" flash outwards, radiating in all directions. "You have been living on the outer shell of your being," a voice intones. "Involution is not bad. The way out is the way in."

The image had both astonished and revulsed me. A worm lives underground, never sees the sun; the cold, belly-white hue of its skin, as if it had spent eons evolving in a lightless cave, gave me the creeps. It seemed a symbol of sickness, bloodlessness, and death.

But I had been amazed by the explosion of light; it had been so bright, I imagined I had awakened with my pupils dazzled to pinpoints.

Its message, "involution"—which I took to mean introspection—had sounded like a terrible idea; it implied solipsism, passivity, and self-centeredness when I most needed to do something decisive. But last Christmas, thumbing through a gift-copy of one of Jung's alchemical tomes, I decided to look up "worm" in the index. The worm, the text affirmed, is an emblem of the Underworld, of all-devouring death. But Jung pointed out that a worm is also a symbol of resurrection: According to legend, when the mythical phoenix is dead, consumed by fire, leaving "only the crude remnants of the flesh," then comes forth "an unseemly worm" which "puts on wings and becomes as new" and, revealing itself as the sacred bird, hastens heavenward.[7]

Involution is also a medical term used to describe the regression of a cancer tumor. It is intriguing that Ainslee Meares' reported cases of tumor regression seemingly resulted from a meditation technique that aimed to produce psychological "regression . . . a return to that state of affairs prior to the onset of the cancer . . . before things went wrong." He postulated this practice helped the normal "homeostatic" or "self-righting" mechanisms of the body to once again "come into play." This healing state, he wrote, is "an atavistic regression to a very simple mode of functioning. The subject may be aware of his existential being but little else"[8]—a state very similar to what many journeyers described to me. (Mitchell May says that healer Jack Gray taught him "healing is the art of doing absolutely nothing. When you learn to do nothing, everything is possible.")

As if in response to this heightened inner receptivity, patients often reported a sense that, in some mysterious way, the world seemed to take on a different spiritual coloration. Instead of the sense reported by many terminal patients of being adrift in an indifferent universe, journeyers often recounted that they felt as if they were now an integral part of a larger cosmic schema. A student of mythology or shamanism might refer to such a perception as "the world navel," the still center of all things, a reenchantment of the world. Patients talked of feeling as if an intentionality were active in the universe—not an anthropomorphic God in heaven, but a perfusion of some higher principle into their lives, something that sounded akin to what medieval mystics called *kenosis,* God emptying himself into the world.

AIDS patient Ken Purcell told me he felt as if an "omniscient playwright" had begun scripting his experience. "Suddenly events seemed to fit together in an amazing way, as if it all had been and would be laid out perfectly. I saw a deer yesterday. The light was just right, and this deer came out of the woods and just looked right at me. And I thought—I know this sounds superstitious and self-centered—but I couldn't help feeling, 'Look what he did for me.' "

Other patients reported entering a state that was like "floating" or "tripping"—a feeling perhaps induced by the body's mood-altering neuropeptides. A somewhat prim-looking, middle-aged survivor of advanced ovarian cancer recalls, "At one point it became, well . . . the only way I can describe it is 'psychedelic.' It was mid-November, in this gloomy, cold, dark northeastern winter, but when I saw a fire hydrant reflected in a puddle on the pavement, it was like Disneyworld multiplied by a million. It made me realize I want to live more than I ever knew." Life took on higher resonance, a burgeoning fertility.

From within this magic circle there was a tendency to see everything as part of "what the universe is trying to say," a piece of a purposeful pattern. Some of the statements reminded me of Alexander Pope's eighteenth-century poem:

> All nature is but art, unknown to thee;
> All chance, direction, which thou canst not see;
> All discord, harmony not understood;
> All partial evil, universal good;
> And spite of pride, in erring reason's spite;
> One truth is clear: whatever is, is right.

This state of harmony and wholeness, so characteristic of mystics, has also been noted in people who are rated as "good placebo responders"—people whose bodies can be most palpably influenced by the power of suggestion. According to one researcher, "Good placebo responders, like good hypnotic subjects, inhibit the critical, analytic mode of information processing that is characteristic of the dominant verbal hemisphere. Good placebo responders will tend to be individuals who are prone to see conceptual or other relationships between events that seem randomly distributed to others. They will inhibit the interfering signals of doubt and skepticism."[9] Such receptive individuals are frequently said to "embroider or elaborate" on the properties of a given placebo drug. This same pattern-making ability is seen in hypnotizable subjects, who also tend to be highly creative in exercises like Rorschach ink-blot tests.

Highly hypnotizable people have also been found to possess unusally vivid recall of childhood memories. One study (by psychologists Theodore Barber and Sheryl Wilson) found that as children they had been more likely to inhabit a world of make-believe. They retained an ability to immerse themselves in fantasy, complete with smells, tastes, sounds, and tactile sensations—fantasies so vivid they often had physical effects (a quality referred to as "mind-body plasticity").

Highly hypnotizable children in general have been shown to have unusual mind-body responsiveness. By using a variety of techniques, they are able to significantly alter their T- and B-lymphocyte activity, to suppress allergic reactions even when they have been injected with antigens, and to eliminate even congenital diseases like ichthyosis (fish-scale skin).

THE HEALING CHILD

Patricia Norris, clinical director of the Biofeedback and Psychophysiology Center at the Menninger Clinic in Topeka, Kansas, notes that "every therapist who uses biofeedback-assisted self-regulation with children knows they are able to warm their hands (increase blood flow) readily, just by thinking about it."[10] She describes one young patient with a terminal brain tumor who first learned to heat his hands, then his feet, then any body part to which he turned his attention, and eventually to modify his heart rate and electrodermal response. The child, who had been given a fatal prognosis, made a remarkable, wholly unexpected recovery. Dr. Norris writes, "Developmentally, children are in a state of close integration of conscious and unconscious processes. . . . Children are naturally able to live in the present, to 'be here now,' to exist easily in a state of being that adults often have to work hard to relearn through meditation, therapy, or some other conscious effort."[11] Perhaps, Norris concludes, "We can look to their strengths to find evidence of a golden thread of healing."[12]

It can scarcely be coincidence that so many patients described the "magic circle" by referring back to the far shores of childhood. Religious and healing rituals across many cultures hold that the first step of renewal is "becoming as a child again." In the Asklepian temple, the patient was "clothed in white linen and wrapped in bands like a child in swaddling clothes."[13] A future Sioux medicine man seeking transformation was lowered into the "vision pit" wrapped in a star quilt tied up with a deer-hide thong, like a papoose.

Such rites are a return to origins, to the still-unformed potential of infancy, where all things are yet possible. Joseph Campbell notes:

> The first step of regeneration is . . . a retreat from the desperations of the wasteland to the peace of the everlasting realm that is within. But this realm, as we know from psychoanalysis, is precisely the infantile unconscious. . . . We carry it within ourselves forever. All the ogres and secret helpers of our nursery are there, all the magic of childhood. And more important, all the life-potentialities that we never managed to bring to adult realization, those other portions of ourselves, are there; for such golden seeds do not die.[14]

Many psychologists have had the greatest respect for the healing power of regression, as in the phrase *reculer pour mieux sauter* ("go back in order to take a leap forward"). The first visiting Spirit to supervise Scrooge's regeneration is, not surprisingly, the Spirit of Christmas Past, which Dickens describes as being

> like a child: yet not so like a child as like an old man, viewed through some supernatural medium, which gave him the appearance of having receded from the view, and being diminished to a child's proportions. Its hair, which hung about its neck and down its back, was white as if with age; and yet the face had not a wrinkle in it, and the tenderest bloom was on the skin. The arms were very long and muscular; the hands the same, as if its hold were of uncommon strength. Its legs and feet, most delicately formed, were, like those upper members, bare. It wore a tunic of the purest white.

This Spirit is marvelously evocative of the qualities of childhood memory; for childhood never *is* simply a memory, but remains alive within us, at once old yet always in "tenderest bloom"; seemingly receded from grown-up view, yet maintaining a powerful, almost supernatural grip upon the psyche. The Spirit—its bare skin and white tunic symbolic of pure, unsullied immediacy—plunges Scrooge into the full sensorium of childhood recollection: "He was conscious of a thousand odors floating in the air, each one connected with a thousand thoughts, and hopes, and joys, and cares long, long, forgotten. . . . The jocund travelers came on; and as they came, Scrooge knew and named them every one. Why was he rejoiced beyond all bounds to see them! Why did his cold eye glisten, and his heart leap up as they went past!"[15]

Such are the emotional and physical sensations that accompany the best of our childhood recaptured. Our vision seems to brighten as we look again at the world through unclouded lenses. There is a surge of energy, buoyancy, unalloyed sentiment; we have for a moment donned a cherished, discarded skin. "If only a portion of that lost totality [of childhood] could be dredged up into the light of day," Campbell writes, "we should experience a marvelous expansion of our powers, a vivid renewal of life."[16]

We might speculate that there could be a more literal truth to Campbell's observations. Mitchell May told me that following his terrible leg injury, he began a daily imaginary exercise of mentally playing Kick-the-Can. "I was immobilized in a full-body cast, but I spent hours recreating this sensation from my childhood—I could *feel* my leg swinging, my toe hitting the can."

Barber and Wilson noted of their highly hypnotizable subjects: "When they remember their very early life, they appear to reexperience the thoughts, emotions and feelings in the same way they did originally. [One] could feel herself sitting in her high chair . . . in her body as it was at that time ('with my big, fat tummy'). Immediately following this vivid recall, she cried out to us, 'Life was wonderful back then.' "[17]

The child within us is a living blueprint for wholeness. At the time they were most broken, many patients found themselves drawn back toward it, as if the "healing system" in its wisdom had accessed the most powerful resource of all. Children have self-healing powers so great that they can sometimes regenerate the tip of a severed finger. Just as an athlete visualizing himself in a race finds his body responding as if he were actually in competition, the evocation of childhood's "feeling-tone" may be a gate to the hidden pathways of healing.

Perhaps the child within is a latent "healing self," a subpersonality with its own psychophysical correlates. Mind-body researchers are showing a renewed interest in people diagnosed with multiple-personality disorder (MPD), who may exhibit an astonishing phenomenon: Sometimes their different subpersonalities have different physiologies as well. Researcher Brendan O'Reagan describes one study in which a person's different "selves" scored differently on eye exams. People with MPD have also been observed to heal from burns with unusual speed.[18]

Michael Murphy, in his book *The Future of the Body*, notes that researchers at the National Institute of Mental Health "compared the massive alterations of mood, cognitive style, and muscular-nervous-hormonal configurations in MPD victims to the dramatic

changes evident in children, who switch emotions with great speed
and flexibility. . . . In becoming multiples, they carry the fluidity of
childhood into adulthood." Murphy notes a study showing that most
MPD sufferers, in fact, express at least one personality that is a child
under twelve years old.[19]

Is it possible that when we "feel like a child again," our bodily
processes—the habitual, interrelated patterns of our organs and
hormones—are also momentarily altered in function? If this were
so, the child within us would be a powerful healing ally. Whether
or not there is a physiological basis for it, many patients told me
of the delight they felt in giving way to almost irresistible urges
to behave "childishly," sometimes for the first time in their adult
lives.

AIDS patient John Davies had grown up as the heir to both family
money and an inflexible, multigenerational military tradition. "I had
lived my life backwards," he says. "I had become an adult first, but
it took getting sick to become a child again. My 'child' does the
things he wants to do. He's not listening to the institutions, the
parents, his mom. He just says, 'Nah, I'm gonna do what I want.' "
John clearly enjoyed expressing what to him, after a stringent up-
bringing, felt like liberating heresy.

Talking to him and others, I recalled the silly delight I had felt
when I left my job and its "grown-up" persona, elated when a long-
suppressed sense of playfulness reemerged. The accounts I heard
were suggestive of a poem, which folksinger Pete Seeger once set
to music, called "Declaration of Independence," written—or, rather,
transcribed—by a man eavesdropping on his six-year-old son's play-
talk:

> He will just do nothing at all
> He will just sit there in the noonday sun
> And when they speak to him
> He will not answer them
> Because he does not care to
> When they tell him to eat his dinner
> He will just laugh at them
> And he will not take his nap
> Because he does not wish to.
> He will go off and play with the pandas . . .

John Studholme found himself drawn back to "the pleasure and
pain" of his youth in order "to pick up valuable pieces and clues,
to retrieve chunks of my goodness that had been hacked away."

Sitting in the stands of a Little League game, wearing an unlawyerly baseball cap and a colorful T-shirt that seemed illegally, deliciously bright in the noonday glare, he observed his two boys with a feeling of profound identification: "Watching them play filled me with a desire to be well, to move as flawlessly as my children. I watched Tom pitching. He had moved his Ozzie Osborne buttons from the front of his hat to the brim, and when he struck out the clean-up hitter for the third straight time—using a pitch he described to me as a 'duck ball'—I began to weep."

THE WOUNDED CHILD

> At first a childhood, limitless and free of any goals.
> Ah, sweet unconsciousness. Then sudden terror. . . .
> the plunge into temptation and deep loss. . . .
> And now in vast, cold, empty space, alone
> Yet hidden deep within the grown-up heart,
> a longing for the first world, the ancient one. . . .
> Then from His place of ambush, God leapt out.

—RAINER MARIA RILKE, "Imaginary Career"[20]

For most journeyers, the return to the precincts of childhood was by no means all innocence and joy. Rilke's verse speaks to the dual nature of childhood as both the source of the pathology-generating wound and a resource for its healing. Thus Scrooge "wept to see his poor forgotten self": a lonely boy, abandoned by family; a preternatural little adult reading by a feeble fire in a bare, melancholy room. " 'The school is not quite deserted,' " said the Ghost. " 'A solitary child, neglected by his friends, is left there still.' Scrooge said he knew it. And he sobbed."

Alice Miller points out that illness can "reactivate the old childhood wound," causing a breakdown of the normal coping mechanisms of the adult ego. Crisis may cause an "emotional awakening to the reality of childhood,"—a reality often thick with negative emotion. But it also offers an opportunity to confront—and perhaps resolve—the secretly tormenting episodes of early life.

Many journeyers reported they had been forced to cope with unusually harsh instances of emotional intimidation, incest, and other physically violative behavior. Scenes of violence toward children often appeared in patients' dreams. One of Dr. Meredith Sabini's cancer patients, "David," had the following nightmare:

> I am in a room, looking out of the window, and see a policeman who is familiar from my childhood. He is leaning over my youngest son [about five in the dream] in a very threatening way, saying, 'Damn you . . . I'll break your jaw!' He smashes the boy with his fist, then picks him up and throws him down. I am struck in the dream by my own detachment and lack of emotional response. Then the policeman starts to attack the boy again. I jump out of bed, shouting to "stop it" and wake up.[21]

David's position is helpless, his natural emotional response suppressed—precisely the position of the abused child vis-à-vis the authority figure of the adult. A similar "detachment and lack of emotional response" was described by many journeyers as the survival tactic they had instinctively turned to in childhood, and whose consequences now blighted adult life.

By the end of David's dream, however, we can see the beginnings of a struggle to defend this inner child. It was important to many patients not only to uncover the wounded child, but to shift their allegiance from the oppressing parent back to themselves. This can be an emotional turning point in the healing process. Dickens paints with great psychological acuity the shift that takes place when Scrooge observes the lonely child he was: "Then, with a rapidity of transition very foreign to his usual character, he said, in pity for his former self, 'Poor boy!' and cried again."[22]

AIDS patient George Melton, afflicted with a lifelong sense of shame and inadequacy, discovered during his illness a similarly new sympathy for his wounded child-self: "If you had a kid and it fell down as it was learning to walk, you wouldn't beat it up. You would pick it up and show it how to do it and how to take the next step. And I started to take that attitude with myself, as if I were a child, and took myself literally under my own wing."

Samantha Coles's childhood was by any standards a domestic horror chamber. She remembers family fights so violent that the police would show up to haul her father away from the house: "There would sometimes even be blood on the floor, but my mother would act like there was nothing wrong. We would just go in and clean it up, and do the dishes. No one whimpered, nobody would say anything, it was all supposed to be normal. No wonder I never learned to trust my own emotional responses, or believe my perceptions could ever be right."

What she calls "the gift that came with illness" was a new ability to honor the crushed and silenced childhood self, which she tenderly nurtured back to life. "Incest really makes you lose this child within. When I started 'talking' to her, I found a real broken kid inside. I did a painting of a naked little girl playing with balloons, and a vicious dog biting the balloons. I called it 'Vulnerability.' The tears started coming up because I'd never learned how to play, only to succeed, to perform. I felt guilty if I wasn't working or doing something productive. I even felt guilty when I signed up for a workshop to learn how to play!"

During her illness, she discovered that this child, its pains and joys intact, was still present inside her—only frozen, as if waiting in a state of suspended animation. For many journeyers, the deep feelings that had been tamped down first by parents, then by society, then finally by the grown-up self became the unlikely soil from which healing grew.

TAKING EMOTIONAL INVENTORY

In the film *It's a Wonderful Life,* we are introduced to George Bailey through flashbacks that sketch a successive attrition of authentic being. Scrooge is taken back to witness the key junctures where he suffered his greatest losses of soul. Former melanoma patient Marilyn Sanders, too, relived an extraordinary sequence of powerful memories during her treatment at a Mexican clinic.

Marilyn's traumatic childhood had left her feeling she "wasn't really important enough to live." She had endured physical abuse— "Sunday punches"—from her mother and desertion by her father. Like many children in intolerable situations, she had in response cut off her feelings and become a classic "little adult." Yet in her bedridden delirium at the clinic, she was plunged into a review of "my entire emotional history."

"As a kid, you get pieces of the picture, but you don't know what's actually going on. I didn't know why my father had left me, for example. But in this experience, it was as if everything was being explained to me. It was like having a big puzzle in the shape of a heart, and each time you slid a piece in the right place, there was this chill of recognition—my God, it fits!—and then, a sudden new warmth.

"Clear as a lightning flash, I'd see my father for a minute in his highway patrolman uniform slipping out the door, and I suddenly knew my parents hadn't loved each other. Then something in me would say, 'Next step,' and I reexperienced my grandmother's death.

I even saw me as a child, which I could never visualize before because I'd always been too responsible for everybody else to ever *be* a kid."

Many patients described a similar process, in which crucial moments seemed suddenly outlined in stark silhouette, each in turn presenting itself for fresh scrutiny, understanding, and ultimately assimilation. Their experience in many ways resembled what researchers of near-death experiences call "the life review."

Some people who have been revived from clinical death describe being "presented" as they are dying with the emotionally salient events of their lives. Similarly, cancer patient John Studholme found himself unexpectedly immersed in a wrenching, sometimes self-critical reexamination of his past. "It was like taking the rind off an orange by scraping it with the grater. But I discovered a surprising sweetness inside." One AIDS patient remarked, "It's important to face yourself, I think; to feel the shame, the fear, the sadness, even the irrational blame."

The appropriateness of blame—of self or others—has become a particularly controversial issue among those who are trying to compassionately grapple with the issues raised by psychological approaches to mind-body healing. It has been said, with some justification, that the current stirring together of disease and personality traits can whip up a poisonous brew of guilt and depression, hardly a healing potion. But psychologist Wendy Miller, who chronicled her own recovery from CFIDS, rejoins that "people who criticize the blaming phase of healing don't understand the process of the larger self. Blaming may be a necessary confrontation with the personality. You're assessing parts of yourself, habitual personality strategies that weren't working very well even before you got sick."

"I'm not into just 'making peace' and attitudinal healing," breast cancer patient Carol Boss told me with a wry grimace. "I think self-acceptance is much more hard-won—and much more valuable."

The health value of such frank emotional self-insight was suggested in one 1988 study of the effects of "disclosure of traumas" on the immune system. A group of college students was assigned to write for twenty minutes a day about "the most traumatic and upsetting experiences of your entire life. . . . your deepest thoughts and feelings." At the end of four days, it was found that the responses of their white blood cells to foreign substances were stronger than a group which had been told to write about "trivial topics."[23]

An ability to hold their hand over the flame of self-insight without flinching is something many healed patients seemed to hold in common. Ji-on says, "I remember a mutual friend casually remarking to me one day when we went out for a walk, 'Oh, there's bad blood between you and the abbot [of the Center].' And when he said that to me I thought, 'That's exactly right.' There *was* bad blood between us, and now I had the 'bad blood' of leukemia in me. It doesn't matter if the two things were connected any more than symbolically. That insight began an amazing process.

"First I went back to reading Shakespeare, Greek plays, all these stories about 'bad blood' between people, about conflict in life and where it leads you. Then, for two weeks, it was as if my whole life up to that point was on a giant movie screen where the movie was playing very slowly, one frame at a time. I spent the entire time watching without doing any editing or commenting, just looking at things as they were. I think it was the first time I gave up my yearning for perfection, which had made me blind to the gap between what I was and what I wanted to be."

THE FIELD OF ANGER

Familiar as she was with the unstintingly frank introspection of Zen, Ji-on was unprepared for what she uncovered within herself: a vast, subterranean reservoir of "pure rage." Resolved as she was to "hang out with whatever arose," she found herself "appalled" at the powerful waves of negative emotions that threatened to inundate her. "It was devastating. I spent five months on that part of the journey, getting acquainted with the 'field of anger,' eventually facing what my responsibility had been for remaining in the dysfunctional situation at the Center. And I remember some days thinking, 'Is this ever going to change?'

"Then came a day I'd been sitting *zazen* one morning for just twenty to twenty-five minutes, doing a very deep inquiry into these afflictive emotions with a commitment to 'no editing,' and I had the distinct feeling of shedding a thin, glasslike skin. I still remember this queer sensation—a brittle glass coating sloughing off my body like a snakeskin as I stood up, hearing it tinkle as it dropped. I think it was all that stored anger. Afterwards, my breathing reached deeper—deeper into my lungs, into my body—than I've ever experienced it."

Though the notion that anger could contribute to the healing process seems counterintuitive—love and harmony seem more valid currencies—its power may be cathartic. In *The Wizard of Oz*, the

Wicked Witch, after cruelly imprisoning Dorothy and maiming her friends, adds insult to injury by contriving to steal one of the child's enchanted silver shoes. The witch is "greatly pleased" with the success of her trick, because the shoe gives her half of Dorothy's yet-undiscovered powers.

At this, Dorothy, who has shown scarcely a flash of anger through all her misadventures, becomes furious.

> "Give me back my shoe!"
>
> "I will not," retorted the Witch, "for it is now my shoe, and not yours."
>
> "You are a wicked creature!" cried Dorothy. "You have no right to take my shoe from me."
>
> "I shall keep it, just the same," said the Witch, laughing at her, "and some day I shall get the other one from you, too."
>
> This made Dorothy so very angry that she picked up the bucket of water that stood near and dashed it over the Witch, wetting her from head to foot.
>
> Instantly the wicked woman gave a loud cry of fear; and then, as Dorothy looked at her in wonder, the Witch began to shrink and fall away.
>
> "See what you have done!" she screamed. "In a minute I shall melt away."[24]

In this parable, the witch, a pathological creature so desiccated of life her very blood has dried up, had managed to steal half of Dorothy's birthright of wholeness. The little girl neither knows how to use the still-dormant powers that remain, nor how to retrieve what is already forfeit to the forces of sickness and death. It is only when, aroused by a simple moment of honest anger, she douses the witch with the waters of pure emotion, that she is able to break the spell and her final healing can begin.

Some psychotherapists who specialize in the treatment of cancer have made a particular virtue of the expression of anger. During a stay at one alternative cancer center I visited in California, we patients—some of us still woozy from drugs and surgery—were led into a room whose centerpiece was a pile of large pasha pillows. The center's therapist, an anxious-looking woman with an edge in her voice, asked everyone to introduce themselves in turn. One patient, a doctor from Toronto I'll call Karen, had scarcely gotten more than a few sentences out when the therapist interrupted.

"You haven't told us how you feel about being *sick*," she demanded, her tone bristling.

"I'm sad," Karen offered.

"Sad," repeated the therapist, sarcastically. "She feels *sad* that she's sick," she said to no one in particular, adopting a wheedling tone and letting her lower lip tremble in mock petulance. Then, turning abruptly to the woman again, she demanded, "What about . . . *angry?*"

Karen nodded, taking her cue. "Yes, I suppose I do feel angry."

"Suppose?"

"Well . . . I *am* angry."

"You're angry," said the therapist with a deep, satisfied sigh. "*Angry,*" she repeated, growling the word and gritting her teeth. Nimble as a cat, she snatched up a tennis racket, placed it on the woman's knees, and stared into her face.

"Let's see some of that anger," she intoned solemnly as the woman leaned away. "Come on," she said, now peremptory. "Would you like to hit the pillows?"

"Yes," Karen said, gamely. "Yes, I *would.*" She stepped up to the pile of pillows, and waggling her hips like a golfer, arced the racket down with an explosive thump that sent dust motes corruscating into the air. As the therapist egged her on, she flailed at the pillows in a fury until, spent, she sat back down.

"Feel better?" the therapist asked, as Karen nodded a little uncertainly.

So it went around the room. I found it ridiculous—contrived, coercive, doctrinaire, a forced conversion to the center's healing gospel: cancer as a disease of unreleased anger, anger bottled up as despair or complaint. *Get angry,* the catechism went, *get better.*

Reducing the journey to such a one-dimensional formula seemed not only simplistic, but distasteful. Still, judging by the testimony of patients I have since met, I have become convinced that in many instances, as William Blake opined, "The tigers of wrath are wiser than the horses of instruction." Many patients reported discovering within themselves great stored reservoirs of anger whose unexpected upwelling seemed to presage a later healing flood.

Joy Ballas-Beeson, who before the crippling onset of arthritis had been chronically intimidated by authority figures, remembers the day on her journey that she turned the tables on an emotionally abusive boss. The man had begun a tirade that relentlessly swelled in volume until the whole office was listening in stunned silence. But Joy surprised herself by leaning across the table and "giving him back exactly what he was dishing out. I felt so conflicted about it, I actually broke out in rashes right afterwards."

A few months later, Joy decided to enroll in a self-defense class. "I was still crippled up from the arthritis. I was wearing braces on my wrists because they were in such bad shape. When the time came to practice with the men, I told them to go easy on me. But when we got into it, I suddenly had so much adrenaline pumping through me I almost killed those guys! I was amazed to find that in that moment, and for some time afterwards, I wasn't in pain.

"A little while after that, my family doctor suggested to me, 'Draw a picture of someone you're angry with.' I drew a picture of my ex-husband. He said, 'Now stamp on it.'

" 'You've got be kidding!' I told him. I could hardly even move! But he just said, 'Do the best you can.' Well, I got into it, and I swear I wonder what the people in the waiting room thought! I yelled and screamed and stamped up and down like hell's fury. But afterwards, for a while, the pain just evaporated.

"When a friend told me she'd learned in a psychology course that some doctors think suppressed anger and arthritis are connected, I had said, 'You're crazy, I'm not angry.' I think I couldn't even feel what I really deep-down felt!"

THE HEALING POWER OF EMOTION

Similarly, it began to seem to AIDS patient John Davies that "this anger I'd clamped down was going to kill me if I didn't do something about it. I began to discover I was angry at my father and mother because they always made me feel I was a chore to them; because they always had someone else take care of me; because they never showed up at school plays or did all the other stuff that's so important to a kid. I felt like I physically had a boiling pot of hot water inside me, heating up, heating up, heating up."

John's linking of anger to heat was intriguing: the physiological heat of fever is a bodily strategy for killing microorganisms, and perhaps even destroying cancer cells. A number of medically well-documented cases of spontaneous remission are known to have occured after infections and fevers.[25] I once spoke with a very relaxed-looking former cancer patient with impeccably frosted hair and a powder-blue leisure suit, the very image of a middle-American suburban matron. "I'm not an angry person," she told me. "I'm the sort of person who takes in stray animals. But around the time before I knew I had cancer, it was like I was possessed. All of a sudden, anger would well up, and then heat would flash up from inside me. I could be doing fine, and suddenly start to sweat and get hot and cry and all the world seemed wrong. Once I had a skillet in my hand and I threw it into the wall. It destroyed the dishrack! I had to literally hold on to the sink to keep from becoming more violent. The heat was tremendous, like in Stephen King's *Firestarter,* like a fire that had hit gasoline, something uncontrollable. I went down to the Army Hospital to see what they could tell me about it, but they just gave me tranquilizers!"

It is certainly possible that her anger was the result of psychological pressure, or even mood-affecting secretions brought on by her yet-undetected disease. But perhaps it was a by-product, or even the catalyst, of an orchestrated bodily healing reaction. The Kung tribe of the Kalahari use the term "boiling energy" to describe what they believe is an intrinsic healing force. Tribal members report that during ritual healing dances, their *num,* or vital essence, heats their bodies to an extraordinary degree. As one tribal healer put it, "You feel your blood becomes very hot, just like blood boiling on a fire, and then you start to heal."[26]

Apprentice Kung healers may experience various frightening physical and emotional alterations from the heating up of their *num.* But they are told that if they can accept these painful changes rather than being dominated by fear of them, they can transform them into vehicles that allow them to heal. It is significant, according to Harvard anthropologist Richard Katz, that such individuals tend to be "more emotionally labile. Within Kung culture, they are said to be more *sga ku tsiu;* that is, their 'heart rises' more, they are more 'expressive' or 'passionate.' During the dance, the healer's emotions must be readily available and capable of quickly changing their intensity and content."[27]

Perhaps the strong emotions described by many patients are also an eruption of the life force, the beginning of the inner movement that virtually all traditions agree is key to healing. One journeyer wrote about the "letting-go sessions" he needed to arrange for himself each day just to cope with the torrents of feeling that would suddenly overwhelm him. He was overcome "by waves of bitter anger, wild grief, and deep desolation—feelings sometimes attached to particular memories, but just as often unspecific and seemingly primal."[28]

Chinese medical theory postulates that a primary cause of disease is the "nontransformation of emotion." Acupuncturists believe that in a healthy person, it is the nature of emotions to change, to transform one into another, to move from organ to organ through the body. According to the theory, when this movement of energy is blocked, illness is thought to ensue. The aim of Chinese medical practice is to eliminate blockages and once more foster the free flow of energy.

Debby Ogg credits this transformation of emotion, not the anger itself, with helping to heal herself. "I only started with rage," she says. "Later I began to realize that rage was the mask for this extreme emotional deprivation I'd suffered. My losses had started when I was five years old, when my parents died, and they just kept happening. I'd thought on some level that I must have deserved it."

In the midst of our interview, she suddenly burst into sobs, as if the dirt on her parents' graves were still fresh, and she were still a child, trying to take in the enormity. "What was under the rage was grief. I just never knew how to get to it before. I'd watch family TV shows and cry, but I didn't realize I was crying about my own life. I was afraid if I ever really let loose, I was going to cry forever. But getting sick somehow made feeling all of this permissible. I would just walk into my therapist's office, sit down and start to cry. I cried for *months*."

Beneath the tears, Debby says, she discovered love, tenderness, and a fullness of being—feelings her inner defenses against early, unsustainable suffering had never fully permitted. For many journeyers, *this* was the inner work of healing: to uncover the heart, layer by painful layer.

Brian Schultz, the former "Tin Woodman" described earlier, says, "It was only when I could surrender to hard emotions that I could experience tiny moments of breakthrough, times the physical symptoms would suddenly subside in a dramatic way. I knew I had to risk expressing my feelings, but this was excruciating, since my family had never allowed it. I could be stewing inside with murderous rage, but for me to even let anyone know I wasn't in the brightest, most cheerful of moods was a life-and-death struggle.

"But I started to make a conscious discipline of exposing my feelings to others, no matter how much sweat it took. I found out that even when I felt scared shitless, I could find a way to just go ahead and do it anyway. First there was only raw pain. Then anger. Then later, beneath that, sadness, guilt, then tears, then love."

THE HIDDEN POWER

"It is precisely because a child's feelings are strong," Alice Miller writes, "that they cannot be repressed without serious consequences. The stronger a prisoner is, the thicker the prison walls." It was because of the sheer force of their early emotional lives that many journeyers had erected vast barriers to feeling—Jericho walls they came to believe had to crumble in order to heal. In *The Wizard of Oz*, the Cowardly Lion feels ashamed because his powerful heart pounds so wildly in the presence of danger. But the Wizard wisely counsels, "The essence of cowardice is not acknowledging the reality of fear. True courage is in facing danger when you are afraid."[29]

Authentic feeling, the story implies, is the real basis of our wholeness. It is our avoidance of who we really are that creates the schism between us and the healthy core we must reclaim. Healing is more a process of uncovering what we already possess rather than manufacturing a "better" self.

To uncover long-hidden feelings may be painful, but most journeyers came to deem the alternative more perilous. The flight from powerful "unacceptable" emotions—which cannot help but imply a flight from the body that harbors them—may indeed be one of the strong underpinnings of pathology. Samantha Coles told me she had put the terrible feelings associated with childhood punishment and sexual abuse "in a little box where I thought it wouldn't affect any other part of my life. But splitting it off from the rest of me probably harmed me more than anything."

The patients I spoke to—like the journeyers in so many time-honored fables of transformation—had to seek out their "living root," and make it bloom in a landscape of devastation. This inner root of health and the roots of illness were often inextricably entwined, for the wound that initiates the journey also may be its destination. Reclaiming our specific emotional history, we take up once again the interrupted story of the "healing self." Then even in the midst of the grimmest ordeal, we begin at last to live the unlived life.

❧ 14 ❧
COMING ALIVE:
EXPLORING THE HEALING
SELVES

The mythological hero is the champion not of things become but
of things becoming; the dragon to be slain by him is precisely the
monster of the status quo: Holdfast, the keeper of the past. . . .
Transformation, fluidity, not stubborn ponderosity, is the characteristic
of the living God. . . . The hero [is] the champion of creative life.

—JOSEPH CAMPBELL,
The Hero with a Thousand Faces[1]

T HE HEALING PATH is made up of the steps we take to enact our
own potential—steps that may lead into every region of our
lives. For if the roots of disease are multifactorial, then healing, too,
must be manifold. If illness tells a story of alienation, then the motif
of the healing drama is relatedness. If sickness echoes through the
concentric circles of our existence, then healing, too, must rever-
berate everywhere.

This paradigm was well known to traditional cultures for which,
as Ivan Illich remarks, "Health care is always a program for eating,
drinking, working, breathing, loving, politicking, exercising, singing, dreaming, warring, and suffering."[2] From this perspective, healing is not just a method of fixing-up, but a way to express the
multiplicity of the soul.

When the Egyptian goddess Isis was called upon to heal her husband, Osiris (the goddess of healing and the lord of Underworld
journeys are eternally wedded), she gathered up his disparate
parts—limbs, organs, head, heart—from the four corners of the
globe. Similarly, those on the healing path discover that they, too,
must restore their long-scattered pieces, those disowned aspects of
identity whose loss has meant a secret diminution.

Former lymphoma patient Arline Erdrich remembers a moment
of childhood that is emblematic of her loss. It was the day her mother

brought home the Green Shoes. "I had very few clothes as a child, usually just hand-me-downs. My mother would go off on extravagant shopping excursions, but only for herself. Then one day, she came home with something for *me!* It was a wonderful-looking pair of green suede shoes, with laces and everything.

"Unfortunately, they were the wrong size, way too small. Still, I never said a word, because I knew if I told her that they hurt, she would just yell at me, or else take them back and not get me any others. So I wore the Green Shoes, even though every step felt like it was killing me."

Metaphorically, Arline had worn her Green Shoes until the day she got cancer. She had continually squeezed herself into emotionally cramped adult relationships and thwarted her most creative impulses, fearing that if she did not, she would not be loved.

In observing the life histories of patients with cancer, psychologist Meredith Sabini writes:

> [T]he image of Chinese foot-binding comes to mind: . . . [T]he metatarsal was bent upward and the toes sometimes fused. The energy for growth had continued to push the foot towards its natural form, but the impediment deformed the natural shape. Is it possible that cancer is like such a growth, taking place incorrectly in the body rather than in the whole being?[3]

We may question how closely such a metaphor can be superimposed on the blind and brutal physiology of disease. But, like many other people I spoke with, Arline believes her own healing could not have taken place if she had not resumed the growth toward her "natural form" that had been impeded for a lifetime.

When I visited her in her New York loft, Arline showed me a self-portrait, the first work in a series she had titled "American Balabusta." Painted before her illness, in a style reminiscent of Edward Hopper, it depicted a woman hunched over an ironing board—"A *balabusta*," she confided, "is Yiddish for *hausfrau*, always cooking, cleaning, straightening"—hair up in a casual topknot, patiently ironing a man's white shirt. A washer and dryer sit stolidly in the background; a nearby chair is draped with sheets awaiting smoothing. The painting is a schematic of domestic pillory. In its far corner is the image of an abandoned easel, its canvas blank, illumined only by faint light leaking through a basement window.

"That was my story," Arline told me, although it was hard to imagine this vibrant woman, elegantly dressed in a blue, Southwestern-style silk blouse, trapped in such a murky half-life. "My ex-husband used to say painting was an indictment of him. 'No,' I'd tell him, 'it's an indictment of me.' I mean, what was I doing? I could have been painting for galleries, but instead I'm ironing his shirts because this is my way to please him. I never really told him how miserable I felt, never took a stand."

As her illness progressed, however, Arline began a fresh series of canvases filled with the urgency of one whose existence has been suddenly telescoped toward finitude. The static, figurative scenes vanished, replaced by thick, energetic swirls. Outgrowing her tiny corner, she took over the entire basement, covering the floor and appliances with plastic, squirting paint from plant-misters to create ever-wilder abstracts.

As her husband, discomfited by her uncontained enthusiasm, began to shrink from her ("He yelled at me that I was messing up the sink," she says, "and I was!"), her canvases grew larger, becoming fierce implosions of luminous color. By the time the marriage ended, Arline was a painter again, this time a real one. At the time of my visit, her loft was overflowing with her latest project, a series of human-sized paintings of the Greek letter *Tau*, the symbol of spirit and life. Her mother's Green Shoes were nowhere to be seen.

Jungian analyst Elida Evans noted that in many of her cancer patients, "The creative life has not been satisfied . . . the regular unfolding of the individual has stopped."

What I witnessed in Arline Erdrich and others I studied was a resumption of that unfolding, a reclamation of what had been lost, or had yet to be found. In the midst of their seeming disintegration, some discovered the larger outlines of the person they were always meant to be. As Dr. Naomi Remen has observed, "In illness, some people go back to their original values, even though they've never lived by them before." Just as the mythical hero often possesses a magical implement (a flying cloak, a pair of ruby slippers, an enchanted staff), its existence forgotten or function opaque until it leaps to hand in a crisis, so patients found healing powers—more, healing *selves*—they had unknowingly carried within themselves for a lifetime.

In *The Wizard of Oz*, it is only on the perilous path that the pilgrims' unsuspected potentials spontaneously emerge. Facing the rapier-clawed, tiger-headed "Kalidahs," the Cowardly Lion tells Dorothy, "Stand close behind me, and I will fight them as long as I am alive." Here is revealed the very courage—*real* courage, not blustering sham—that he is consciously convinced he lacks. Similarly, the Scarecrow, who fancies himself brainless, under duress proves himself a master strategist. Our delight in the characters' transformations stems from our own surprised assumptions: We, too, cannot believe our own power could be so close at hand, residing in the very places we feel most wounded.

SEEKING POWER

As sages from Epictetus to Emerson have noted, we are often made uneasy by our own deepest truths, for these resist all conscious contrivance, insisting we embody without compromise the unlived yearnings of the soul. The inner self, once awakened, demands ever-wider life. Lawrence LeShan in his book *You Can Fight for Your Life,* describes the case of a successful thirty-five-year-old lawyer who discovered that he had a massive, inoperable brain tumor. Ignoring his doctors' predictions that he had a few scant months to live, the man entered intensive psychotherapy, gradually realizing over years of treatment how much his success had been predicated on others' terms. Sorrowing that he had purchased love only at the expense of his own deepest longings, he eventually divorced, and returned to his earliest passion, music. Later, he went on to play with a professional symphony. The brain tumor disappeared, and was still not in evidence when LeShan saw him twelve years later. In another research team's study, which included the similar case of a man with a brain tumor who resumed a singing career and made a remarkable recovery, so-called "Category I" self-healers were found to be "receptive and highly creative," scoring high on indices like "nonconformity."[4]

Jung once wrote in a letter to a colleague, "Whatever you do, if you do it sincerely, will eventually become the bridge to your wholeness, a good ship that carries you through the darkness.[5] Several supposedly terminal patients I met had decided to set out on heartfelt voyages that had seemed to some of those around them the height of irresponsibility. Several found ways to undertake long-postponed personal pilgrimages. One AIDS patient bought a truck, painted RECOVERY on its side, and took off across the country. Carol Boss packed her precious herbs in her suitcase and set off on a trip to China's Wu Yi mountains, long the refuge of Ch'an Buddhist sages and Taoist monks. "I'd always wanted to go there. I figured, Why not now? I wanted to climb the mountains by myself. The route was long and hard, and I got lost a few times. I was pretty weak— the mountains looked like the Himalayas to me, and felt like them, too. But with every step I was affirming my own strength, strength I didn't even know I had before."

Similarly, Samantha Coles, ostensibly dying of malignant melanoma, impulsively decided to travel to Europe. "The strangeness, not being able to speak the language, not telling anyone else on the tour I was sick, was completely liberating," she says. "My mood changed one hundred and eighty degrees. I felt like a different person."

Healing springs from what instinctively vivifies us; what causes movement and change; what "turns us on," "rings our chimes," penetrates unexplored territories of the self. When the longing for fuller life arose within him, analyst Albert Kreinheder, suffering from rheumatoid arthritis (and later, cancer), embraced it. Though health seemed only a distant pinprick of brightness in a black void, he found himself instinctively turning toward whatever gave off a glimmer of "power. Wherever I went, whatever I did, I was always seeking the power. Some life experiences had it and some didn't. And it was a completely individual thing. What was power for me might be nothing at all for someone else. If a person, an object, an activity had no power for me, I was completely bored and I turned away."6

I, too, recall turning away from, even being repulsed by, people and circumstances that once would have sufficed but suddenly felt dangerously inert. At the same time, I was drawn toward relatively insignificant things that had unaccountable juice. Ill and unemployed, with time and little else on my hands, I cruised local rummage sales, passionately buying up oddball furnishings—gold-specked, Formica-and-chrome kitchen tables; old fans with sinuous forties grillwork; bulbous, useless toasters; Dali-meets-Ozzie-and-Harriet lamps from the fifties. It was dopey stuff, some of which—like a junked, three-hundred-pound red mystery machine blazoned with cryptic silver letters that read VITALIZER—I madly lugged with me from move to move over the next few years.

For reasons as much pecuniary as aesthetic, I bargained for floppy thriftshop gabardine suits and heel-worn cowboy boots, cultivating for the first time a rudimentary personal style. Looking back, I think I was, in some small but tangible way, changing my identity; planting evidence to win my own conviction the past *was* only prologue. A cinderblock bookshelf-and-bluejeans-type since college, I had always disdained fashion, furnishing, and anyone who paid them unwonted attention. Now they became crucial conjunctions between the inner and outer world, ways to visibly honor my own oddity of heart. I would sit and let my eyes rove from my broken World War II alarm clock to the plaster eagle with the missing foot and feel I had, in some way, brought an invisible world to life.

I also began to use my voice. Though music had been a brief first career, I had never really performed any of the songs I had written. That was for center-stage preeners with "good" voices, while I'd chosen a dignified but wistful vantage point in the wings. Now I began sneaking into the back of a local Baptist church just to hear my own thin tenor meld with the congregation's gospel harmonies. Once at a party, I got up and sang what everyone later agreed was a dreadful a cappella. I didn't care. I composed and then howled into a cheap mike a series of barely listenable demo tapes, thrilled when one record producer I played them for cautiously allowed that I had "a real serviceable rock 'n' roll voice."

That my own peculiar expressive noise could rise up unapologetically from my belly, rattle my breastbone, and spill rough from my throat delighted me beyond reason. Singing was a tangible metaphor for speaking, without shame, my own ungilded truth.

Dr. Richard Moss recounts how he uses special singing exercises to push patients closer to new, yet undiscovered sources of healing energy. Most people, he says, at first stop short, "as if they sense that going further requires a far deeper trust and self-abandonment. . . . They sing songs that they know, over and over again, rather than trusting a new song to emerge. Most of us do the same things with our lives, with our repeated attitudes, our repeated routines. We perpetuate our identity by unconsciously barricading ourselves in behaviors that limit our aliveness."[7]

I count it as no accident that so many patients described the crucial role that music seemed to play in summoning a healing response. The Greeks were convinced that music had a divine power to counteract sickness. The mythical musician Thaletas was said to have rid Sparta of a deadly epidemic by playing surpassingly upon his *aullos,* or flute. Chiron, the centaur instructor of Asklepius, insisted that physicians master the art of music, the confluence of feeling and thinking, heart and breath, the rhythms of the body and the surging of the soul.

Neurologist Oliver Sacks describes how music helped to stimulate his recovery from a nerve injury that had left one of his legs utterly without sensation. At the lowest, most seemingly hopeless point in his journey, a friend brought him a recorder with a cassette of Mendelssohn's Violin Concerto. Though never a Mendelssohn fan, Sacks was amazed at the profound effect this "charming, trifling piece of music" had upon him. From the moment the tape began to play,

> Something happened, something of the sort I had been panting and thirsting for, something that I had been seeking more and more frenziedly with each passing day, but which had eluded me. Suddenly, wonderfully, I was moved. . . . I felt, with the first bars of the music, a hope and an intimation that life would return to my leg—that *it* would be stirred, and stir, with original movement, and recollect or recreate its forgotten motor melody . . . as if the animating and creative principle of the whole world was revealed . . . that our living moving flesh, itself, was "solid" music—music made fleshy, substantial, corporeal.[8]

Sacks's injury had left him feeling disembodied, disoriented, sundered in half. His problem, he saw in a flash of insight, was as much one of harnessing flesh and spirit in tandem as repairing the gross neurological defect. "What was disconnected in me was not merely nerve and muscle but, in consequence of this, the natural and innate unity of body and mind. The 'will' was unstrung, precisely as the nerve-muscle. The 'spirit' was ruptured, precisely as the body. Both were split, and split off from one another."[9]

REDISCOVERING THE BODY

According to the late Tibetan lama Chogyam Trungpa, this sort of disconnection is the fundamental root of both physical and mental pathology. When we think in one direction, feel in another, and act in yet another, the competing strains of disharmony are echoed in our level of health. "When body and mind are not synchronized, sometimes your mind is short and your body is long, or sometimes your mind is long and your body is short." Similarly, the Greek Gnostic Plotinus suggested that sickness results when the body loses contact with the soul and finally "no longer resembles it."

Joan Halifax, a field anthropologist who experienced the healing of her own serious illnesses at the hands of shamans and Buddhist teachers, found in the practice of meditation an indispensable tool for reconciling spirit and flesh. She writes lyrically:

> The body and mind ride the ebb and flow of breath. The mind and body begin to recognize each other; they have long been

> partners but turned their backs on each other long ago. The mind began to push the body about like an animal trainer who does not consider the well-being of his charge. The body's desire or aversion began to create patterns of craving or dislike in the mind. The reunion between body and mind is sewn with the thread of breath in the light of concentration.[10]

Surely Chiron the centaur, the progenitor of Western medicine, was himself a symbol of this principle: human (consciousness) and horse (body) undivided, inextricable, smoothly and powerfully intermeshing in a living whole. For the healing agenda is not only to repair the mechanism of the body, but to restore communication between psyche and soma. "The purpose of treatment," write Drs. Laurence Foss and Kenneth Rothenberg in *The Second Medical Revolution*, "is to heighten the patients' mental-emotional sensitivity, to make them aware of the events taking place within them—'to listen to their own skin.'"

To "listen to their own skin" meant for many I spoke with a new acknowledgment of the body, for it is through the body that we "live out the soul's meaning and intentions," as Albert Kreinheder put it. "The psyche manifests itself physically. It wants to be part of our bodies and part of our concrete empirical existence."

The body is our very presence in this world, the space only we can occupy, the place where the self's private story is given breath, tongue, visible limbs. It is the body which often speaks most loudly for authentic being, confronting us not with how we *should* feel, but how we actually do. When we say we feel "self-conscious," we mean those very moments when our mouths parch, our voices choke, our faces flare hot with embarrassment—moments when our bodies bear unimpeachable witness to the movements of the soul.

The body, in a manner of speaking, *is* the soul. As Nietzsche declaimed: "'I,' you say, and are proud of the word. But greater is that in which you do not wish to have faith—your body and its great reason: that does not say, 'I,' but does 'I.'" The body, the repository of emotion, is ever threatening to speak a deeper, more spontaneous truth beyond ego's control. The young soldier tries to ignore the turning in his gut when he does not "have the stomach" to kill. The put-upon office manager attempts to run roughshod over his body's plea for respite. The hurting child smothers the searing grief and rage she feels when a parent crushes her feelings.

In *The Wizard of Oz*, the Lion seeks to deaden his body's palpitating, high-strung responses to danger. But the Wizard is insistent upon the wisdom of the flesh: the Lion *feels,* he tells the beast, because he is a "living thing."

But to the Lion, to be alive means the conquest of feeling. The state of ill-being is a dictatorship that seeks to suppress dissent, whether it comes from the body or the "shadow" side of the psyche. Indeed, the two are sometimes interchangeable. The psychologist John P. Conger writes:

> The body is the shadow insofar as it contains the tragic history of how the spontaneous surging of life energy is murdered and rejected in a hundred ways until the body becomes a deadened object . . . [I]t holds the record of our rejected side, revealing what we dare not speak . . . bound energy that is unrecognized and untapped, unacknowledged and unavailable.[11]

In particular, the "disease-prone personality," for whom the body often has been the producer and receptacle of dangerous emotions, may tend to respond to the body as an alien Other, to try to silence it rather than straining to hear what it is saying. But disease drives us inescapably toward the body, toward both its perils and potentials. Dr. Jacob Zieghelboim says that he realized the extent to which he had gotten used to "overriding my body's cues rather than respecting them. I had become numb to my basic thresholds—biological, psychological, emotional, spiritual. I began to look at both illness and healing as coming into touch with the real forces of life."

EROS

Many journeyers reported that the "real forces of life" sometimes took the form of powerful erotic feelings. I, too, was startled when in the midst of my illness I began feeling an almost overwhelming sense of eroticism. Like several other male patients, one of whom told me he felt like he "was fourteen again," I began to have copious adolescent wet-dreams. I was surprised at the powerful sexual imagery they contained, and at the free-floating desire that began to permeate my waking life.

It is a special irony that patients are usually relegated to the sexless category. Illness (a diminution of the life force) and desire (a hypertrophy of it) are assumed to be mutually exclusive. Yet, while illness is usually regarded as a fading, a weakening and trailing away of primordial forces, it also may be a bursting forth, a freeing of the body's powers just when it has become our darkest prison. It is as if disease, by forcing our descent into the flesh, also activates its possibilities. Sexuality, aside from disease itself, is perhaps the strongest intersection between psyche and soma. Our bodies feel flooded with consciousness, while our minds are anchored in physical experience. We feel an onslaught of sensation from the very basis of our beings.

The Hindu saint Gopi Krishna, in the grip of the strange illness that preceded his enlightenment experience, remarked in bafflement: "I could not fail to take notice of such a startling development in the sexual region. . . . The agitated condition of the hitherto quiescent are now in a state of feverish activity . . . as if forced by an invisible but effective mechanism, not in operation before."

Perhaps the "mechanism" he describes is part of the "healing system" that sometimes seems to awaken in the crisis of disease. Sexuality and healing seem to have been strongly associated in the Greek mind. Paintings in the cupola of the *tholos* at Epidaurus, the largest Asklepian healing temple, show two figures, one a feminine deity representing "sober drunkenness," or intoxication of the soul, and the second Eros, holding a lyre in place of his bow and arrows.[12] Even the sexual god Priapus was considered a healing god, characterized by the adjectives "life-giving" as well as "light-giving." And in the central healing temple of Asklepius at Cos there was, according to Cicero, a prominent statue of Venus, the goddess of love.

Arline Erdrich recalls a period during her treatment for lymphoma when "my sexuality increased dramatically. I actually went a little berserk." Looking back on it, she says, "I suppose it was partly that I wanted to be reassured that I was still sexually attractive. But I also felt this incredible welling up of energy. Men were responding to it, being flirtatious. I wound up in a few pretty torrid affairs— even once, briefly, with my *doctor*. People would tell me there was something about me that gave off this glow. I used to say kiddingly, 'It's the radiation!' But I think what one gives off is life. It's like a new light, this aura that shines around you."

Albert Kreinheder, too, felt powerful stirrings, the arising of a long-deferred desire to be a "lusty, hearty person who's alive in the body." He wrote in his journal, "I go on day after day, plodding, worrying, conforming, making no waves, receding into the scenery as if I am nothing. Yet here is Kundalini, bottled up inside of me. . . . What is there to fear? Shall I open the bottle and find out? Someday, someday before it is gone forever, we must take the risk. We must live before we die. If it is too much, let us find out."

Using the technique of "active imagination," he encountered the figure of a beautiful woman, "the lady within." She instructed him to "open the bottle. . . . But do not ask me how. Feel the energy. Let it stir you. Always it is with you. Do not let it go. Carry it. Let it move you. Honor it. Love it. Worship it. Let it be expressed in all you do. It is yours to live with. You do not know how it will express itself, but you know that life is nothing without it."

Kreinheder's eroticism was in reality a longing to consummate life itself, to merge with "everything that was the opposite of my life to this point, everything feminine, everything sensuous and emotional, all those things I had left behind in my overemphasis of the masculine and the intellectual."[13] In his earlier life he had held back the most vital aspects of himself. His desire was not simply for sex, but for Eros, the principle of union; for love in Plato's profoundest definition: "The desire and pursuit of the whole."

THE HEALING SELVES

The "soul-approach" calls for honoring what the poet William Blake called "the Four Zoas" that comprise a human being: Tharmas (the flesh), Urizen (the intellect), Luvah (the emotional life), and Los (the creative spirit); or body, brain, heart, and imagination. Each must be invoked for the healing task, as well as for the art of living.

But the disease-prone personality in particular may have a tendency to have split off aspects of the self. Earlier in this book, Samantha Coles echoed the predicament of other journeyers I spoke with when she reflected, "Because of what I went through as a kid, I never really hooked up the analytical and the feeling parts of myself. My body was there, but the emotional component was somewhere else." The syndrome she describes is known in the psychological literature as "dissociation." A child exposed to physical or emotional trauma often learns, in the words of University of Connecticut researcher Kenneth Ring, to "selectively 'tune out' those aspects of his physical and social world that are likely to harm him by splitting himself off."

The dissociative personality, as Ring and a number of commentators have remarked recently, can be a double-edged sword. On the one hand, it is a defensive response to the childhood traumas that misshape the personality. But Ring finds that such people may be "unwitting beneficiaries of a kind of compensatory gift in return for the wounds they have incurred growing up." Among those gifts, he maintains, is an ability to "focus one's attention on the figures and features of one's inner reality," a greater capacity to draw on powers of imagination and visualization and to enter with relative ease into states of "psychological absorption" like hypnotic trance— all of which have been correlated, interestingly, with phenomena such as placebo healing.[14]

The most widely known case of exceptional placebo-response, reported by Dr. Bruno Klopfer in the late 1950s, is that of a patient he called "Mr. Wright." To quickly summarize a story that has by now become a popular staple of mind-body lore:

Mr. Wright came to the hospital with a generalized terminal lymphosarcoma. His neck, groin, chest, and abdomen had tumor masses "the size of oranges." So many large cancers blocked his thoracic duct that several quarts of milky fluid had to be withdrawn from his chest every other day to enable him to breathe. At most, he had weeks to live.

Mr. Wright read in the papers one day about a new wonder drug, Krebiozen. When he insisted on being treated with it, Dr. Klopfer dubiously complied. To the physician's surprise, Mr. Wright's tumor masses "melted like snowballs on a hot stove, and in only these few days, they were half their original size!" Mr. Wright walked out of the hospital "practically symptom-free." The man who days before had frequently required an oxygen mask even resumed flying his private plane.

When news reports shedding doubt on Krebiozen began to circulate, however, Mr. Wright's symptoms quickly recurred. This time his doctors administered what they told him was a double shot of "improved" Krebiozen, but which in fact was only sterile water. His tumors again seemed to magically evaporate and his recovery time was even more dramatic than before. But when several days later the A.M.A. officially pronounced Krebiozen "a worthless drug," Mr. Wright reentered the hospital, succumbed to his affliction, and died.

Mr. Wright's attitude did not "cause" his death. But apparently his beliefs had been so powerful as to stave off for a time the ravages of advanced disease. How could such an implacable condition undergo such almost capricious alchemy? According to Dr. Klopfer, in a little-noted comment, one of the keys to both the fragility and the power of Mr. Wright's healing response was his "floating ego-organization." The patient's sense of self, Klopfer reported, was unusually fluid, undemarcated. His dissociative personality made him more susceptible than normal to both negative and positive suggestion, which in turn seemed to translate more readily into alterations of bodily state.

The most exotic, extreme, and crippling example of such "floating ego organization" is multiple-personality disorder (MPD). Here the entire notion of identity undergoes an agonizing series of refractions into "subpersonalities" or "alters." But as we noted earlier, people diagnosed with MPD may also exhibit startling bodymind abilities. I once met a person whose multiplicity extended to carrying business cards for his various selves. "Several of us," Edward (not his real name) informed me excitedly, "are even collaborating on a children's book." One of his female subpersonalities—a talented artist, he said—was doing the illustrations, another the writing, and yet another was the agent!

Edward, an amiable, nondescript man whose constantly darting gaze was a little unsettling, claimed he was a puzzlement to his doctors. Sometimes, he told me, one of his subpersonalities would get a disease that the other ones didn't have. One of Edward's female subpersonalities had developed an hysterical pregnancy (pseudo-cyesis) and was rushed to the hospital with a grotesquely distended abdomen. When another personality took over, however, his/her stomach returned to normal.

As I have mentioned earlier, some cases have been reported in which "multiples," by "switching personalities," have instantaneously shut down severe allergic reactions; nullified the effects of powerful drugs; and eliminated symptoms of diabetes, third-degree burns, color-blindness, and, according to some reports, even epilepsy and tumors.[15]

Thus, though multiple-personality disorder presents itself as a manifestly fragmented condition, it may also produce a peculiar form of bodymind integration. How could this occur? One "multiple" named Cassandra averred that her unusual self-healing powers came from something she refers to as "parallel processing."

> As she explained, even when her alternate personalities are not in control of her body, they are still aware. This enables her to "think" on a multitude of different channels at once. . . . Whereas normal people only do healing imagery exercises two or three times a day, Cassandra does them around the clock. She even has a subpersonality named Celeste who possesses a thorough knowledge of anatomy and physiology, and whose

sole function is to spend twenty-four hours a day meditating and imaging the body's well-being.[16]

Thus, a divided form of selfhood may paradoxically prove, from a bodymind standpoint, remarkably congruent. Cassandra's case recalls the experience of self-healer Alice Hopper Epstein, with her multitude of subpersonalities ("I am Amanda the Builder. I am strong. Kill the cancer"), in her case consciously invoked. Epstein wrote in her autobiographical book, "[M]y subpersonalities . . . represented feelings and information that were not available to me in any other form. This is because each subpersonality represented a unified emotional and action potential . . . I believe that these images were close to the higher self. . . . They may not seem to have been higher in terms of their subject matter, but they were *higher in their authenticity*" (my italics).

As Epstein proceeded on her healing journey, she increasingly allowed her subpersonalities to come alive. Like the shaman or the artist, she creatively integrated her inner life with her outer one. Unlike the multiple-personality sufferer, who is painfully trapped in a condition of fragmentation, she began to delight in her multiple aspects. One morning, she relates, she decided to "become" one of her subpersonalities: "I would be 'Little One' for the day in order to feel what it was like and to give her the freedom she longed for so much. She liked physical contact, so I played hard with the dog, who had a grand time. I hugged and pushed [my husband] Sy in fun and I said exactly whatever came into my mind. I had a ball. My theory was that she should have a time to express herself before we talked about that 'integration' word. It was strange because at one level she wanted to be integrated, and at another the word was anathema to her. How confusing."[17]

Epstein's explorations led her to a central paradox of wholeness itself: that our ego identity is only one portion of a much larger circumference of being; that we have not just one but many healing selves. Perhaps her experience also contains a key insight: When the controlling ego is provisionally relinquished, parts of the self that contain greater "unified potential" and "authenticity" may emerge.

As I have previously suggested, those who are most vulnerable to diseases where the psyche seems to be a co-factor may develop a powerful, if displaced, connection between body and mind. I have wondered if these same factors may conceivably predispose them to be better self-healers. A more dissociative personality that tended to "somaticize" unacceptable thoughts and emotions might also, like Mr. Wright, more readily somaticize healing. Recall Arline Erdrich's comment that as a child she could "create" high fevers to get her mother's attention; Joy Ballas-Beeson's weeks-long rashes in response to forbidden feelings of anger; or Niro Asistent, the self-described "black swan" of her family, who could "paralyze" her legs in order to get out of school—a paralysis so convincing that doctors could produce no reflex in her. Alice Epstein, too, reports that she would break out in fever blisters during childhood in response to extreme emotional tension. Her last severe outbreak, some years before her cancer, was on the day that she told her parents she wanted to marry the man they disapproved of.

Referring to such physical reactions caused by emotional complexes, Jung noted that "it is as if that particular complex had . . . a sort of body. . . . [I]t behaves like a partial personality."[18] Could such "partial personalities" heal as well as hurt? An emotional complex, writes analyst Albert Kreinheder, "has more power than seems to be logically explainable. [It is] where the blessed ones can enter— as well as the monsters of the deep." (Indeed, one "personality-attitudinal" study of long-term cancer survivors concluded they tended to have "more expressive and sometimes bizarre personalities.")

Dr. Hans Schilder, a researcher at the Helen Dowling Institute in Rotterdam, Holland, undertook a detailed study of seven cases of spontaneous remission (SR). Schilder, who sports a mop of blond hair and is lanky to the point of elongation, is attempting to identify specific psychological changes that might precede seemingly miraculous regressions—searching, in effect, for a tumor necrosis factor of the mind.

One case, a woman with terminal breast cancer, her weight dwindled down to ninety pounds and near-comatose, had been moved to a hospice because her husband felt incapable of caring for her. But realizing she had been relocated to a place to die, the woman suddenly became pugnaciously assertive. "From a neat and well-educated woman," says Schilder with wry amusement, "she changed into a woman who was cursing, singing dirty songs, making dirty jokes. She carried on like this for three weeks—although she still waited until people left the room to do it!" Inexplicably, her tumor began to regress. Ten years afterward, the woman remained in a good state of health—"still very tidy," says Schilder, "but now very earthy as well."[19]

Schilder noticed in his SR cases a quality cited by other researchers: an emotional "ambivalence" (which one colleague termed "hostility without loss of control"). Psychologist Al Siebert has observed that survivors of human ordeals like the Bataan March seemed to have personalities he labeled as "biphasic" or "paradoxical"—able to be both angry and loving, selfish and unselfish, self-confident and self-critical. I once interviewed a man named Peter Hettel, who had experienced a remarkable spontaneous healing of terminal neuroblastic sarcoma. Peter, a former executive in a Florida software company, told me, "I used to feel very conflicted. All my life, I had flip-flopped back and forth between 'left brain' and 'right brain' mode, feeling like I had to cover over my intuitive side with strict, military precision. When I got sick, I began to see it's not that one state of mind is good and one is bad, but which state is appropriate. When you can shift easily back and forth between them, you don't get stuck."

The Kung Bushmen have been studied by anthropologists intrigued by their healing traditions. (More than half the men and 10 percent of the women become healers.) Kung healers seem to be able to draw on many facets of the personality rather than being wedded to a rigidly fixed identity. They seemed in a sense less tied to a limited ego organization, more able to bring forth other "selves" and an ever-changing spectrum of feelings. According to the results of the draw-a-person and thematic apperception tests that anthropologists administered, Kung healers had "a body self-image determined more by their own inner states than by external anatomical criteria. . . . Healers emphasize the central importance of fluid psychological processes and transitions that break out of the body's ordinary anatomical boundaries. [They have] easier access to a rich fantasy life . . . an openness to the unfamiliar and a primarily intuitive and emotional response, rather than a logical or rational one."[20]

As the indeterminate, multifaceted god Hermaphroditus would no doubt concur, the line between pathological dissociations like multiple-personality disorder and unusual powers of integration is perhaps not as stark as we might think. Michael Murphy writes: "Like certain religious adepts, multiples alter their flesh and consciousness through highly focused intention, hypnosis-like trance, and the retention of childlike mutability, though they do so in a dissociated and psychologically destructive manner. Further studies of their self-transformative strategies, conceivably, could reveal more practices that they share—however perversely—with people who display well-integrated forms of extraordinary functioning."[21]

But evoking the healing energies is not an ability limited to MPD sufferers, shamans, and saints. As Dr. Kenneth Ring points out, "We all dissociate to a degree."[22] To some extent, too, we are all capable of great fluidity of consciousness; the notion that we possess an invariant identity is, as both mystics and cognitive psychologists are wont to insist, something of a convenient fiction. Jung went so far as to maintain that "the ego itself is only a centralized complex which is not in full possession of the body, but is more just a focus. . . . In principle there is no difference between the ego complex and any other."

Dr. R. Fischer maintains that many, possibly even most, people live a form of multiple existence "by living from one waking state to another waking state; from one dream to the next; . . . from one creative, artistic, religious, or psychotic inspiration or possession to another; from trance to trance; and from reverie to reverie."[23]

His reference to trance may be particularly relevant. Physician Dr. David Cheek and several other mind-body researchers have proposed that hypnosis occurs spontaneously at times of severe stress.[24] And in a hypnotized state, Ernest Rossi notes, "the transformation of thought into action, sensation, movement, or vision is so quickly and so actively accomplished that the intellectual inhibition has no time to act."[25]

His description recalls that of the Kung healers and their more uninhibited "lability" of emotion and enactment. Trance and other altered states of consciousness are apparently more accessible to healers and dissociative personalities—as well as to those under the stress of illness. According to some theorists, trance is an *intrinsically* healing state "in which the patient can reallocate and reorganize his inner psychological complexities."[26] Perhaps it is through this reassociation that the "real forces of life" are enabled to move through us once more, animating us in new and unexpected ways. The Zinacanteco Indian notion that we have "thirteen souls," each of which must be kept healthy, implies there is a vital place in our lives for our complexities, our multiplicity, our unresolved issues and nascent potentials. The healing self seems to be not singular but ever changing, shifting, flowing from state to state—ever coming alive.

From this standpoint, disease-proneness begins when we cut off parts of ourselves that do not fit—those selves that speak too loudly, move too clumsily, shine too brightly, desire too ardently. But there is a law of conservation in the psyche—energies are never destroyed, only transformed. If these shadow parts cannot grow with us, they may grow against us—or, if given a chance, may emerge from the shadows to help make us well. As Alice Epstein discovered,

"Mickey," the subpersonality that seemed most intent on destroying her, was the very one most needful of love, and ultimately the one that bore the most magnificent healing gifts.

To come alive is to meet selves we do not yet know, selves we cannot yet love. Disease may bring them clamoring to the surface, for each part of our personality, each "soul," seeks its own authentic being. In crisis, dissociated parts of ourselves may struggle to be born again, to be accepted for what they are, to fulfill their own deferred dreams and destinies.

In *The Wizard of Oz*, the journeyers have been deprived of access to their real powers, leaving them with only pale imitations. The ersatz Scarecrow, the Woodman who chops himself to bits, the Lion with the phony roar are, in the words of one critic "three different ways of writing 'eunuch' "; three creatures (representing mind, emotion, and body) depotentiated, unable to fulfill their authentic being-in-the-world. Each inwardly mourns the severed connection to his own true feelings. Each attempts to replace the spontaneous, diversified energies of being with a falsely constructed "as-if" personality. Each slowly comes to understand that only by honoring the insurgent feelings that cause them such shame can they become whole. The Lion's pounding heart, as the Wizard points out, might be perceived not as a mortification, but as a powerful sign of aliveness. His counterfeit roar may not conceal his cowardice, but his courage: The disease-prone often siphon off what is strongest within themselves to effect a deadening parody of real being. We may find the clue to our authentic self in that which we do most frantically to hide it; in our defensive guises we may glimpse ephemeral, distorted images of our true face.

THE EMERALD CITY

In *The Wizard of Oz*, this notion of disguised good can be seen in the description of the Emerald City itself. As it turns out, it is not really an Emerald City at all; it only appears so because the inhabitants have had green glasses locked onto their heads with golden bands since its very founding. In spiritual parables, cities and buildings are often metaphors for the self. (St. Teresa of Avila spoke of the soul as an "interior castle . . . made of very clear crystal in which there are many rooms.") The Emerald City—not crystal (which admits all colors) but, in effect, one big monochromatic green room—represents but a small portion of being; a persona whose uniform grandiosity is, in the end, as monotonous as Dorothy's depressed, uniformly gray Kansas.

In the Emerald City, nothing can be appreciated in its uniqueness, but must be subsumed under one all-controlling emerald regime. We are told in the book that the sky is green, the sun is green, popcorn is green, lemonade is green. This city/self's external "colorfulness" has leached all life's *real* colors away. It is a situation reminiscent of the bright but ultimately superficial life strategies so often adopted by emotionally wounded people: always good, always "on" or "up," always talented, generous, busy, vigilantly paving over their vulnerabilities lest more dangerous and unpredictable realities of the self break through.

Ironically, as the journeyers later learn from the Wizard, Oz without the designer sunglasses is really "a beautiful place, abounding in jewels and precious metals, and every good thing that is needed to make one happy." The emerald world—undifferentiated, invariant, rigidly enforced, an artificial caricature of identity—has blinded its inhabitants to the vibrant multiplicity that is literally right before their eyes.

The suppression of our own real wealth of experience, of those primary feeling-colors that are, in Alice Epstein's words, "higher in their authenticity," distances us from our own idiosyncratic healing powers. To reclaim them, our emerald glasses, locked in place from the outset to protect its residents from the "glare," must be removed. For beyond both depressed inner Kansas and the inflated, manic Emerald City lies a magnificent kingdom with buildings of multi-colored gemstones (as well as earthy, ordinary brick)—only waiting to be fully inhabited.

🌺 15 🌺
THE SOCIAL FABRIC AND THE LOOM OF THE SELF

Destiny has summoned the hero and transferred his spiritual center of gravity from within the pale of his society to a zone unknown.

—JOSEPH CAMPBELL,
The Hero with a Thousand Faces

THERE ARE MANY other "emerald cities" along the path of healing—other people, with their own distorting glasses and potential for wholeness, each of whom can profoundly affect our progress. Of all the strands in our personal "web of existence," none are so crucial, or so vulnerable, as those that bind us to other people. Illness is a radical disruption of patterns of family, friendship, and community, a "disturbance in the Force" bearing unpredictable consequences. Our social connections may grow stronger, leading to new levels of intimacy; or they may fray, or snap altogether.

As we have seen, patients are often plunged into a process of profound personal change. They may begin to give vent to difficult emotions; grieve unreconciled losses; insist on different family roles. Those who know them best may feel they no longer recognize them—perhaps the reason social isolation is a recurrent theme in so many narratives of the healing journey. People in crisis may suddenly seem like strangers. Those around them feel at a loss where to place the "new" person within the existing social constellation. Journeyers can threaten the social structure itself, which may have secretly relied for its cohesion on allegiance to a sick-making status quo. Merely absenting themselves from their usual place in the order of things may reveal just how precariously that order has been balanced. A social fabric painstakingly woven over many years may unravel when a person struggling on the healing path yanks on a loose thread.

In *The Healing Family*, Stephanie Simonton counsels sick patients to focus more on their own needs, even if it means acting in ways their families consider selfish or greedy. The resultant behavior can seem shockingly out of character: The ever-accommodating Mom may refuse to play the docile wife and homemaker; Dad, previously an island of stability, may founder in waves of long-deferred tears or volcanically explode in rage. Issues long papered over may become painfully transparent, and their resolution suddenly seem essential to getting well again. Journeyers may find that they can no longer play their accustomed part on the social stage if the cost of a continuing role is an abandonment of the self.

This scenario is played out by the self-sacrificing George Bailey of *It's a Wonderful Life*. Since childhood, George has submerged his heart's urgencies in favor of everyone else's—his mother, father, brother, and uncle. As a result he is profoundly ambivalent about family ties. In his oddly stilted courtship of his wife-to-be, Mary, he at one point shouts at her in near despair, "I don't want to get married to anyone! I want to do what *I* want to do."

Their eventual union becomes an outwardly ideal marriage—virtuous, well-behaved children, self-sacrificing wife, upstanding husband. But just under the surface lie the dormant energies of George's long-suppressed selfhood. His role as family provider, pillar of the community, and curator of the downtrodden has failed to sustain his soul. His stoic acceptance hides a congealing depression, beneath which is a deep well of unexpressed anger. No wonder when his unconscious strategy of adaptation—George the All-Good—shatteringly fails, he goes on a rampage, barely restraining himself from beating up his alcoholic "Uncle Billy," yelling at his children's "stupid teacher," angrily demanding of his wife, "Why do we have to have all these *kids*?" Mary, who has never suspected his inner abyss, recoils in horror. She has chosen to ignore the cost of his social persona, and can be of no help when it finally shatters into pieces. It is only when George's inner guide, the guardian angel Clarence, orchestrates his journey of creative disintegration that he is able to recover his authentic self.

A RENT IN THE FABRIC

When one person undertakes a healing journey, it may affect not only his own body, but the "social body" as a whole. Traditional cultures recognized the powerful interplay between the sick person and society: The healthy individual was conceived of as an unbroken unity of self and social relations; the ill one, a symptom of imbalance in the "individual-cultural-environmental *gestalt*."[1] It would be useful, suggests one medical anthropologist, if we, too, recognized that our bodies, in sickness or in health, are the "terrain where social truths and social contradictions are played out, as well as a locale of personal and social resistance, creativity, and struggle."[2]

But we do not expect to bump up against "social contradictions" when we become ill. We assume that should sickness strike, we will quickly find ourselves at the center of a tableau of solace. Family will gather, encircling the sickbed in warm, protective wings; friends will materialize, offering service and succor. If any have cared about us in the past, love us now, or wish us boons in the future, surely they will come with caring multiplied a hundredfold in our hour of greatest need.

This is sometimes the case, and there is no shortage of moving stories of how families and sometimes entire communities join hands and hearts to help an ailing member. But from my own experience and that of others I talked with, the reality is often different, strewn with the unexpected obstacles to healing. In account after account, the journeyer finds herself adrift in a strangely reconfigured social matrix, cut off from familiar interchange, uncertain of others' responses. The archetypal nature of such dilemmas can be seen in the book of Job: Job's friends not only refuse him real comfort, but even castigate him as he sits helpless in the dust. And it is hard to forget George Bailey's dismay when shadow-world versions of his friends and loved ones not only fail to offer their hands, but push him roughly into the street.

Dr. Oliver Sacks trenchantly conveys his feelings as one of the afflicted during a day on the hospital grounds, watching the healthy shrink back from the invisible boundaries of the kingdom of the ill.

> Nothing gave me such a sense of the social caste of patients, their being out-cast, outcasts, set apart by society: the pity, the

abhorrence our white gowns inspired—the sense of a complete
gulf between us and them, which courtesy and ceremony served
only to emphasize. I realized how I myself, in health, in the
past, had shuddered away from patients, quite unconsciously,
never realizing it for a moment.[3]

This response to illness may be far less common in aboriginal
cultures, where healing typically becomes a community-wide affair.
But for most of us, sickness is to varying extents a plunge into radical
aloneness. The world of social norms may appear intact, yet feel
strangely disjunct. We are suddenly like a leaf in a rainstorm, bat-
tered from the common branch, eddying away. We try to communicate to those who are closest to us, hoping they can share our
burden, but our suffering remains maddeningly private. As one
patient said, "My friends and family were around, but it was like
they were all in a club I no longer belonged to, the Club of the
Living."

From within this isolation, reassurances can sound attenuated, as
if bouncing off a distant satellite—or perhaps it is we who are ca-
reering from the orbit of the social system into a bleaker quadrant
of interpersonal space. Arline Erdrich echoes the experience of
many: "At first, everyone rallies to your side. The energy's running
high. Friends, husband, children—they're all going to fight as a
unified front against this horrible disease, shoulder any load, endure
any hardship.

"But then things grind on, weeks turn into months, and then it
starts to wane. Your husband is getting irritated because he's tired
of doing the shopping after work every day. The kids are miserable
because they have extra laundry chores. Everybody starts wanting
it to be over.

"But you know it's not going to be, and they *see* it isn't going to
be, and the original overshowering of love and attention begins to
subtly dry up. They start conserving their own resources, and you
start to feel very, very alone."

Illness also can bring other people's primal issues to the surface,
revealing parts of *their* psyches that are normally obscured by the
patina of accustomed routine. Particularly in families that are skewed
towards narcissism and "co-dependence," patients may find themselves forced to deal with others' emotional demands while their
own desperate needs remain unmet. A medical student in San Francisco told me that when she haltingly informed her mother that she

had melanoma, "My mom got furious and screamed with accusation in her voice, 'You're going to die and leave me!' "

Annie Nathan, a rehabilitation counselor, recounted a conversation with a best friend who had recently injured her knee. At the time, Annie's cancer had just recurred, but her friend steamrollered all talk toward her own upcoming orthopedic surgery. "Finally I told her, 'Look, don't you realize that my *ass* is on the *line*? That I'm afraid I'm going to *die*?' We didn't talk for five months after that. When we finally did, we had this screaming battle. She kept saying, 'You weren't there for me for my knee!'

"Later, I learned that in her family, whatever she was going through was never considered important by her parents. So she wound up reenacting this childhood drama with me at a really inopportune time."

Suddenly, the world can seem topsy-turvy. Those we count on most may disappear or fall apart. Our own pain may evoke more conditional fear than unconditional love; our needs may intensify our loved ones' festering sense of deprivation. We reach out, but we are not sure anyone is there.

ALONENESS

See me. A physical wound may be an implosion, driving us toward the reality of our existential separation from each other. Once, when I was trying for the umpteenth time to convey to my girlfriend the specific texture of my suffering, she wearily interrupted me. "What you have," she said, measuring her words, "is a particularly vile distillation of the basic human condition. But you're not unique. *Everybody* suffers." Intellectually, I knew she was right. But I still wanted her to somehow crawl into my skin, to viscerally know my specific anguish, so I could escape for a minute my desperate solitude.

Feel me. I recall a conversation with a young San Francisco heiress dispatched by a well-meaning friend to look in on me after my surgery. She had dropped in on a particularly bad day. As I grated out my story, trying to describe the horror I felt at losing a vital organ, her baffled look suddenly resolved into an expression of empathy. "I know how you feel," she said. "I once got this really *terrible* haircut, and there was nothing I could do . . . "

Touch me. When she had solicitously placed her hand on mine, it was hard to know whether to laugh or cry. Maybe her coiffe-from-hell *was* the most physically dismembering event she could recall on the spot. Perhaps from her own cosseted reference point, she was doing her best to be responsive: Her attempt to break through the helplessness we all feel in the face of the irremediable was, in some sense, as touching as it was ludicrous.

Heal me. In the midst of conflagration, we hope fervently to be rescued, to be carried from the burning building of our body in the fireman's arms of those who love us. We may instead encounter a terribly human response: They may feel both angry and afraid in the face of something they feel helpless to change.

Those who become ill may be surprised to be confronted with another manifestation of human vulnerability, reproach, when they most expect the world to rally to their defense. "It's what we refer to as 'The Just World Hypothesis,' " a sociologist friend confided to me. "People may feel sorry for someone who's gotten sick. But they also feel threatened: If so-and-so, who hasn't really done anything wrong, is being 'punished,' then the world is intrinsically unjust. If that's true, it means *I'm* vulnerable. In order to keep clinging to my safer, more benign view of reality, I may have to blame you for your sickness, or start edging away so I don't have to face the fact that *you* could easily be *me*."

Job's friend Eliphaz, witnessing his sudden fall from grace, frets that such misfortune could befall him, too, for no one is "blameless against his Maker." Eliphaz sighs complainingly to Job that now he, too, is having nightmares: "In my thoughts during visions of the night . . . fear came upon me, and shuddering, that terrified me to the bones." Meanwhile, Job's friend Bildad can do little more than chirpily recite a Biblical Hallmark card—"Once more will he fill your mouth with laughter, And your lips with rejoicing"—counselling Job to imagine a more halcyon future.

Job is furious. More than promises of brighter days, certainly more than anxieties and condemnations, he wants his feelings to be heard and his pain acknowledged. But his friends, momentarily cantilevered over the abyss, can think only of backing gingerly to safety. Job lashes out: "Your reminders are ashy maxims,/Your fabrications are mounds of clay./Be silent, let me alone! that I may speak/and give vent to my feelings."[4]

What ensues is mutual incomprehension. "What do you know that we do not know?" Eliphaz demands of the now raging Job. For his part, Job can only restate that he knows, in the most intimate way possible, the impenetrability of suffering.

Job's predicament is not necessarily due to his friends' character flaws, for the ill can be frustrating conundrums. They want support; they want to be left alone. They want to receive love; they want to let out their anger. The dynamics are well expressed by former melanoma patient Chuck Kelley. "I'd been a 'loner' all my life, convinced I had to be in control and do everything myself. When I got sick, I became aware of wanting very much to give up the role. I wanted to be dependent on someone and be taken care of, but I also still needed to be independent and in charge. It was probably a little confusing."

Dr. Jacob Zieghelboim, flying up to Palo Alto each week for radiation therapy, found himself alone for the first time in years. It felt as if an engine that had been thrumming, impelling him through life for as long as he could remember, had suddenly fallen silent. He spent the week doing whatever he liked, reading the paper, going to the movies every day, walking aimlessly around the pretty college town.

"It was a period of gestation," he says. When he got back to UCLA, he carried his newfound aloneness back with him. To his shock, the life of being an immunologist at one of the world's great institutions suddenly looked as flat and washed out as an old mezzotint. "I walked in for my checkup and realized that nobody cared what was going on inside me, how I was really handling being sick, or was even curious about something so simple as what kind of diet I was following. The personal interactions suddenly seemed mechanical. How was it possible none of these things mattered to them? I began to question further: Why did this tumor develop? In what way was I different from everybody else?"

A REMINDER TO FRIENDS

Solitude may sometimes be integral to healing, a vessel in whose dark recesses new insights may germinate. Part of me wanted to be surrounded by helpers and supporters; longed to be rallied around as I fought what I then believed was a toe-to-toe, pike-against-broadsword battle with death. But I also craved isolation, time to explore strange and purely private terrains. I was feeling a compounding of vulnerability and exhilaration, of poignancy and fright, that I was unsure anyone from the bright climes of the healthy could comprehend; still, I was not prepared to formally renounce my citizenship for the protectorate of the ill. "You were sending out such mixed messages," a friend told me recently, "we were never sure *what* you were really asking us for."

I was asking them just to *be there;* instead they receded from view. Until I heard other patients describe it, I assumed my isolation was pure personal circumstance. I had come to a strange city, where I knew no one, and been confined for eighteen months in an isolated corner office trying to sustain a rickety enterprise. While I thought I had established relationships with a few other editors, I soon found that they had regarded me more as a beleaguered executive than a friend. And I felt mortified to want help from those whom I had tried—with less success than I had imagined—to impress with my capacity to solve all problems with unilateral aplomb. It was hard to admit I needed—needed with a terrible urgency—the hands-on caring of those around me.

It seems clear to me now that my life, particularly my relationships, had been ailing long before my illness. I had ignored messages from increasingly irritated friends, lovers, and family members. When I finally became sick, their frustration over years of not being heard came pouring through the sudden breach in my defenses. Expecting open arms, I instead found people bristling with unassuaged resentments and overdue I-told-you-so's. My illness became in effect an unaccepted apology. One writer-friend told me years later, "You struck me as this person who wanted to sing their own aria and be applauded for it, not enter into a dialogue and hear what someone else had to say. You were living at a self-dramatizing, operatic pitch for so long, you'd worn us out."

As my sociologist friend had described so well, one person's illness also can be an unwelcome reminder to others of how fundamentally fragile their own lives are. "My brethren are undependable as a brook," Job laments about his friends. "They see a terrifying thing and are afraid." John Studholme describes a friend he used to see once a week who vanished like a ghost. "I saw him twice that whole year, once when he waved weakly and crossed to the other side of the street before I could reach him."

Annie Nathan, a vivacious woman who radiates a warm concern, had worked in psychiatric centers for twenty years. "I did ten years with 'acting-out' adolescents, mainly in 'recreational' therapy and 'reparenting,'" she says. "I loved it."

But when she was diagnosed with breast cancer, her colleagues at the youth center—people with whom she had felt the camaraderie born of toiling, understaffed and overstressed, for idealistic goals—responded "as badly, as bizarrely, as you can imagine. No one could manage to talk to me directly, but there was this steady undercurrent. In one staff meeting, someone said, 'You know, it feels like there's just not enough milk to go around, like someone cut off a breast or something.'

"At the time, I was facing a mastectomy! I said, 'If anybody wants to talk with me about my health . . .' but they all quickly said, '*Oh, no, nothing to do with you.*'

"The arrogance of the healthy!" she exclaims, remembering a close friend who didn't call her for more than a year after learning she was sick. Finally, she got a Christmas card with a small note: "Trust all is well."

"Annie!" he said when she phoned him. "I have spent *thousands* of dollars talking about you!"

"What do you mean?" she asked, baffled.

"In *therapy.*"

Annie cracks up as she tells it, though his unavailability had been a harsh blow. "I just said, 'Listen, next time, save the money and just call *me.*' "

By contrast, the smallest gesture, the most random act of kindness, can seem magnified a hundredfold. The ill are like cameras set at their widest aperture, sensitive to the tiniest shard of light. While staying at a cancer center, I had a brief affair with a young woman who had been operated on for a liver tumor.

"It was a year before I let anyone touch me," she said as I gently traced the hard, rutted surgical scar than ran like a second spine from her sternum to a point below her navel. Being with her was the first chance I'd had to really compare notes with another patient, and I was amazed that she, too, had so quickly found herself alone. "It was strange," she told me. "It was the janitor at the elementary school where I taught—a guy I'd only nodded to a few times in the hall that year—who became my closest friend. He was the one who took it upon himself to bring me soup, read poetry to me. Even when he just sat by the bed, I could tell by his posture, by the angle of his head, that he was feeling what was inside me."

Many patients reported that people who had been most marginal in their lives "came through" when those they counted on receded. It did not take grand gestures to make a difference. John Studholme still remembers how far a single act by an old friend went to give him hope: "After my second chemo series, I was weak, nauseated, and exhausted. I could barely keep my head from falling on my plate over lunch. But my friend was insistent we walk over to a photo gallery because there was something he wanted me to see. We climbed up the stairs and he pointed out a black-and-white portrait of a young woman in an old tattered slip, her hands curled on the top of an overstuffed chair, looking away from the camera. The tone was so calm, like the moment after orgasm; like she was waiting for her lover to bring her a cigarette.

"I loved my friend for showing me this. He was telling me that I was still a man, not some sickly sonofabitch who could never again dream of putting himself in this scene. A week later, I bought the photo for him as a gift."

TESTING RELATIONSHIPS

The vagaries of friendship were not nearly as hard for journeyers to negotiate as the changes that took place in relationships with lovers and spouses. Marriages that had seemed stable for decades sometimes cracked along concealed faultlines. It sometimes seemed to me that the relationships that best weathered the storm were, ironically, those tethered to the shortest anchor chain of common history.

Some time after her divorce, Annie Nathan had begun a romance with the man who was to become her second husband. "We were going together for only nine months when—boom!—I get cancer. I told him, 'Look, you didn't bargain for this. If you need to, you can get out now and I'll understand.' He just put his hand on his heart. It's a ritual we still do. He stayed with me every second, through everything."

Debby Ogg, too, had just begun a new relationship. "Oscar and I had only known each other a year; we got married, and this disease happened." But "Oskie" was able to stick it out where others she had been closer to had not.

"I mean, even my own sister—who I'd lived communally with for years, who'd been mother, daughter, best friend—was just terrified beyond words. So she withdrew, muttering about someone she knew who had tried to heal herself and had *died*.

"It wasn't so much that she didn't believe in holistic medicine— she'd lived her life around it—but she couldn't bear the thought of me dying. And I was *enraged* with her. We spent a good month living in the same house not speaking ten words to each other.

"But Oskie, this relatively new person in my life, was there for me in this incredible way. I would ask him, 'Is this going to be all right?'

" 'Yes,' he would say.

"And I would say, 'Do you really know it, or just think it?'

"And he would say, 'I know it.'

"Of course, later on, when I started getting well, he told me he had been scared shitless!"

Often these new relationships came at the turning point that sometimes precedes the appearance of illness. As I have suggested, disease may be discovered at a significant juncture, when an old life strategy has reached a dead-end, or a new road is opening. In times of personal change, old relationships sustained by unsuspectedly fragile cobwebs of habit may finally shear away. Some people, like Samantha Coles, were forced to the painful realization that her closest relationships had been built on sand. "I think I've spent a lot of time unconsciously manipulating others to get my needs met. I'd always used relationships addictively, as a distraction to get away from my own pain. When they didn't work out, I'd get to feel abandoned, but would manage once again to avoid the deeper issue of *why*. I guess I attracted people all through my life who were manipulative and needy. No wonder they couldn't tough it out."

REPEATING FAMILY DYNAMICS

Samantha's observation is a key to understanding why the path through the social realm is often paved in broken stones. Particularly in the case of the disease-prone personality, relationships have a tendency to mirror the dysfunctional family dynamic. Ties may be based less on healthy mutual respect than on raw need, fear of abandonment, and the mechanism psychologists call "repetition compulsion"—the tendency to recreate the original family neurosis in a futile, unconscious attempt to heal it.

Samantha had always wanted a "normal family, like on TV." But the horror of incest had ruined the picture. Her social life, before she was diagnosed with melanoma, had consisted of "crazy relationships you'd need an advanced geometry degree to figure out." At the time she was facing her first operation, she had been dating a married man at the same time as she was living with someone else. And she was still enmeshed in the incest-tainted triangle with her parents, who, rather than joining together to give her support, used her predicament to score points against each other.

The entire cast of Samantha's personal soap opera showed up at the hospital after her first surgery. "Both my men were in the room, acting totally hostile to each other. My mother as usual was playing the Drama Queen, staging her own little vignette in the waiting room, using my being sick to get sympathy for *herself*. And the closest my dad has ever come to intimacy is to ask, 'How's the car running?' Here I am all bandaged up, the two boyfriends starting to fight, my mother screaming and yelling, my dad in his own automotive universe, and I have to send them all home. And then here I am again, alone, with no one to love me."

Abandonment was the last thing Samantha wanted—it had been the recurring motif of her life. When she mounted her first graduate art exhibit, her parents were no-shows. Gallery after gallery had opened and closed on her paintings with no sign of the people she was really doing it all for, the people she wanted to be proud of the high-achieving, twenty-four-year-old daughter who was already a university professor.

It was maddening. "You've performed as best you can," she says. "Done it the way you thought *they* thought it should be done, and you *still* can't get their approval."

Samantha had several times considered suicide to resolve "that trapped feeling" of wanting something so utterly unavailable. *After I'm dead, they'll care*, she'd fantasize. But then she would catch herself, thinking ruefully, *Drama Queen*.

Now that she was ill, "playing the Death Scene," she thought her parents might finally give her the love she still craved. But to her dismay, her illness changed nothing. Later, well along in her own psychological explorations, she tried to talk to her mother about their family life, only to receive an angry denial that there had ever been any problems: It was all in her head. After that, Samantha didn't speak to either of her parents for nearly two years. "If you didn't get the approval from your biological family, whatever you wangle from other people never quite works. I had been willing to *die* to get my mother into my life. Now, finally, I'm beginning to own my past, to heal my relationship with my inner parents, instead of trying to get love from my real ones."

A cascade of self-help books has lately made clear that such families are a poor foundation for subsequent life partnerships. Many of the journeyers I interviewed had laid the cornerstones of their relationship without ever considering if the building would be a soaring, light-admitting home or a dank gothic castle—so long as the roof kept out the lonesome rain. Often partners had been subconsciously chosen for their perfectly interlocking neuroses. Life together was a potato-sack race; as long as each had one leg, things might hop along. But if illness caused one person to lose his footing, the relationship toppled over sideways when it most needed to stand firm.

Sometimes when the person who had been playing the role of prime nurturer got sick, the partner who had come to depend on their unceasing bounty reacted with more petulance than sympathy. Arline Erdrich's husband became what she described as "a hypersensitive basket case. One of the first things he said to me was, 'If you die, what will I do? How will I take care of these kids? How will *I* survive?' He was so focused on himself, which was typical of the marriage. My getting sick just exacerbated it."

Because the quest to enact the authentic self inevitably produces a demand for authentic relatedness, the personal changes that accompany illness may also threaten the partner. A patient's wanting to become who she truly is sometimes proves an unacceptable premise. Arline describes a scene from her marriage:

> When I was sick and low, my husband could be nurturing. But when I was at a high point on the healing rollercoaster, he almost seemed to resent my sudden enthusiasm for living. One day he looked me right in the face and said something that will stay with me forever: "I wish you had died. It would have made all the suffering worthwhile."
>
> What he meant was, if I'd died, he would have suffered, but he would have been a hero, because everyone would have acknowledged him as this attentive, long-suffering husband who had done his level best. He could have mourned and it would have been over.
>
> Instead, I'd get back from the hospital and do my best not to just get healthy but *better*. He became convinced I was exercising to maintain my youth, so that I'd be attractive to others. He accused me of painting large canvases just to get attention. But I was fighting like the devil to not just fall back into old patterns. I was pulling away as a separate being. I was saying, I am not an extension of you. Together we make a team, we have similar purposes and goals, but we are not one, we are two.

Arline's newly emergent sense of self created a demand for *change* in her relationship, a crucial factor noticed by almost all researchers who study exceptional recovery. The Japanese researcher Ikemi noted that the "dramatic change of outlook" which preceded all remissions he catalogued had caused "the reconstruction of the patient's relationship with his human environment." He cites, in his famous report on spontaneous remission, the case of a fifty-eight-year-old farmer's wife who had married early into virtual bondage to a "strict" mother-in-law and a "bossy and self-centered husband," who between them had made her life as "bitter as death." After she was diagnosed with terminal stomach cancer, her family underwent a radical shift, their previous "demanding and indifferent approach" turning into a "warm and sympathetic concern." Ikemi refers to the work of fellow researcher Sir David Smithers, who wrote that a key contributing cause of cancer was the "traumatic interaction between the patient and his human environment," while a crucial healing catalyst was an "intentional or accidental" change for the better.[5]

What constitutes positive change in the social equation of illness and health can vary wildly. Charles Weinstock, a former clinical professor of psychiatry at New York's Albert Einstein College of Medicine, compiled a list of examples from medical literature and spontaneous remissions seen in his own practice. It included such social sea-changes as "a sudden fortunate marriage by a woman of forty; a nun's experience of having the entire order engage in intercessory prayer for her; the fortunate death of a decompensated addicted spouse who had blocked the patient's musical career by his dependency; unexpected, enthusiastic praise and encouragement from an expert in one's field."[6]

In Arline's case, her marriage, too shaky to weather the buffeting, eventually landed on the rocks. For a long time, she resented her husband for not having changed along with her as she had begun at last to come into her own. After they separated, Arline came to a realization: "I figured out why he couldn't love me; he really couldn't love himself."

FORGIVENESS

Despite a lingering bitterness, Arline managed what she felt to be a surpasssing emotional feat: She and her former husband became friends. "He even boasts about my painting career now," she says with a laugh. "I learned to accept responsibility for my part in what went wrong. I've healed that relationship, repaired it. It's quite phenomenal, but I learned to forgive him."

The ripples spread by the healing of relationship can become powerful healing currents. Forgiveness and healing in particular are often said to be peculiarly related. The very word *remission*, the term for the regression of disease, also means, according to the dictionary, "relinquishing, surrendering; forgiveness, pardon as of sins or crimes."

But the realm of forgiveness, too, has its own tricks of terrain. "Genuine forgiveness does not deny anger but faces it head-on," writes Alice Miller. She criticizes "the religious notion that a 'gesture of forgiveness' will make you a better person," preferring to champion the patient's right to explore emotional trauma without pressure to renounce the "anger, rage, impotence, despair that may accompany it." Only then can anger and hatred be transformed into sorrow and finally sympathy. Only then is forgiveness truly a form of grace, appearing "spontaneously, when a repressed (because forbidden) hatred no longer poisons the soul. The sun does not need to be told to shine. When the clouds part, it simply shines. But it would be a mistake to say that clouds are not in the way if they are indeed there."[7]

Wil Garcia had no doubt about the presence of dark social thunderheads in his life. All he had to do was feel his own fulminating resentment at the sight of the co-manager at his office, a woman who had become his archnemesis. Wil was in dire straits. The acrobatics of juggling his computer job with doctors' appointments and sick care for his lover, George—to say nothing of the stress of concealing his own AIDS diagnosis from his co-workers at the brokerage firm—were taking their toll. Weekends and nights were the only times Wil could make up the work he was missing, and even then, he was shuttling back and forth to his apartment, checking on George. Once, late on a Saturday night, he left for an hour. His co-manager was furious. What followed was "one for my personal annals of nastiness. I was so professional usually, I'd lived my life under such rigid rules, that I couldn't even use vulgar words. All I can remember of my argument is saying 'Woman' when I meant 'Bitch,' while she kept calling me 'Mister,' whatever she meant by that!"

After that, work became a snakepit. The air throbbed with tension every time he passed her in the hall. "I started thinking: if I can forgive this woman, I can forgive anyone." Wil made up a mental exercise based on a chapter in a self-help book he was reading. "I visualized her sitting calmly on a stage. Suddenly wild wolves would come in and tear her to shreds. The image was really bloody, and she'd just be mangled completely. Then I'd imagine her fired from her job, humiliated and abandoned. I wouldn't bother to stifle my emotions, because I'd figured out that if you don't express them, nobody's going to express them for you."

Down would come the curtain on Wil's grisly playlet. But then it would come up again, and Wil would visualize his enemy as "beautiful, healthy, wealthy, loved, with everything she's ever wanted in her life. I'd allow that part to go on as long as I could stand." Then the curtain would fall again, this time rising on Wil, now similarly radiant with health and fulfillment.

Whenever he would see her in the hallway, feeling his rage mount, he would run to the bathroom and "start visualizing like mad. This would happen two, three times a day—I'm sure she thought I had a problem!" But he noticed that every so often they would make eye contact, have a trivial conversation, even occasionally talk.

One day, suddenly, unexpectedly, the clouds parted. "She said to me, 'Wil, there's something I have to tell you. For the past two months I've been sending you love.' It turned out she'd been doing for me the same thing I was doing for her! It also turned out that she had her own burden of suffering: she had just lost a dear friend to AIDS, had broken up from a long-term relationship, and had been having serious problems with her seventeen-year-old son."

Soon afterward, Wil told me, shaking his head in amazement, the same woman became an integral member of his "healing circle" of friends and associates.

SOCIAL HEALING

Our culture tends to assume that the ordinary social web is resilient enough to support the enormity of illness. But Wil and many of the people I studied stressed the critical importance of mobilizing extended family, networks, healing circles, and support groups to help them on their path.

Few traditional cultures could conceive of individual healing as separate from community life. In their worldview, one person's illness affects the whole social corpus, and therefore all share responsibility for helping the afflicted person to heal—perhaps healing themselves and society in the process. In the face of our society's tendency to isolate the sufferer, journeyers' efforts amounted to an attempt to resurrect this older order of collective caring. For a number of them, it was as if some social gene, already encoded with knowledge of these ancient bonds, had suddenly switched on.

Carol Boss found that the informal network of friends that coalesced around her was almost miraculously able to integrate her illness into their lives. At first there was a shockwave—she was the last person anyone had expected to fall sick. But somehow, everyone around her seemed to join in a rhythm of transformation, as if she had unwittingly provided the catalyst for their latent longings for wholeness. "The people who wanted to heal me started healing them*selves*. The fact that I was doing my 'work' made others take *their* medicine, whatever it was. The tendency when we're ill is to close ourselves off, not let people know. But I don't think we can go off in caves and heal by ourselves. In some mysterious way, it's a communal experience. I think healing is contagious, just like infection."

This is an intriguing observation in light of the Kung tradition of communal healing. Richard Katz points out that *num*, or healing power, is not sought for its own sake, but for the individual and the group simultaneously:

> There are no restrictions in the access to *num*. In egalitarian fashion, all receive healing. *Num* is shared throughout the community. It is not meant to be hoarded by any one person. Perhaps it never can be. There is no limit to *num*. It expands as it boils. Healing is directed as much toward alleviating physical illness in an individual as toward enhancing the healer's understanding; as much towards resolving conflict in the village as toward establishing a proper relationship with the gods and the cosmos. A healing may be specifically directed toward one of these focuses, but the healing in fact affects them all.[8]

Deena Metzger came to almost identical first-hand conclusions about the social dimensions of illness and healing. It became clear to her, she wrote in an essay titled "Cancer Is the Answer," that

> healing takes place in the larger body, in the body of friends and loved ones that gather around the patient. Just as one person often carries the illness for the rest of us, for the family and small circle, as well as for the body politic, so the body politic, the small circle, and the family, by healing themselves, by attending to illness, can begin to heal the patient. In fact

there exists only one world and one body, and illness or health in one part directly affects the others.[9]

The social body, like the human body, seems to possess an innate healing power. Dr. Dean Ornish originally set up his heart groups as a way of helping people stay on their rigorous programs of diet and exercise. But what he found, he told me, is "the support groups are probably the most powerful therapeutic intervention of all. We create a place where people feel safe enough to show who they are beneath these masks they wear. Even in our own families, with our own spouses, we have trouble letting ourselves be seen."[10]

An individual's social role may have profound effects on her or his level of wellness. I was struck by how many of the "self-healers" I spoke with turned out to be the sort of service-oriented "givers" who wind up in caring professions, take on others' problems, try to save the world. In dysfunctional-family gospel, such people often suffer from a crippling need to rescue others while ignoring their own needs, a linchpin of the disease-prone personality.

It may be that such people *were* drawn into their social pursuits by a low sense of self-worth or "soft ego boundaries." And certainly, do-gooding too often has a psychological shadow—the public saint may privately loathe himself, the great community benefactor may browbeat his family. But it was striking how so many journeyers, even in the midst of their own struggles, turned toward helping.

Evy McDonald was a classic giver who worked for years as a nurse and high-powered hospital administrator. But in September of 1980, she was diagnosed with a particularly rapid form of incurable amyotrophic lateral sclerosis (ALS), in which the muscles of the body simply waste away. (Stephen Hawking, author of *A Brief History of Time*, is a tragic and luminous prisoner of this condition.)

Evy was given at most one year to live. Sitting in her wheelchair, she writes her article, "A Healing in the Theatre of Life," she was overcome with a "single passionate desire . . . In my last months of life I wanted to experience unconditional love." With her flaccid body withering at an alarming rate, unable to brush her own teeth, she began with herself. Looking down at a body she realized she had always hated and now found "disgusting" and "intolerable," she devised a series of radical exercises. Sitting naked before a mirror, starting first with small, halting self-testimonials—"I have lovely hands;" "my hair is truly pretty"—she gradually learned to accept as "aesthetically pleasing . . . soft, sensuous" the "bowl of Jell-O" she had become. Coincident with her discovery of this "fresh new experience of self," her ALS mysteriously reversed its course.[11]

In lectures, Evy repeatedly stresses that her physical healing was not a sought-after result, but a "by-product" of the deep, wrenching personal changes she wished to make before she died. Many of these changes, she told me, had to do with her relationship to the world. She began to realize that her social self and inner self had long been severed by "a life of hypocrisy" in which she was ostensibly helping others, but secretly felt trapped in a spiral of competitive achievement. "I had declared my life was devoted to service to those around me," she told a gathering of ALS health-care workers in Italy after her unprecedented recovery, "but I was soon forced to admit this was not quite true. Yes, I did charitable things, I became a nurse and cared for others, I acted with kindness, but it was all done with an expectation of something in return. . . . not out of the joy of giving."[12]

During her illness, she had repeated to herself a catch-phrase: "You can accomplish anything if you are willing to take credit for nothing." This mantra was not a sugar-coated petition for a miracle but "a program for me to stop all of my pretenses, drop all my masks." She learned, she says in her soft, firm voice, the difference between "people-pleasing, helping others for recognition or out of duty, and the spontaneous upwelling that comes from the soul." No wheelchair, no handicap, no disease, she insists, can render this "place of upwelling" inaccessible. Health, she concludes, "is not only soundness of mind and body, but soundness of social connection."

THE COMMUNITY OF AFFLICTION

Dean Ornish confided to me his suspicion that *giving* support in a group might play as large a role in the healing process as receiving it. "I think one of the reasons that people get better in our studies is the very fact that they know they're part of a project that could be important not just for them, but for other people. It's healing to them to have this role of making a difference to other people." Perhaps the crucial factor is the sense of belonging to the human community that a giving interchange creates. "The literature indicates," says Dr. Ornish, "that even just being a member of a church or a synagogue seems to reduce mortality from heart disease by forty or fifty percent." Even in cell studies, a strong positive correlation has been found between natural killer cell strength and the social adjustment of the donors—the sense of "fitting in."

Some of the patients who fared best, however, struck me as somewhat desocialized people. They might have rejected (or been rejected by) their families, or tended to swim upstream against social norms—particularly while pursuing their quest for healing. But perhaps this route was necessary when to be a "well-adjusted individual" had meant fitting into an unhealthy social milieu: "Normal" life, for some patients, may have itself been pathogenic. An interlude of "not fitting in," of leaving familiar moorings, sometimes led to a community of like-minded people with whom a deeper healing could be shared.

Sometimes the strongest sense of community developed among those similarly afflicted. During the first few days of my week-long stay at an alternative cancer center, I felt myself resisting any identification with the other "sick people." But I soon discovered the great relief of sharing humor, anguish, hope, jargon, and gossip with people of your own genus of suffering, or encountering those who were further along the road of healing. And seeing those worse off than I was knocked the props out from my own self-pity. As in the ad hoc community of afflication formed by Dorothy, the Tin Woodman, the Cowardly Lion, and the Scarecrow, the healing journey can be enhanced by companions on the path.

Dr. Oliver Sacks, commenting further on his experiences in a rehabilitation wing full of patients with similar ailments, writes:

> I was no longer confined to my own, empty world, but found myself in a world peopled by others—*real* others, at least in relation to each other and me: not just role-players, good or bad, as my caretakers had been. Only now could I exorcise the fearful words of the surgeon to me: "You're unique!" Now, speaking freely to my fellow patients—a freedom made possible precisely by fellowship, by the fact that they were, *we* were, brothers together, under no status pressure to conceal or distort—I learned that my own experience, my "case," was far from unique.[13]

Today, no matter how exotic the disease category, any moderate-sized community boasts a plethora of self-help and support groups. A few residential retreat facilities have sprung up around modern scourges like heart disease, AIDS, and cancer, and there are any number of outpatient counseling organizations, such as Santa Monica's Wellness Center (made famous by the late "Saturday Night Live" star Gilda Radner), Denver's QuaLife, and New Haven's ECaP (Exceptional Cancer Patients), the latter founded by the holistic guru and surgeon Dr. Bernie Siegel.

I saw Dr. Siegel at a $15-a-ticket talk at the cavernous Denver Coliseum not long ago. The place was packed to the balconies, and Bernie was omnipresent—on TV monitors, on T-shirts (where he was represented by a rose), on audiocassettes and videotape boxes. Brimming baskets of lavender flowers were laid like oblations before the podium. Red, corpuscular helium balloons jostled overhead to strains of the ubiquitous Pachelbel's Canon. When the short, bald man in the dapper blue suit mounted the stage, I expected the six-thousand-strong crowd—most of them patients and their families—to take up a full-throated athletic-event chorus of "Ber-*nie!* Ber-*nie!*" Such gatherings are Chatauquas of psychoneuroimmunology. The audience, the majority of them patients and their relatives, had come together for an evening of inspiration and information, for a small moment of respite, or salvation; they gazed longingly at the figure at the podium, his shaved pate gleaming in the spotlight.

Other longer-term communities of affliction have developed, from farflung, losely affiliated networks to full-blown subcultures replete with their own mythology, terminology, social rituals, and even political clout. Perhaps none has formed with more visible and sometimes noisy cohesion than the AIDS community.

During a visit to Los Angeles, I attended a gathering for several hundred people with AIDS (P.W.A.'s), held across the street from the city's famous "Big Blue Whale" Pacific Design Center. I was amazed, after the isolation I had felt as a cancer patient, at the warmth and camaraderie in the crowded room. "P.W.A. dance at Oil Can Harry's," boomed a lanky man with a gray ponytail. "Come in drag, jeans, C&W, disco, whatever you want."

There were "energy tables" for massage, "sharings" at the microphone, help lines and carpools. A tough-looking black man whose close-cropped "fade" sported an intricate pattern of furrows announced he had come to try to forgive the cousin who had molested him as a child. The cousin, he said, his voice trembling with an inconceivable mix of emotions, had just died of AIDS. A woman stood up and choked into the mike, "I love my gay son," then sat down to sustained applause. Others spoke of not being able to afford drugs like AZT or DDI, or of the struggle to live in a society that considered them lepers.

Street people, an unusually high percentage of whom have AIDS, had been invited to the gathering. A man in cheap orange sunglasses and stained blue chinos sat on a folding chair in the back, fastidiously cleaning his bare feet with a towel while a speaker called the disease "the ultimate vulnerability. My healing has been in tearing down the wall around my heart that isolated me from other people." I felt a moment of disorientation. Was it AIDS Woodstock? The disease, the speaker was saying, will change the medical system, lead to new cures for other ailments, heal families of their emotional ills. It was a proposition of Plague as Panacea.

Perhaps because the dark stain of AIDS has spread within a cohesive community of relatively young people, or because there is as yet no hint of a cure—or even because AIDS is a quintessentially interpersonal disease—there has arisen among some PWA's an inclusive, almost salvationist evangel: We can heal through love and self-acceptance, and through that, we can save the world. "We need to reorient from self and competition toward cooperation," said a speaker. "We are all cells on this planet. If a cell in the body goes its own way and says, 'Screw you!' it's cancer."

But if cancer is a disease that has lent itself to Cold War metaphors of battle lines and borders, civil war and subversion, AIDS is an Information Era disease, global and borderless, a malignly replicable glitch in the cellular software. It is seen as breaking down the touchstone of biologic individuality, the immune system, which distinguishes "self" from "other"—suddenly rendering boundaries between gay and straight, between nations, between cell walls infinitely permeable.

"We carry within us the power to end all the fighting," another lecturer intoned, "to put up the white flag. It's not giving up, but surrendering to the universe. It's the one flag with nothing on it. It says, 'I forgive myself and those I thought were in conflict with me.' "

"This plague may take our lives," added a final speaker, "but it cannot take away our dreams." Indeed, the AIDS epidemic often has been compared to the Great Plague, the fourteenth-century Black Death. But while medieval Europeans saw their symptoms, as signs of "God's terminal disappointment in his creature" (in the historian Barbara Tuchman's phrase), many AIDS patients I spoke with saw theirs as a chance to take up a different banner, the one once hoisted by William Blake: to dethrone the God of Judgment within oneself, and replace him with the God of Forgiveness and Healing.

In place of the fourteenth-century Dances of Death with their phalanxes of bloody self-flagellators, many AIDS patients have created "Circles of Love," in which as many as six hundred gay men and a sprinkling of straight friends and relatives pack into rented gymnasiums to sway together to the strains of "Spirit Am I" ("Spirit am I/Freed of all limits/Spirit am I/Safe, healed, and whole/Spirit am I/Free to forgive/Spirit am I/Free to save the world").

At the gathering I attended, a final speaker said, "Like the Black Death, AIDS will probably go away when it's done its job." That job, he claimed, is not punishment but feedback, a "planetary metaphor" for the human species' collective rush toward self-destruction. In its time, the Black Death, too, was thought to be a mirror of the imminent fate of the earth, of tempests and earthquakes then widely reported to be resonating through the macrocosm, of a planet groaning beneath the weight of accumulated sin.

Similarly, I have heard various members of the AIDS community juxtapose the disease with the ravaging of the environment, as if AIDS were a reflection of industrial society's destruction of the "planetary immune system" (the ozone layer), of the earth's living cells (the biota), bloodstream (polluted oceans and streams), lungs (the burning forests), and very flesh (toxic waste dumps).

SICKNESS AND SOCIETY

Such notions are largely a function of how people "come to use health, illness, and healing as expressions of their concerns for meaning, moral order, and individual effectiveness and power in their daily world," as one study of alternative health groups expressed it.[14] But epidemiologists have suggested that at least some of our current "diseases of civilization" may well be linked to what we are doing to our world. (Indeed, some biologists have suggested that the increase in harmful ultraviolet rays from our industrial society's depletion of the ozone layer could result in a global increase in immune-related disorders.)

The "big picture" view of disease is often ignored in the microscopic search for genetic single causes and molecular magic bullets. Our dominant medical-scientific efforts could be viewed from one standpoint as attempts to keep the human components of the engines of commerce functioning in an increasingly toxic environment; to sweep the real effects of industrial culture under a diagnostic-therapeutic rug; to find a technological quick fix for diseases that barely existed before the ecological abuses of technology.

"We act as if we can look at a gene and say, 'Ah-ha, this gene causes this disability,'" says Harvard biology professor Dr. Ruth Hubbard, "when in fact the interactions between the gene and the environment are enormously complex. It moves our focus from the environmental causes of disabilities—which are terrifying and increasing daily—to individual genetic ones."[15]

It was long theorized that African-Americans had a genetic predisposition that accounted for their cancer rates 6 to 10 percent higher than those of whites. According to *The New York Times*, however, a recent reexamination of the raw data suggests that a root cause is *poverty*: substandard living conditions (often including more polluted air and water), bad nutrition, and poor access to health care.[16]

Heroically and at great social expense, doctors try to save one person at a time from death; but unlike shamanic healers, few address the wider significance of the disease. By treating illness as a personal or at most familial tragedy, we effectively shield ourselves from awareness of the larger patterns of disharmony. As a result, a larger, more embracing "cure"—putting a brake on a system that is willing to trade a mounting toll of misery to maintain a consumer economy—is viewed as impractical and romantic.

"An advanced industrial society is sick-making," the philosopher Ivan Illich writes. "People would rebel against such an environment if medicine did not explain their biological disorientation as a defect in their health, rather than a defect in the way of life which is imposed on them or which they impose on themselves."

It is perhaps worth reciting here the litany of some of the grosser impositions: 40 million Great Lakes residents exposed to concentrations of toxic chemicals in water and fish; 42 million Louisianians living along "Cancer Alley," a center for petrochemicals, toxic landfills, and industrial waste dumping in the Mississippi River; 50 million U.S. residents drinking pesticide-contaminated water; every U.S. citizen potentially exposed to the 2.6 billion pounds of pesticides applied each year on lawns, parks, forests, schools, homes, and at every link of the food chain; 135 million Americans living in areas with unsafe levels of ozone and carbon monoxide; more than 2 million plastics workers exposed directly to vinyl chloride . . . and the list goes on.[17]

Clear evidence emerged in 1993 that common pesticides are likely co-factors in the staggering, three-decade rise in breast cancer. The same chemicals that quell insects and stifle weeds can, it turns out, also mimic the effect of estrogen, the hormone associated with higher risk of breast cancer. Mary Wolff of New York City's Mount

Sinai Medical Center discovered that women whose blood contained high concentrations of DDT residue were four times as likely to get breast cancer. "The numbers are terrifying, really," she says. "I still can't believe the risk is that high."

If the studies are confirmed, said one article, "it would mark the first time that a direct environmental cause has been established for breast cancer, and the focus of the nation's multi-million dollar battle against breast cancer could shift to prevention, instead of diagnosis and treatment."[18]

The Quollahuayas, a Bolivian tribe known as the "lords of the medicine bag" for their use of a sophisticated healing system dating to 700 A.D., believe their health is irrevocably linked to that of a nearby sacred mountain. Since sickness is thought to result from disharmonies between land and people, the mountain, Pachemama, must be cared for like a living creature. Healers periodically gather at special points corresponding to its "organs" to give it medicines to restore it to health.

This strikes us as merely a quaint animism. But what would be the result if we, too, looked upon our environment as our own body, considered its sicknesses our sicknesses, its regeneration our cure? Would we tolerate the effluents flowing into our water-arteries, or the chemicals poisoning the rich loam of our flesh? Would we not rush out to clean up the toxic waste-dumps that are not only festering chancres in our planet-body but sources of carcinogens that may one day lodge in our own bones? Would not, in other words, treating the "diseases" of nature make us collectively less sick?

One-third of humanity died during the plague of the Black Death. Today it is projected that one out of every three Americans will get some form of cancer. Not only our fragile environment but our own fragile bodies bear witness to the slow-motion catastrophe that is the underside of our astounding civilization.

Our tendency is to ignore the wider symptomology until it appears at our doorstep, on our dinner table, or inside our bodies. Even at that point, we are likely to avoid dwelling upon the implications lest we face the necessity for disruptive social change.

Medical anthropologists Nancy Scheper-Hughes and Margaret Locke write:

> All of us can be open and responsive to the hidden language of pain and protest . . . or we can cut it off by relegating our complaints to the ever-expending domains of medicine ("it" is in the body) or psychiatry ("it" is in your mind). . . . Once safely

medicalized, however, the social issues are shortcircuited, and the desperate message in the bottle is lost.[19]

Our current social order may be implicated in illness to a degree that we have not yet measured. It may even be that our contemporary social life itself is squeezing us into boxes too small for the bodymind. *Homo technologicus* is a mere fingernail paring in the long reach of our species' upward climb. Recent studies have shown our body-minds are still best suited for hunter-gatherer diets, for life in tightly knit communities, for living according to the rhythms of seasons and diurnal cycles. The "workweek" of our tribal ancestors has been estimated at only twenty hours; the rest of the time, judging from the lives of contemporary tribal peoples, was spent in conversation, grooming, song, dance, ceremony, and play.

In 1967 Senate testimony, industrial-policy experts predicted that by 1985, the workweek would be reduced to twenty-two hours as a result of labor-saving devices and more efficient postindustrial technologies. Harried modern humankind would go back to the Garden. Instead, the average workweek is now forty-seven hours (eighty hours or more in some professions), and leisure time has continued to shrink. "Stress has become one of the most serious health issues of the 20th Century," said a 1993 report by the UN's International Labor Organization. Our workday permits no siestas (which we consider lazy and unproductive), even though human biorhythms mandate daily periods of rest. Should it not tell us something that, during our end-of-the-workday ritual of the nightly news, we are bombarded almost exclusively with ads for stomach-pain and headache remedies?

The Japanese shamanic healer Ikuko Osumi states that one of the main causes of illness is "the accumulation of tiredness due to the overuse of nerves and body functioning, resulting from unwise ways of living and working." But our society as a whole seems to be running out of the time and space to properly nurture the bodymind. The Japanese refer to a new and deadly affliction called "hurry disease." A successful American architect quoted in a recent magazine article said ruefully, "Technology is increasing the heartbeat. The pace is so fast now, I sometimes feel like a gunfighter dodging bullets." It is almost superfluous to point out the correlation between this level of stress and the excess release of cortisol and other hormones that are implicated in disease formation. In 1922, Emily Post counseled that the proper mourning period for a mature widow was three years. Fifty years later, Amy Vanderbilt advised the bereaved to be about their normal business within a *week* or so, although current studies show decreased immune system reactivity in the blood of surviving spouses for up to a year following a partner's death.

Human societies, as social psychologist Erik Erikson observed, tend to create through their child-rearing methods the personality types on which they place the most functional value. In our culture, the narcissistically wounded child becomes an adult willing to barter hypertrophied patterns of labor, consumption, and material accumulation for love. The Tin Woodman, who tries to chop clean and strong with his sharp blade, under the Witch's spell winds up cutting off his own limbs and replacing them with metal; the perfect adaptation to the industrial megamachine, he becomes a machine himself.

And so, from the family to the schools to the corporation and eventually the hospital, we hear the drone of self-forsaking persuasion. The "loss of soul" is pandemic, attested to by all the measures we take—substance abuse, exploitative relationships, workaholism, overeating, and a mass appetite for vicarious entertainment—in trying to fill the void within.

The Greek mythological character Procrustes always greeted visitors to his island with impeccable hospitality, supplying them with intoxicating libations and holding stupendous feasts. But as night fell, he would exact a fearsome toll: He would lay his unfortunate guests one by one upon an iron bed. If they were too tall for it, he would lop off their limbs to size; if they were too short, he would stretch them on a rack until they fit perfectly. The Procrustean nature of twentieth-century life needs no further confirmation than our "diseases of civilization," the running tally of the hidden cost of what we have built and paid for—and continue to operate, maintain, and consume—in the name of a better life.

AN ANATOMY OF PROTEST?

In the midst of such a mass cognitive dissonance experiment, we must wonder if those who find the music of society's clashing spheres most excruciatingly out of tune are not those most likely to fall ill— if they are not the canaries in the coal mine, warning of impending breakdown. In an imaginary history of the twentieth century, Deena Metzger suggests that the most disease-prone among us are those least adaptable to accepted levels of societal "mayhem . . . [those]

who could not tolerate the culture and so succumbed, psychologically, spiritually, and then physically."[20]

The sick person may in fact be a component of the social machine that has broken under the strain of the manufacture of pathology. Some of our illnesses might be seen as a form of a passive revolt, a bodily protest lodged against the toxification of the environment, Procrustean social compacts, and the sheer pressure of living out agendas that are personally inauthentic. We tenants of modern industrial society find ourselves forced into ever smaller rooms as more of our common house becomes walled-off and uninhabitable. Cornered in the world we have collectively created, something must give way. Sometimes, in a way known only on our deepest level of being, physical breakdown may be the only avenue out.

Perhaps it is as the Kung believe: Sometimes the ill bear witness to the disruption of the larger community of life. The evidence, if we care to examine it, shows clearly that we are living through an era when many are sick at heart, sick in the head, sick to their stomachs; sick in the family, the community, the biosphere. But sometimes, when the individual breaks down, for one brief second the machine must halt. When the part is returned to operation (or perhaps, from one), it is no longer the same. Some odd, crucial difference—a change in gear-ratio, an adjustment of tolerances—may change, in some infinitesimal yet immeasurable way, the machine itself. The return of the journeyers from the realm of disease may have unpredictable consequences, not only for themselves but for the society. Ironically, they may become reminders of what it is possible for human beings to become.

❧ 16 ❧

THE RETURN: TREASURES
FROM THE DARK

Return: After a time of decay comes the turning point.
The powerful light that has been banished returns. There
is movement, but it is not brought about by force . . .

—I CHING

Reintegration with society, which is indispensable to the
continuous circulation of spiritual energy into the world
and which, from the standpoint of the community, is the
justification of the long retreat, the hero himself may
find the most difficult requirement of all.

—JOSEPH CAMPBELL,
The Hero with a Thousand Faces

THE PERSON WHO begins on the path of healing is not the same
one who returns from it. He or she has experienced terrors—
and sometimes wonders—that are hard to communicate even to
those they know best. They have knowledge of the body's perils and
potentials born of experiences that the healthy cannot imagine. Because of the depths they have plumbed within themselves, the reen-
try into society, to "normal life," can itself be a risky passage.

" 'Uneventful recovery!' " exclaimed Dr. Oliver Sacks. "What
damned utter nonsense! Recovery was a 'pilgrimage.' . . . Every
stage, every station, was a completely new advent, requiring a new
start, a new birth or beginning. One had to begin, to be born, again
and again."[1]

In *The Wizard of Oz*, Dorothy's journey back from the land of Oz
is no simple click of magic heels, but a traversing, on foot, of a
menacing series of borderlands. She must make her way through
"the Dainty China Country," where china milkmaids milk china
cows, and a china princess prettily explains how her people fear

winding up on "mantle-shelves and cabinets and drawing-room tables." Dorothy must step carefully through this domestic realm, lest
she shatter its inhabitants. "They are all so brittle!" she exclaims.

Surely this is how ordinary existence must sometimes appear to
patients as they return to their friends, relationships, and jobs bearing tales—and scars—that confound superficial discourse. Arline
Erdrich says, "I see my body like a car that gets a dent in it and
then gets a not-so-hot repair job. It still runs great. But it's surprising
how hard it is for some people to deal with. I was dating this very
handsome man, an Air Force pilot, who had pursued me with great
ardor. But when he first saw me without my clothes, he suddenly
got up, showered, and got dressed. I'll never forget him sitting on
the edge of the bed, moving his tie up and down, this cool guy
suddenly a fumbling idiot. It was as if he was afraid of contamination
from touching a person who'd touched Death."

DARKNESS BEFORE DAWN

Not merely touched it, but traveled on foot through its night-black
realm. Before Dorothy ever reaches the Dainty China Country, she
must first pass through a dark forest full of deadly trees that reach
out and threaten to engulf her. Similarly, for many of those I spoke
with, recovery was preceded by a dark passage, a final confrontation
with annihilation. Medieval mythology refers to this juncture as "the
Castle Perilous"; St. John of the Cross called it "the dark night of
the soul." The theme of darkness just before the dawn is a common
thread in initiatory journeys: The hero, writes Joseph Campbell,
must "arrive at the nadir of the mythological round, and . . .
undergo a supreme ordeal" before he can finally "re-emerge from
the kingdom of dread."

We can arrive at this nadir at any point on the healing path, often
when we least expect it. These are moments in which hard-fought
ground is sudenly lost; the sun is swallowed up; the long and arduous journey suddenly ends in a cul-de-sac. It may seem that we
have gotten well only to plummet back into the original abyss of our
suffering—more deeply than ever, for once we have been flung from
a hard-won purchase, faith seems pointless, and the universe a love-
less void that cares nothing for our individual survival.

In the Bhagavad-Gita, the Hindu hero Arjuna, in the dark hour
before his victorious battle, has a vision of the god Vishnu, his

"tusked and terrible mouths" flaming, ransacking friend and enemy alike, devouring all the worlds. Human life, the deity tells the quailing warrior, is foreordained to be impermanent. Human beings can live fully only by confronting the knowledge that they are "already slain."[2]

Likewise, before the joyous bells of Christmas toll Scrooge's rebirth, he must encounter his final, most awful night visitor, a "solemn Phantom, draped and hooded, coming, like a mist along the ground, toward him . . . shrouded in a deep black garment." The spectral harbinger of Death imposes on Scrooge a prevision of his own dissolution, forcing him to watch as his worldly goods—the mainstays of his former identity—are plundered down to "a pair of sleeve buttons, a pair of sugar-tongs." The tokens of success Scrooge had clung to so tenaciously are revealed as mere scraps for the scavenger's shop, tossed away atop a pile of "old rags, bottles, bones, and greasy offal."

Here is Yeats's "foul rag-and-bone shop of the heart;" here the charnel ground where Tantric yogis meditate upon the final emptiness of ego-centered existence; here the place of shamanic dismemberment, in which the outworn carapace of the initiate's old self cracks away; and here the soul-testing, purificatory crucible of Ezekiel ("Heap together the bones and I will burn them in the fire"): Before rebirth must come a surrender, an acknowledgment that the old adaptation of the self cannot cross the threshold.

I once asked an old Buddhist monk if he was afraid of death. "How could I be?" he asked, grinning broadly. "I have been preparing for it for sixty years!" He went on to observe that death occurs constantly throughout life. Each time a friend is lost, a cherished possession broken, a job terminated or a belief irrevocably shattered, our rigid sense of identity is carried away with it like ice in a swollen spring stream. Rather than clinging desperately to what we cannot retrieve, he explained, we might try to let go; for pain, loss, and emptiness carry with them a possibility for renewal.

DEATH'S DOOR

At the crescendo of her healing experience, Alice Epstein's visualizations filled with horrifying images. She saw "Baby Alice" walking along a path lined with pikes topped with skulls, twirling screaming skulls with ragged black hair about her head like a lasso, tugging behind her a red wagon brimming with bones. But these evocations of finality marked the beginning of "wresting power and spiritual healing" from the darkest part of herself. They also coincided with a dramatic reduction in the size of her remaining tumor. Her experience supports psychiatrist Charles Weinstock's observation that a "favorable inner change occurs upon facing death (and subsequently deciding to live differently and more constructively)" in people who undergo spontaneous remission.

A number of former patients told me that confronting death had been a critical turning point on their healing path. When Winnie Scott refused diagnostic surgery for two suspicious spots on her lungs, her husband and doctors concluded that she had become incapable of facing the potential lethality of her ailment. "To see if I was in denial like they said I was," says Winnie, "I practiced dying." She visualized the doctors gathered around pronouncing her dead. She placed herself in the position of all the people she cared about as they were told that she had drawn her last breath. The exercise was sobering: "I realized all their lives would go on. *Oh, no,* I thought, *I'm the bottom line only for me!* But I felt stronger knowing I could face my own end."

Wil Garcia undertook a similar mental exercise: "My healing began when I imagined what it would be like to die. I visualized my deathbed, saw who was going to be there, what issues were still left unsaid between myself and my parents, between myself and George and other loved ones. I pictured clearly my own passing, the whole dying process. Then I thought, *Why wait until my death? Why wait to say it? Why not start healing those relationships now?* I think that's when I began to live."

Dr. Jacob Zieghelboim, the oncologist whose personal struggle with cancer had triggered a series of radical life changes, told me: "My sense is that any time there is a serious disease, there is an impending death. That's part of the initiation, the passage. A death needs to occur. It will be either in the psychic arena or the physical, or both; but certain patterns sometimes have to come to an end— my own had survived for thirty-seven years!—as part of our life-process."

Before my operation, I dreamed I was burying in a deep grave "a Volkswagen that revved in all gears." I at the time took this as a warning of literal death. But I have since wondered if the dream wasn't urging the interment of a self-destructive identity—one so incapable of slowing down, it was burning out its own engine.

This interweaving of meaning between the "death" of the old self and literal death is discussed by the Jungian analyst Marie-Louise von Franz, who notes that "all of the symbols which appear in death dreams are images that are also manifested during the individuation process."[3] Literal death and metaphorical ego death have elements in common: Both are the end of a particular organization of the self; both insist that change is inescapable; both force the journeyer into the soul's territory, because there is no longer anywhere else to go.

Mark Pelgrin's first symbols of death approached him on the night of Easter Sunday. Twenty-four hours before the first symptoms of his disease had appeared, he had a vivid dream of his wife, who had died of cancer five years before. In another dream shortly before that, a doctor, repeating his words for emphasis, had told him that he had only "six to eight years" to live.

During his subsequent bout with pancreatic cancer, Pelgrin traveled what he called "the path of the wholly new, the wholly untried commitment to the paradoxical, irrational side of the universe." His night-world was crowded with numinous dreams. He reexperienced for the first time the trauma of his mother's early death from a fever in a South American mining camp, and rediscovered a trove of "strange, wild" childhood memories that filled him with a sense of piercing beauty. He communed with his young children, and walked with "the Presence" that overtook him when he was alone and silent—a feeling, which he still questioned as "mystical nonsense," that he was pure "Being, as the leaves or the birds are being." Before his death, seven years after his six- to eight-year "dream prognosis," Mark Pelgrin had come to a profound understanding of life. He had suffered and loved, deeply, through unendurable pain, grief, and joy; he had struggled all the while to find "a treasure in the darkness."

In one of Pelgrin's dreams, death was a "stately, dark, silent woman" who appeared in the company of Love. *Is it the death of the self, or the death of the body?* he wondered. Another time, he dreamed of "a black coffin with a white rose upon it. A tall man with dark eyes hovered there, with a red rose between his teeth. The rose became a fire at the end of a large corridor. Shadow figures moved up and down near the fire, endlessly circling in a solemn ritual. 'In my end is my beginning,' they were saying."

Stephen and Ondrea Levine, in their book *Healing into Life and Death*, have proposed that facing death, even real death, is sometimes a beginning as well as the end of a cycle of human growth. The Levines cite the case of a man named Bill, an AIDS patient who had come to their meditation retreat brimming with shame and a deep sense of failure. He had been told by doctors that his illness was terminal; by the intolerant that he was being punished for his sins; and by those he called the "pseudo-hip holistic" that since he had created his disease in the first place, he could "uncreate" it. The Levines' work, however, is based on Buddhist-influenced "acceptance of what is," in which they counsel patients to "send your heart into your pain." Though their approach could not alter the fatal spiral of his disease, Bill discovered it profoundly affected his outlook.

Shortly before he died, Bill wrote an open letter in which he announced that "a great healing" had occurred. After months of medical treatment, both traditional and alternative, after long periods of spiritual meditation supported by his friends, his lover, and other helpers, he felt that he had faced his worst enemy—fear—and become "free."

> For many months, my idea of healing was that of curing my body. I gave it my very best shot and I am proud of that fact. I was even given several months of relative health and energy. At that time, I often expressed my certainty that I could heal my own body with my own powers. I still believe these healing powers exist, but as my physical health reached a point where optimism would have had to become self-denial, I realized the need to accept by own impending death.
>
> I realized that self-compassion meant feeling in my heart that even physical death was not a sign of weakness and failure. This seems to be the ultimate act of self-acceptance. . . . An open heart is a much greater blessing than death is a tragedy.[4]

THE PITFALL

Bill's final confrontation with death had been expected and prepared for. But sometimes the dark night occurs when a patient has begun the return to life, only to find that the disease has suddenly reappeared. These are junctures known to all horror movie fans. They have sat, eyes wide, heart palpitating, pressed against the seat back, as the hero battled and finally triumphed, however gorily, over seemingly unconquerable demonic forces. Despite their better judgment, they breathe a sigh of relief. Seconds later, the monster bursts out of its grave for a final all-out assault.

Describing patients' reactions to the recurrence of cancer, Michael Lerner writes:

> They may have suffered through rigorous courses of therapy, or made profound and sometimes arduous changes in their life, or carried out deep explorations of self-inquiry, or felt certain that they were successfully combating their illness, and then suddenly, often after a new psychological or physical shock, the cancer recurs. . . . The key to this transition may be to explore fully the despair over the recurrence so that the grieving can be completed. Often, new levels of awareness then emerge.

Just as she had begun painstakingly to recover from crippling rheumatoid arthritis, Joy Ballas-Beeson's world was plunged into darkness. She was raped by two men. The experience added horrifying insult to injury: She had been in slow recovery, with one arm still in a sling, and the assault proved a devastating blow to her nascent healing process. She described it as being "betrayed by every guardian angel I'd ever had. I'd always had so much faith, but now I'd go into the bathroom and yell at God at the top of my lungs, 'How could You let this happen?' "

Soon, Joy's condition worsened drastically. Her pain honed itself to an excruciating knife edge that kept her from sleeping for more than an hour at night. In the middle of one such night, nearly maddened by fatigue, she felt a murderous rage consume her. "I swear if the men who had raped me had been there, I would have killed them. It wasn't directed just at them, but included all the suppressed anger I'd been holding back at my ex-husband, his dad, other men. Oh, was that painful!

"I decided to kill myself at that point, because I started just *feeling* so intensely—the physical pain, the emotional pain, the anger at myself for letting myself get into abusive situations. I started planning my suicide, thinking of how to do it so it wouldn't be messy for my mother and father. These thoughts shocked me, because I'd always been so full of life.

"One night, at the absolute bottom, I made an inner declaration— I don't care if I die or if I get well, but· I'm not going to stay somewhere in between. I just refuse to live that way. The next day, I asked my doctor for some Prednisone so I could get a little sleep. I think if I had gone one more night without sleep I wouldn't have made it."

Joy started "signaling for help." An acquaintance who had unexpectedly volunteered to help her with the most basic tasks of life—cooking, cleaning, making the bed, opening car doors—took her one evening to a Church of Religious Science meeting, where Joy had an "ego-smashing thought."

> I said, "Look, God, I'm obviously incapable of healing myself, you're gonna have to take over." There was this great relief to give up, to admit I could not *make* myself well, that I wasn't in control. And there was this instant mental shift. I don't know how, but that final giving up helped me feel the healthy parts I still had, rather than constantly expending all my energy fighting the disease.
>
> It seemed to have a physical effect, too, because somehow later that week, without any assistance, I was able to drive myself to my doctor's, sit down, get up from the chair by myself, and walk into his office. He was shocked, not only by my mobility, but at the test results. When I'd last come in, my sedimentation rate was one-twenty. Now it had gone down to twenty, the normal level. The hemoglobin rate was down to normal. My pulse rate, which had been very, very high, was normal; blood pressure, everything. It did seem a little miraculous.

Joy Ballas-Beeson's recovery would still be a succession of hills and valleys. But what changed, she believes, was that she had "surrendered." "Before, I was saying I was so powerful, I was going to *force* healing to happen, right now. But it wouldn't. I think I had to totally fall apart, give up, reach the very end—the tip!—of my rope before I could regain my connection with any kind of healing energy."

SURRENDERING HOPE

A similar act of surrender coincided with the extraordinary remission of a man named Everett Paul.[5] A taciturn, fifty-five-year-old Idaho farmer ("lentils and winter wheat, mostly"), firstborn in a family of six and a lifelong member of the fundamentalist Church of the Nazarene, Everett had joined the Peace Corps when he was twenty-three, and was dispatched to Kenya. "The draft was the main reason," he states simply. "I didn't want to go to Vietnam and shoot anyone."

After two homesick, overworked years overseeing a crew of sixty workers constructing water reservoirs, Everett noticed a persistent pain in his right leg. He was sent to a Nairobi hospital and then to what is now Wymann Park Hospital in Baltimore. There, a reticulum cell sarcoma—an aggressive disease with an only eight-month prognosis—was found in his right pelvic bone.

Refusing experimental chemotherapy and radiation, he opted to return to Idaho, where "the local doctor told me there was no point going back to Baltimore and dying in a research center. I might as well die at home." By the end of a year, his deteriorated pelvic bone had cracked from a visibly protruding, half-grapefruit-sized tumor. He was in such agonizing pain he could neither sit nor lie down. His lanky, five-ten frame had shrunk to 100 pounds. "I was good as gone," he recalls. He sometimes had to sleep upright on crutches, he says, with his mother maintaining an all-night vigil to ensure he didn't tumble over.

Through it all, Everett maintained a simple faith. "I was trying to trust God wouldn't allow me to suffer more than I could bear." Members of his church stopped by regularly to pray with him. His mother prayed with him daily. "Ideally it would be nice if we were close enough to God that we'd really know how to pray. But I was doing my best. I wasn't demanding He heal me. I didn't know what He wanted." One day there came a turning point. "I told God if He wanted me to die, I was ready to go. From then on I started living one day at a time."

On a Sunday night service four days later, standing in the back of the Church, Everett remembers, "I don't know why, but I just sat down. I hadn't been able to for a month." The next day, he recalls, he was able to "sit comfortably and read a book." By Wednesday, the lump was nearly gone, the swelling began to leave his legs and hands, and the pain had diminished "by ninety percent." New X rays, taken a month later, showed the cancer inexplicably receding, his pelvis recalcifying, and the cracked bone beginning to knit. During the next three months, the skeletal former invalid gained ten pounds per month. By August, harvest time, he was able to drive the big combine on his father's farm. By September, he was hefting hundred-pound sacks of seed wheat. In the nineteen years since his remission, Everett has married and fathered two children. No sign remains of his illness save a slight localized numbness from the original diagnostic biopsy.

This simply devout, laconic farmer, driven beyond hope, even beyond despair, did not attempt to mentally redirect the flow of white blood cells, or visualize the behavior of cancer cells. Like another case he strikingly resembles, the much-documented

Lourdes *miracule* Vittorio Micheli (whose hip bone, disintegrated by cancer, mysteriously regrew after bathing in the sacred grotto), Everett somehow got out of the way, allowing an unknown spiritual, neuroimmunologic, or biopsychosocial grace to flood through him. He had no visions, heard no voices, saw no white light, felt no blazing heat. No matter how much I prompted, he could recall no memorable dreams. He cannot explain why he, out of millions of sufferers on this planet who surrender themselves daily to the divine, praying to God, Allah, Brahma, and the Buddha for surcease and healing, was elected to be made whole.

All he can say is, "God's timing isn't our timing. He can use things for our teaching if we allow it." His viewpoint is reminiscent of the Japanese researcher Ikemi's cases, one of whom told him, "Faith to me is not attachment to life, just wishing to be saved, but the gratitude to god [sic] who saved my spirit. I had begun to live a real life . . . " Said another, "Whatever should happen will just happen." They embraced a perspective, particularly prevalent in Japanese culture, called *wabi, sabi*: "an existential sense of unavoidable death and its positive acceptance."[6]

A surrender to the blunt reality of one's immediate, unavoidable experience can be therapeutic in itself, even if it does not cause dramatic medical change. Dr. Jon Kabat-Zinn cautions patients who enter his program at the University of Massachusetts that meditation "will not necessarily cause tumors to regress or change T-cell helper-to-suppresser ratios." He advises that instead of putting all their energy into wishing for a cure, they try to cultivate "an attitude of not-striving, the notion that they're already well, even in the midst of illness. The body is constantly decaying and dying, and it's also being built up. The best chance for coming into harmony is to just allow yourself to be where you are, in the 'don't-know mind.' You don't know where you're going, and you don't know how long the body is going to last; but in accepting that fact—whether you have cancer or AIDS or heart disease—something profoundly healing takes place."

"Be still, and wait without hope/" wrote T. S. Eliot, "For hope would be hope of the wrong thing; wait without love/For love would be love of the wrong thing. . . . /Wait without thought, for you are not ready for thought. . . . " This was the stanza that neurologist and author Oliver Sacks says sustained him during his crisis. Trapped in a strange physiological deadlock he was powerless to alter, Sacks despairingly chose to become an "*explorer* of the abyss."

All the cognitive and intellectual and imaginative powers which had previously aided me in exploring different neuropsychological lands were wholly useless, meaningless, in the limbo of Nowhere. I had fallen off the map, the world, of the knowable. . . . Intelligence, reason, sense, meant nothing. Memory, imagination, hope, meant nothing. I had lost everything which afforded a foothold before. I had entered, willy-nilly, a dark night of the soul.[7]

It was a predicament that struck at the very roots of his identity as an athletic, hard-driving staff physician at his professional peak. "I had to relinquish all the powers I normally command. I had to allow—and this seemed horrible—the sense and feeling of *passivity*."

Paradoxically, the moment of utter defeat can be the traditional turning point in the journey. It is the moment when all conscious stratagems have failed, the ego abdicates, and deeper forces of life may make their appearance. St John of the Cross, in describing "the dark night of the soul," points out that it was only when Job lay "naked upon a dunghill, abandoned and even persecuted by his friends, filled with anguish and bitterness, and the earth covered with worms" that "the Most High God . . . was pleased to come down and speak with him there face to face . . . in a way He had never done in the time of his prosperity."

Likewise, in pagan European mythology, the Green Man descends into the bleak Underworld in winter, only to poke up through the hard ground with glorious shoots and flowers in spring. Sacks, broken, sunk into the lightless depths of his own psyche, found that "mysteriously, I began to change—to allow, to welcome this abdication of activity. . . . The watchword at this time was, 'Be patient—endure . . . wait, be still. . . . Do nothing, don't think!' "[8]

THE TURNING POINT

For Sacks, and for others, this moment was the turning point:

I had had the foundations of my inner world shaken—nay, I had had them utterly destroyed. I had experienced "reason's scandal," and the humiliation of mind. I had fallen into an abyss, with the breaking apart of my tissues, my perceptions, the natural unities of body-soul, body-mind. And I had been lifted from the abyss, reborn, reaffirmed, by powers beyond my understanding and reason.

From despair, joy; from great darkness, greater light. The experience, Sacks says, "humbled me, horribly, took away hope, but then, sweetly-gently, returned it to me a thousandfold, transformed."[9] The return, whether it takes days or years, is often characterized not by simple restoration of what was lost, but a sort of multiplication of boons.

Thus as Job emerges from his private hell, all those who were absent during his travails draw near. "All his brethren and his sisters came to him, and all his former acquaintances . . . and condoled with him and comforted him . . . and each gave him a piece of money and every one an earring of gold." No fewer than ten new children were born to him, and his flocks prospered. The Lord "blessed the latter days of Job more than his earlier ones." In *It's a Wonderful Life*, George Bailey returns from the netherworld to be showered with the love of family and community, as well as enough "earrings of gold"—contributions ladled into a basket by friends and family—to thwart forever Mr. Potter's evil designs. The creatures in *The Wizard of Oz* not only receive the exalted gift of inner wholeness, but each is elevated to the status of ruler of a realm.

Joy Ballas-Beeson, after her plunge into a dark crevasse and subsequent "giving up to Spirit," found herself mysteriously embraced by life. "People would pay me back money I'd loaned them years ago, just spontaneously, out of the blue. As Joy began to recover, not knowing what she would do to support herself, she discovered "a sort of universal bank account of goodwill where I could make withdrawals." She felt as if she had come back to a world that functioned by other rules than she had previously assumed. She began avidly to explore new directions, went back to school to take classes, and eventually began a personal study of metaphysics and healing. "I used to think I had to be an overachiever to justify my existence, even to survive. I was used to working eighty hours in the restaurant, doing a side job to help the family over rough times, tending a quarter-acre garden, keeping a corral full of animals, chauffeuring two children around different places—good grief! I thought that if I loosened my grip, or did what I really wanted to do with my life, I'd perish."

Instead, Joy and other patients who had once felt they had to continually pump up the bicycle tire of life to keep it from deflating found their return occasionally supported by wheeling spokes of grace. It was as if their wounds had made an opening, so that now the energies of the self could finally flow out into the world, and the energies of life—life beyond the ego control they had assumed was indispensable to survival—could flow in.

Rather than defining themselves by what they could acquire or achieve, many learned they also could measure success by the riches of simple being. "Sometimes I look out and I see every single leaf as if it were outlined," Art McGrary told me. "When the sun shines it's like I can see each individual ray. I feel as if maybe I'm blessed with this opportunity to be really grateful for being alive."

In *A Christmas Carol*, Scrooge, returning from the world of the Spirits, runs to the window, thrusts out his head, and discovers a wealth that had eluded his endless accounting: "Clear, bright, jovial, stirring, cold; cold, piping for the blood to dance to; Golden sunlight; Heavenly sky; sweet fresh air; merry bells, Oh, glorious . . . Glorious!"

For Scrooge, the slate has been wiped clean by a classic spiritual metanoia, a profound change of heart. On the one hand, he has reclaimed his long-abandoned selfhood; on the other, a new person—one who is more, in Kung Bushman terms, *sga ku tsiu*, whose "heart rises" easily—has been born of the journey: "I don't know what day of the month it is! I don't know how long I've been among the Spirits. I don't know anything. I'm quite a baby. Never mind, I don't care. I'd rather be a baby. Hallo! Whoop! Hallo here!"

In Brazil a few years ago, I witnessed a ceremony of the Candomble sect, whose rituals have roots deep in African Yoruba culture. It was a wild, swirling dance in which initiates directly encounter their spirit-archetypes and are swept into the Otherworld. One initiate, holding a red flower on his head, his face radiant as obsidian, his entranced eyes shedding light, was gently led into a back room. I was told that after such a priest-to-be has been seized by the gods, he will often emerge "like a little child," and for weeks afterwards will have to be dressed, fed, clothed, taught how to speak, and shown how to behave in society. It is a graphic rebirth, a reforming in which the person can grow up all over again, begin a new life, and create a new self.

WELLER THAN WELL: THE WISE BODY

Many patients insisted they felt better than they had before the journey had begun. On some level, whether spiritual, physical or both, they had become, in Karl Menninger's term, "weller-than-well."

Part of the aftermath of illness, Winnie Scott told me, is a new sense of mind-body integration—"a connection with the power that keeps your eyes moist, your food digesting, your hair growing. You reclaim your connection to the universe with each breath."

At the same time, there is a realism about personal limitations. "We are embodied beings in the physical world," says Jay Simoneaux, "and part of the fun, and the horror, of being embodied is you don't have total control over what happens. In the physical world, trees fall down, cars crash, airplane engines blow up. Same with the body. Bad things happen, amazing things happen. The important thing is to work with it all. That's what makes it interesting."

Many journeyers described having developed a deep awareness of the body, a respect that gave them new tools for physical health. "You become sensitive to the body," says Joy Ballas-Beeson. "You're more a partner with it, instead of it being separate from you. You can't abuse it like you used to. And you *never* take it for granted. I've discovered that if I get off track I get new reminders, like allergies, which tell me my immune system is getting out of whack. Then I know I'm supposed to take better care so I don't get crippled up again."

The sense of separation from the body, so common in what I have referred to as the disease-prone personality, is replaced by a greater feeling of psychosomatic unity. "I used to not want to have anything to do with my body," says Debby Ogg. "I was always fat as a kid, so I always wanted to hide it, didn't want it to be seen or touched. When I got cancer, I realized I needed to demonstrate, to myself, that I could care about me, whole body and all.

"I learned to pay attention to my diet, to exercise, to my emotions, to every layer of my being, all wrapped up together. Now there's nothing in my body anymore that seems too minute. I can feel when it's getting out of balance, when I'm getting out of control. I used to stay in situations that didn't make me feel right. Now I can act more on literal gut feelings."

Many former patients report a sense of psychosomatic wholeness below the threshold of consciousness. "I have not had one single cold in over three years," says Arline, "when everyone around me has had flus and bronchitis. I think that says something." Science has discovered the immune system is educable; it gains its immunity by "remembering" past encounters with pathogens. Is it possible that the encounter with serious illness creates new mind-body pathways, sets up new lines of communication—early-warning systems—that persist even after the illness is gone?

A number of journeyers volunteered that they felt in some ways physiologically more robust than they had before the onset of illness, as if the healing process had become so strongly mobilized that it had in a sense overshot the mark. When Brian Schultz's ankylosing spondylitis was first diagnosed, he had developed a condition known as *lordosis*, a misshaping of the spine. Now his disease has not only stopped progressing, but his spine has regained a normal form. "I went to a chiropractor a few weeks ago," he says, "because I wrenched my back a little playing Ultimate Frisbee, and this guy looked at me and said, 'You have a spine which looks like you never had ankylosing spondylitis.'

"I feel it's more than a remission. Remission in medical terms is just a way of saying, 'Your degenerative process has stopped temporarily and we don't know why but we're not going to say you've actually moved in the direction of healing.' Instead, it seems I've gotten to a point where I'm actually healthier than I was before it all started."

HEALING NEVER ENDS

Brian was one of many former patients who carefully reiterated that health was not an end product, but a continual process. "People think that once the symptoms are gone, you're all well. But the healing goes on and just gets more intense."

"Healing isn't something that you do and put away on a shelf," said another. "It's a dynamic equilibrium that has to be maintained daily, in every decision and every conversation, and it can be jeopardized by every choice you make. I'm no longer challenged by bodily symptoms, but I'm constantly being challenged by the body of my life."

John Studholme recalls his feelings after his doctor walked into the treatment room with an X ray showing that the tumor had shrunk "beyond anyone's wildest expectations." His doctor credited chemotherapy; John attributed the result in part to his meditation and imagery. Whatever the cause, John said he was filled with "amazement at the power of healing. I began to hope I could rid myself of other less tangible illnesses. I could win the cancer battle and at the same time, exorcise some of my other *dybbuks.*"

The great Lakota Indian shaman Lame Deer once remarked,

"The find-out, it has lasted me my whole life." Anthropologist Joan Halifax observes, "It isn't like you have one rite of passage, one death-rebirth experience and then, You Get It." Niro Asistent, whose HIV antibody status reversed from positive to negative in 1985 (an extremely rare medical event called seroconversion[10]), told me in even more simple terms: "Healing never ends. My symptoms are gone, but now I'm healing a whole emotional part of myself. And I don't know what I'm going to heal next. My definition of healing now is not just getting well, but reaching your own maximum potential. If I've done it physically, now I'm going to do it with something else and something else and something else. It's a continuous growing process."

Once they cross the threshold of return, journeyers often find themselves beginning a new struggle to heal an entire pattern of life. It is as if the bodymind, having taken on the healing agenda, now insists on presenting all pathologies for inspection. "Unless a sort of death of the old self takes place," Dr. Jacob Zieghelboim believes, "then even if the cancer is cured on the structural level, the disease may remain in the deeper sense and can express itself in another form, at another time, in another place." How people reconstitute their lives without falling back into habits, relationships, and attitudes that contribute to getting ill, has profound implications. Many journeyers concluded that wellness required a continuous restoration of balance. The perspective is shared by traditional cultures. One anthropologist writes, "The Kalahari Kung dance is part of their continuing effort to prevent incipient sickness, which they believe resides in everyone, from becoming severe and manifest."

Alice Epstein returned to psychotherapy after a two-month hiatus, "not with any pressing issues to discuss, but with an understanding that I was not yet well, not yet whole. I knew if I neglected any finishing touches, I might succumb to a new illness sometime in the future. I had to . . . sweep away the seeds of some new bloom of self-destruction."[11]

After his healing, Jay Simoneaux came to the painful decision that it was necessary to separate from his wife. They had had a sustaining intimacy during his cancer journey, but he felt strongly that he needed to find "the source of my own power. To friends I seem crazy, breaking up this happy arrangement. But I feel, if I'm going to avoid a recurrence, I have to really develop my own creativity, step aside from guilt and fear and express what I need to express. I know now that my emotional and spiritual issues are issues of life and death. They're that important. I can't compromise them the way I used to."

LIVING THE SOUL'S PURPOSE

One commentator compares the dark forest that Dorothy must traverse in *The Wizard of Oz* to the dire wood of Canto XIII of Dante's *Inferno*, where suicides have been turned into fruitless trees tormented by Harpies who gnaw at their limbs—symbols of the distortion of life that grows from a rejection of one's own creative powers. The psychologist Paul Roud, who investigated the cases of eleven "incurable" patients who had unexpectedly recovered, says that all had learned during their illness to "follow their heart's passions. Living this way was so satisfying that they did not regress to old patterns once they recovered." One former patient left his job as an encyclopedia salesman to became a jazz musician. Another moved from the frenetic city to a farm. On the whole, they stopped trying to please others, and began to live according to their deepest inner biddings.

Carl Jung, too, suffered several bouts of severe illness that transformed his life. In *Memories, Dreams, Reflections*, Jung wrote: "It was only after my illness that I understood how important it is to affirm one's own destiny." As was the case for other journeyers, this period also marked the beginning of his most creative work.

Dr. Jacob Zieghelboim says, "If somebody had told me six years ago, 'Look, when you are forty-two this is what you are going to be doing,' I would have said they were absolutely crazy. I would have considered it very childlike behavior to change careers, to follow your own star or whatever without knowing in advance where it would lead you. My path has led me back to practicing medicine, but in a different form than anyone ever told me was possible, or permissible. When I say, 'I'm doing transformative work with cancer,' my colleagues look pretty incredulous."

Several patients talked about returning from illness with a pressing sense of personal destiny. After an experience of "overwhelming love" during a meditation, Alice Epstein "became obsessed with the idea that I had been saved for some important work in the world and that I would receive a message about my future direction. But "the 'answer' I sought never came." Instead, "poised at the crest of a mountain, searching for my path with heart," she spent time in a holding pattern, doing volunteer work for the Audubon Society. After considering a career as a healer, she realized that she could best heal by example, not intervention: It was necessary to her own health, she concluded, to "reduce my extreme empathy for others." At the end of her book, she was just beginning to seek out "a rewarding direction" for the rest of her life.

Jay Simoneaux did become a healer for a time. "I was counseling people with cancer, people with AIDS. I can foster someone going into their own process, coming up with images and following where they lead. But I realized it was becoming more than I could handle to take on everyone else's problems, getting so close to people and then sometimes seeing them die. I could feel I was starting to shut down."

Instead, Jay began to work with a friend who had a carpentry company. Soon he found he was looking foward to going to work each day. "The issue for me after all these years of dealing with consciousness and the ephemeral nature of reality was really mastering the physical world, becoming someone who was competent. These days, if ill people come into my life coincidentally, I'll work with them, but right now I just hang out in the building trade."

SELLING WATER BY THE RIVER

Simply by discovering how to live more authentically themselves, many journeyers inevitably wind up affecting the society around them, sometimes even becoming agents of social change. Perhaps in one sense the carrier of the wound has taken into him- or herself a portion of the collective pathology. Their healing process may similarly extend beyond their own individual lives into a larger community.

Arnold Mindell suggests in *Working with the Dreaming Body* that disease may create a breach through which unexpected messages may be transmitted to society at large:

> The ill person needs only to know that transforming himself means coming up against interiorized cultural edges. If this transformation is to occur, he will have to disturb the status quo of the world around him as well. The person in the midst of an individuation process must know that when his symptoms disappear, a new kind of pain is likely to arise: conflict with the history of the world, of which he has been an integral part.[12]

The ill may return feeling that they bear boons, but they also may find they disturb the status quo. They often discover they cannot go back to "going along to get along," for they have changed too deeply. They navigate less by outward approbation than by inner cues. When Scrooge returns from his healing journey, "Some people laughed to see the alteration in him, but he let them laugh, and little heeded them; for he knew that nothing ever happened on this globe, for good, at which some people did not have their fill of laughter at the outset."

Joy Ballas-Beeson now lectures insurance underwriters on the efficacy of nontraditional healing. Sometimes she faces ridicule, but often she finds enough receptive ears to continue what has become a personal mission. Debby Ogg, whose story was made into a successful TV movie-of-the-week, wondered how she had the "big-mouth audacity" to turn such a profoundly private experience into a mass-audience broadcast.

"But it suits me," she says. "I decided I wanted to be on the prevention side of things rather than just dispensing first aid, and this was a way to get the word out. Now I'm back doing local social work, but this time on my own terms. I plopped myself down in boots and a parka into an extremely conservative professional community. I didn't hide the fact I was using techniques they would consider really 'out there.' I was sometimes pretty abrasive—I need to work with that energy in a more positive way! But in the end, they accepted me, because they could sense I had a certain integrity."

THE WOUNDED HEALER

Some descriptions of the legacy of illness resembled those of near-death experiencers (NDEer's), who often report profound changes in outlook. Many journeyers described their own changes in terms nearly identical to those of researcher Kenneth Ring's NDEer's: a new sense of spirituality, greater self-acceptance, and deeper empathy.

Before Art McGrary's passage through illness, he had possessed, like Job in his respected old age, all the hard-earned material blessings: "a pension of four thousand dollars a month," he says, ticking off the litany of the Good Life, "four cars and a boat and an RV and a spa and a swimming pool and a hundred-fifty thousand in the bank."

By the time he had arrived at his own castle perilous, Art—who had once charged out of burning buildings carrying smoke-inhalation victims on his back—had become a 125-pound husk, unable to take half a flight of stairs. At his darkest moment, his second wife left him flat, absconding with his life savings and "everything from my cufflinks to my old uniforms. I thought about suicide at that point. Why go on? I'd saved enough pills for my exit. I took them out of the drawer a few times and looked at them, then said, 'I'll give it a few more days.' "

Art had cut himself off from his family, but his daughter from his first marriage heard about his travails, tracked him down, and showed up unexpectedly on his doorstep. "When I saw there was someone who cared," he says, "that was the turnaround." He moved back to his hometown and, continuing on a strict health regimen (the so-called Gerson Diet), began a new existence from the ashes of the old. His life blossomed into what he calls "my second adolescence. There are a lot of single women in my age group, and I found that old guys like me are a rare commodity. I was dating two or three gals. It was amazing, terrific, better than when I was a teenager.

"In the midst of all this, I was having my prostate cancer checked all the time by this doctor in Santa Barbara. One day he said, 'Hey, the lump is gone, there seems to be some scar tissue, but the gland is almost back to normal size.' It still is. He still won't say the word 'cured' after all these years. He just says, 'controlled.' When I go to other doctors now, I don't even tell them."

McGrary, who recalls disparagingly, "I used to be a big man with a gun in my hand," finds that his healing has been accompanied by a puzzling change of personality: "If I had to explain it—if I *could* explain it—I'd say that the feminine side, the caring side, has been allowed to come out. I had picked a job where your feelings had to be buried. Who could take the most pain, who could eat the most smoke, who would stay in the most hellish place longest. . . . It was idiotic, insane. I mean, if I saw a child who was burned or smashed, I might turn away and feel like crying, but I couldn't let anybody see me. I've learned how to cry since then."

His newfound access to his emotions has left him with an almost overwhelming urge to help others. Without any detectable vanity (and in fact with faint embarrassment), he paints a picture of a life transformed: "The guy next door went blind from an eye problem, so I mowed his lawn for six weeks. Recently, I had a job I liked that was paying very, very well. A lady who worked there had health problems, no insurance. Someone had to be laid off, so I volunteered because it seemed to me she needed it more.

"It's my way of saying, 'Thank you, God or whoever, for letting me live.' It's not so much helping the world at large. I'm no hero. I never was. When I was a fireman, it was more trying to prove myself. It was a selfish thing, it wasn't a giving thing. Now, I'm much better one-to-one."

Niro Asistent, too, has discovered a growing sense of purpose that she attributes to her passage through disease. She explains in her music-inflected Belgian accent, "For me, a few months before I got the AIDS diagnosis, I was wondering what my purpose was in being alive. Much later, after I started getting well, the question came up again, and then the answer came: Work with dying people. I noticed the doctor, the nurse, the relatives, get afraid of AIDS. But they cut themselves off from an incredible gift! P.W.A.'s [People With AIDS] are living in almost another dimension. When I work with them, I feel like I dissolve, like the boundaries between us disappear.

"Once I was holding the hand of a guy who had only hours to live. He was gone, in what the doctors call 'dementia.' Suddenly, he just sat up, grabbed his blanket, and said 'Niro! Did you see the light under the chair?' And his face was in bliss. Then he described for me how now he was playing on the beach with his dead father. Then he said, 'Now, you take good care. Take good care.' And he lay down, and he was gone. A lot of people are afraid of this, but for me, I feel grateful. I want to do more."

Once a Tibetan lama I studied with described for a rapt lecture audience the characteristics of the Buddhist saint, or *bodhisattva*—impeccable compassion, selflessness, illumination, joy. A student raised his hand and asked, "Does this mean the bodhisattva no longer feels *dukha*, the suffering of existence?" "No," he answered. "The bodhisattva is a magnet—a vacuum cleaner!—for *dukha!*" Then my teacher, himself severely crippled from an auto accident, burst into contagious laughter.

Commenting on the Yacqui Indian teachers she has studied with, anthropologist Joan Halifax explained to me, "The training of the shaman entails a complete humbling, losses of all kinds. A lot of medicine people actually seek experiences of suffering so that they don't forget. It's what connects them with their work, their job, their capacity for compassion, for feeling what others feel. The wound makes medicine people more permeable, more able to access other realms. In a sense, for them the wound *never* heals."

Many patients said that as they returned to the world, they were almost subconsciously drawn to others' pain. Margaret Green told me of watching a vivacious woman with her family several tables away in a restaurant. "I was so struck by her, I actually followed her to the ladies' rest room. I had imagined they were celebrating their anniversary and were blissfully happy. But she told me her daughter had just been diagnosed with cancer. On the outside, she looked serene, but her life was coming apart, and I subconsciously sensed it. I gave her my phone number, and I think I've been able to help just talking to her. I seem to attract this kind of thing nowadays."

A surprisingly high percentage told me they felt they had acquired an almost unavoidable ability to empathize. "Since my illness," Debby Ogg says, "I can *feel* what's happening in other people. It resonates in my body, like electricity. It influences me." When she is doing therapy and "the client starts crying about something sad or gripping, I start crying, too. I'm not afraid of their feelings, or my own for that matter—I just go right with them."

Their experiences accord with the view of many shamanic cultures, which hold that a person is not fully healed until he becomes a healer himself. *The Medicine Buddha* text enjoins the meditator to use his own sicknesses to increase his compassion: "Because of his own illness, he should take pity on all others who are sick. . . . He should become a king of healing and cure all ills."

For many, it was only a short step from compassion and helping to actual hands-on healing. Joy Ballas-Beeson says, "I started to develop the ability to feel where others had emotional pain with my hands. I'd put my hands on their chest, then out of my mouth would come something I sensed about them, and they'd start to cry. I didn't always know what I was telling them, but they'd thank me later and tell me I was right.

"I think it's all about opening up a channel for healing to come through. I step aside and this healing energy goes through me to them. I'm not personally taking on their pain and disease, but they're getting benefit and I'm benefiting as much as they are from this energy flow."

Arline Erdrich says, "I was always able to make my kids feel better without medicine when they were little, just by stroking their heads or whatever. They used to call me 'The Doctor.' Lately, though, I've been able to touch them and within minutes, the hurt part seems to start healing.

"One time, my daughter Karen hit her elbow on an arm she'd already damaged in an accident. She couldn't bend it. I just spontaneously put both my hands around her elbow, and she said she could feel her arm actually getting hot. After I let it go, I asked her to try to raise her hand, and she was shocked she could do it without pain. She said, 'It was like you sent energy into my arm.'

"My son Bill was hurt in a motorcycle accident. His stitched-up ankle blew up like a balloon. But I could literally feel the swelling going down under my hands. Each time I did something and something happened, I wondered, *My God, am I really able to do this?* I think there's a force we are all capable of, that we can channel to people at certain times."

But those who have walked the healing path also know there is a dimension to healing that cannot simply be conferred from the outside. After two extraordinary healings from cancer, Ted Lothammar's reputation led patients to seek him out. "They'd send people to me—relatives, aunts, uncles—because here was this guy who pulled off this cancer miracle. I did counseling for about a year, telling them to do what I'd done, to eat healthy food and all that. Then I realized, *Bullshit.* Because the main thing that cured me was a decision I'd made one Thanksgiving just to live. I've had to make that choice many times since then. Sometimes I can almost tell who's going to make it when they come to see me. Some come in saying, 'Help me, save me, tell me what to do, chemo or macrobiotics, anything.' Outwardly, they look like they're fighting it, but they haven't decided to wrench their lives around."

Journeyers have a first-hand knowledge of the challenge of transformation. "You can't expect to have some insight and just change," Lothammer says. "That would be like sticking a piece of shirt cardboard in the Colorado River and expecting to divert its course. The river's been going over and over this same piece of land for millennia. It's not so easy to reroute your habits."

Carol Boss, who had been given a prognosis of several months for metastatic breast disease, managed to live a rich and difficult seven years beyond her doctors' predictions. The last time I saw her alive, she was insistent that the terms of sickness and healing must be stripped of all language of failure and success. "It's great to get well," she said, "but it's not the main thing. All human beings have limited resources. Technically speaking, I'm still in critical condition; technically, we *all* are. The main thing, I think, is to find a way to live so that your life has real *meaning*."

WALKING THE PATH OF HEALING

What remained for all those who traveled the path of healing was the quest for meaning. In some sense, meaning *is* healing. At the conclusion of the journey, the Wizard unfastens the Scarecrow's head and replaces the straw with a mixture of bran, pins, and needles ("proof that he is sharp," puns the Lion). He takes a pair of tinner's shears, cuts a small, square hole in the Tin Woodman's chest, and inserts "a pretty heart made entirely of silk and stuffed with sawdust." The Cowardly Lion is given a courage potion from a square green bottle. The Wizard is dispensing potent metaphors as medicine. As in shamanic initiation, the dismembered self is restored in a symbolic "operation" aimed at finalizing a transformation of consciousness. The anthropologist Mircea Eliade relates that in the initiatory visions of the Dyak shamans of Borneo, "In order to achieve insight into healing, their brains are washed and restored into their heads. Gold dust is inserted into their eyes to empower them to see souls that might wander off. Their hearts are pierced with arrows to enhance their ability to sympathize with the sick and suffering."[13]

The Tin Woodman tells Dorothy that his new heart is "a kinder and more tender heart than the one he had owned when he was made of flesh." But what is the real meaning of these strange replacements of natural parts with sacred totems? Perhaps it connotes that the body now includes the artifacts of mind; the flesh has become enmeshed in the workings of the soul. Purely unconscious, automatic life has come to an end. In the journey back to vitality, a permanent alteration has occurred within the bodymind that cannot be undone.

Those who shared their stories with me came, perforce, to honor this journey, awful though it had been. None would be so glib as to claim they would not have avoided it at almost any cost. But not one expressed the desire to forget the hard-fought route by which they had come. All asserted that they would not be who they were now if they had not traveled its path. In *The Wizard of Oz*, Dorothy is shocked to discover that she had the power all along to get back to Kansas, had she but clicked her heels. But her companions—symbols of mind, heart, and body—protest that they might never have discovered their own potentials:

"But then I should not have had my wonderful brains!" cried the Scarecrow. "I might have passed my whole life in the farmer's cornfield."

"And I should not have had my lovely heart," said the Tin Woodman. "I might have stood and rusted in the forest 'til the end of the world."

"And I should have lived a coward forever," declared the Lion, "and no beast in all the forest would have had a good word to say to me."

Alice Epstein writes that her healing path allowed each piece of her own totality to reveal itself at its own pace, to get as much emotional support for change as it needed. "I really had no choice but to allow the subpersonalities to proceed as they wished, because I never understood or could predict their paths until they were fulfilled." At the end of her journey, Alice found, somewhat wistfully, that they had all grown up. Even "Baby Alice" became "a young woman dressed stylishly in white, with shoulder-length brown hair cut blunt and turned up," a wife who now had a husband and twins! When Alice tried to engage her in dialogue, she replied that now Alice didn't need her any more: "She was perfectly nice, but as always she had her own agenda and was eager to return to it."

The emergence of wholeness from brokenness is a mystery of nature, even in the inanimate world. Even nonliving crystalline structures, when too great an energy surges through them, sometimes come apart only to knit together again. Belgian physicist Ilya Prigogine received the Nobel Prize for discovering how, when some crystals exposed to increased energy disintegrate into a seeming jumble of chaotic elements, a new structure can arise almost phoenixlike from the ruins—one that is capable of utilizing the greater flow of energy that had nearly been its destroyer. Writer Marilyn Ferguson described this renascence in terms suggestive of the healing process itself: "The elements of the old pattern come into contact with each other in new ways, and make new connections. The parts reorganize into a new whole. The system escapes into a higher order."[14]

Those who have been subject to the powerful energies of illness and healing, who have undergone the ordeal of being shattered and reformed, sometimes also give the impression of having "escaped into a higher order." But theirs was not an airy ascent into ethereal light, but to a ground of being that is "higher in authenticity," as

Alice Epstein remarked. Such a place supports little commerce in easy answers, or in visions of a life free of ambiguity. In the aftermath of her healing, Alice writes, "Instead of seeing everyone as all good or all bad, I understood that each person has both."

Mark Pelgrin reported that his wife had a final dream just before her own journey through life ended: She was sitting on a small island in a great sea, beside a dark man who was braiding strands of bread. The man turned and said emphatically, "The dark and the light must be braided together." Oliver Sacks, who experienced "blazing joy" and "the gaiety and innocence of the newborn" when he recovered, was appalled to find "after the exalted, lyrical sentiments I professed . . . sudden floodings of bile." Sacks, too, came to understand wholeness as a braiding of dark and light: "How can I claim that my goodness, my lofty feelings, constitute the 'real me,' and that my rancor and malice are just 'sickness'?"

Amid the chaos of profoundly disturbing events, paradoxical truths become imperatives. At the place where things fall apart, a greater center may obtain. Struggling with disease, disability, even death, the deepest questions of existence suddenly demand a personal resolution. Here the rules of ordinary logic must be suspended: The ugliest creature we can imagine may carry in its mouth a golden key. The crop that falls to the ground may yet fertilize a more abundant harvest.

At some unavoidable juncture in our lives, we each will be called upon to accomplish the most elemental of tasks: to embody our unique human potential. Perhaps the great knowledge that journeyers snatch from the dragon-realms of illness is a recognition that the work of wholeness has just begun.

❧ 17 ❧
EPILOGUE:
A SECOND BIRTH

> *Choose life instead of those prisms with no*
> *depth even if their colors are purer,*
> *Instead of this hour always hidden, instead*
> *of these terrible vehicles of cold flame. . . .*
> *Choose this heart with its safety catch. . . .*
> *Its scars from escapes, Choose. . . .*
> *The life of being here, nothing but being here. . . .*

—ANDRÉ BRETON, "Choose Life"[1]

SEVEN YEARS have passed since I emerged from a second birth; almost a stillbirth, for something—some spark of joy, capacity for love, motility of imagination—seemed for a time to have died in me.

But the force of life is a relentless, unsentimental pursuer. It seizes upon agendas that are wholly its own. It intrudes upon the heart—sometimes with delicacy, other times with a clarity so bright that it swallows both shadow and perspective. The Still Small Voice, my Bible teacher used to call it, as if all God could now muster was a cricket squeak of conscience, not the rank roar of lions. As if the primeval, upthrust landscape of the soul had been safely paved over for Sunday driving. As if the ancients had been credulous, trembling children, their empire of visions all sand-drowned ruin, their world of wonder and terror dismantled, tagged, and stored away in museum basements.

As if dreams didn't matter.

In *Perceval, le conte del Graal,* the last of Chrétien de Troyes's twelfth-century Arthurian romances, the knight-errant Perceval embarks on a quest for Christendom's most sacred relic, the Holy Grail. One day, as the sun is beginning to set with no shelter in sight, he encounters a fisherman who directs him to a castle where he might find welcome.

Arriving at the castle, Perceval is surprised to find the same fisherman, now attired as a king, recumbent before a gigantic blazing fireplace. Though the Fisher King has suffered a terrible wound on his thigh which prevents him from standing, he proves a gracious host, giving Perceval a sword sheathed in gold Venetian embroidery and seating him by his side at a sumptuous banquet.

As the young knight partakes of the feast, marvel after marvel unfolds before his eyes. A squire passes before him with a white lance from whose tip springs a freshet of blood. A damsel, holding a Grail emitting a brilliant light, appears and vanishes with heart-stopping grace down a corridor.

Not wishing to appear rude, however, Perceval neglects to ask the Fisher King about these miraculous displays, planning instead to interrogate one of the squires the next morning. He bids the King good night, stumbles to his quarters, and falls instantly asleep. But upon awakening, Perceval finds the castle deserted. He rides across the drawbridge to seek out its inhabitants, assuming they have gone into the forest to tend to the royal traps and nets, but none are to be found. When he glances back over his shoulder, the deserted castle is fading away in the distance.

Riding deeper into the wood, he happens upon a maiden and breathlessly describes to her the strange events of the previous night. The young woman, quizzing Perceval in the manner of an analyst eliciting a dream, tells him that the Fisher King had surely done him a great honor to bid him sit by his side. When she learns of the white lance that bled, she demands to know if Perceval had inquired as to *why*.

"I said nothing about it," he replies. The woman, looking pensive, listens as Perceval describes the appearance of the Grail. Indeed, she affirms, this was the true and eternally sought relic. When she discovers that he again failed to ask a single question, she can contain herself no longer.

"So help me, God," the damsel bursts out, "learn, then, that you have done ill!"

She explains to the baffled youth that had he but asked the Fisher King *whom* the Grail served, and *why* the lance bled, "You would have cured the maimed King, so that he would have recovered the use of his limbs and would have ruled his lands and great good would have come of it." But because of Perceval's lack of curiosity, the Fisher King, and the land itself, would remain blighted and infertile.[2]

Perceval's night in the vanishing castle may be seen as a "big dream," what the Irish refer to as an *echtra*, a journey through the Otherworld. The Fisher King is a ferryman of the soul, a wounded healer trawling the waters of the psyche to find nourishment in its teeming depths. Perceval's failure is clear: He does not actively inquire of his psyche when it is resplendently before him. At a holy feast where the meaning of the wound and its cure might be found, he does not pose a single penetrating question. Perceval, the brave knight who never flinched from rescuing damsels or fighting dragons, falters at direct engagement with his own inner life.

The pattern is hauntingly familiar. I believe that I went into the hospital in part to avoid the questions posed by my own dreams. I have come to learn that without a process of inner inquiry, it is difficult, if not impossible, to find the Grail of wholeness. Without asking the source of our own still-bleeding wounds, without serving our own purest light, we cannot be participants in our own destiny, and our inmost fields will remain fallow.

However accounts like Perceval's—like all stories of initiation—vividly portray the dazzling power of the visionary world, they are not necessarily the heart of the path of healing. Even in cultures where visions are honored, an anthropologist friend reminded me recently, "Someone still has to make the coffee. The shaman is often a working stiff, a farmer or hunter, not some guy always bumping his head on a cloud."

Perceval later redeems himself not through revelation, but through a life of service and prayer, the venerable ground-game of the spirit. I, too, have found that healing is grunt-work, having to do more with carpooling than charisma; more with the sometimes maddening drip of water on stone than with freeing the sword Excalibur. I try to remember there is nothing that is not path. Daily practice, no cramming; consistency, not crisis.

The task of becoming whole, say the Buddhists, is a case of quantitative leading to qualitative change—"polishing one's tile into a gemstone" or "churning the milk of mind into the butter of *dharma*"; manual labor which—if the polishing and churning are consistent enough—may work a strange alchemy.

I've been reading the occasional inspirational book lately, the kind with bearded, anorexic-looking Christs on the covers, stretching forth their hands in colorblind green and yellow: "A man's mind may be likened to a garden. If no useful seeds are put into it, then an abundance of useless weed-seeds will fall therein, and will continue to produce their kind." I need these homely, unerring truths, these Dick-and-Jane primers of the spiritual life.

Not that there is any unerring formula for healing. In a recent article, Naomi Remen polled her peers to ask which emotions they believed were most conducive to wellness. "All had worked with loving cheerful people who died, grieving people who lived, angry people who never became ill, and humorous people who were unable to heal themselves." But it doesn't matter. I plant my variegated seeds anyway, always alert for herbs among the weeds.

I have the visceral certainty we live in a reflexive universe. Each monopole of love or hate seems to whirl through my system like a charge in a particle accelerator, redoubling itself, returning to me mysteriously magnified, imbued with velocity.

Meanwhile, my outward velocity has slowed. In the seven years since my operation, I have been living a life that would once have been inconceivable to me. I turn off the phone in the morning, rarely skip breakfast, occasionally miss deadlines, or even turn down work if it starts to take too much from me, or takes me too far from those I love. There is much I still want to accomplish, but my old ambition feels like glorified running in place. My career, which I had fixed on as an unassailable virtue, now seems like a bit of a con. "Wherever you go, there you are." Where did I think I was going?

Recently, while visiting friends in Aspen, I was invited to a small party given for a well-known movie star. I surprised myself by passing it up: What in the world, I thought, would I have to say to her? And, as faint as those signals that radiotelescopes occasionally detect from distant pulsars, I receive confirmations in my now infrequent dreams:

> Bluesman Muddy Waters has given me a harmonica just like his, but it needs a tiny battery to bring up the volume.
> I have the smallest mansion in a mansion district but, I am told, "The interior decoration is what counts."
> I have inherited from my grandfather "the world's second-best guitar," and am slowly, haltingly teaching myself how to play it.

The dreams echo a conversation I once had with a Korean martial arts master. After sizing me up for a fraction of a second, he pronounced curtly, "Your kind of person always have to be Number One." I smiled at what I took to be a compliment. "No!" he fairly shouted. "If you don't want get sick again, you better learn be Number *Two!*"

Not surprisingly, being Number Two has produced undeniable twinges. During my years-long healing journey, an old friend and collaborator has won three Academy Awards. Other colleagues have written important books, started successful magazines. A surprising number of acquaintances from my media days have attained the national recognition I used to imagine as a supreme haven, a honeyed land warmed by an ever-beaming sun of attention. Seeing their names in print once would have thrown me into secret paroxysms of tire-biting envy, but those feelings are now, if not wholly absent, strangely blunted. Jung once said that the only real events of his life were those times when "the imperishable world irrupted into this transitory one." In some way that I have no control over, I feel the same way.

There is a price for this attitude. For uncomfortably long intervals, I've been a member of the New Poor. But even then, there have been compensations. For a few years, I moved in with friends, which netted me a place with a view of the mountains, cheap rent, and the added bonus of ready banter when I felt the walls close in. I didn't have a car, so I walked miles every day, sucking in freshets of reasonably clean air, bumping into neighbors. I still can't afford many long-distance calls, so my relationships are chiefly local, person to person.

My surgeon was wrong, I think, when he said my illness was not a spiritual problem. But I was equally wrong to think that my healing path ended when I had surgery, or would have been made smooth if a miracle rather than medicine had cured me of cancer.

I have kept up on occasion with all those I met on my own journey. A few have died; a few others had recurrences of their diseases. Whatever the treatment or lack thereof, a remission can unpredictably last five years, ten years, or a lifetime. For myself, my Grail turns out to be a trick cup—a dribble glass—that keeps miraculously refilling with the help, in part, of a refillable prescription. The occasion each day when I take my pill is a private *auto-da-fé;* an act that says whatever I've done is worth living with, what I haven't is worth living for. Faith is, after all, also eating what's on our plate; is only our clumsy, human embrace of the inevitability of molting and seasons.

The moment of faith is a daily occurrence. Sometimes it tolls like an iron gong, banging aside compromise, waking the neighborhood, demanding that we come along without proper goodbyes, with no provision but blind, unjustified trust. Other times, it is the tip of a branch we thought we heard graze the windowpane just as we were falling asleep. It is the moment Yeats described: "One lifts a flap of paper to discover both the human entrails and the starry heavens."

At some point, I am certain, each of us will come face to face with precisely that which we most fear. At such times, says a Roman proverb, *Fata volentem ducunt, trahunt nolentem:* Whoever is willing, the fates will lead; those who are not, the Fates will drag along. So I try to practice the higher form of fidelity, obedience to awareness. I've been taking the advice of a Brazilian friend: "Your job is only to live your life from the inside out—let the universe take care of the paperwork."

And indeed, unexpected opportunities have begun to present themselves. Last year I was asked to write a global environmental broadcast that the network producers, with some hyperbole, claimed was beamed to a potential audience of a billion. The show, like all shows, was ephemeral; it came and went. But I was gratified we had decided to cast kids to deliver the message: In their words, I scripted in the plangency of my own childish heart.

On the day after my operation, Susan wrote me to say she had dreamed I had a major heart operation. My surgeons had lifted out the powerfully beating organ, pulled out some "black stuff," and then replaced it, saying, "This is a good heart." I catch myself hoping she was right, for there could be no greater healing. When I miss the crystalline dream-realms that held me spellbound, I think of Saint Paul's warning about putting too much stock in the other world's shining baubles: "If I speak with the eloquence of men and angels, but have no love, I become no more than blaring brass or crashing cymbal. If I have the gift of foretelling the future . . . but have no love, I amount to nothing at all. . . . It is the one thing that still stands when all else has fallen."

Susan, however, is long gone. I reread the letters she wrote me in Boston, suddenly seeing the loneliness between the lines of her anecdotes and pep talks, the longing at last so much my own that I am sometimes tempted to mail them back signed with my name. But the rules are clear: no postage to the past.

She has gone back to school. When we meet for lunch, she talks to me about Dante and Derrida, an earnest, slightly inflamed light in her eyes. She wears a monk-like cowl, collects Anunciation reproductions, gives occasional public readings of ironic tone-poems about bad boyfriends. "You dope," she wrote in a card some time back. "I always knew it would take an ending to convince you of the reality of love."

My daughter, Leah, put it more gently in a poem, with instructions to hang it over my desk: "If you have no love in your life," it begins sonorously, "then the silence of life will be banging." In the silence, though, I can hear: I had used love more than given it, another Grail that was harder to grasp the closer to it I came.

When I interviewed the radical psychiatrist R. D. Laing in London a few years before he died, he had been, he told me, "doing a great load of cogitating about love."

"We are all other to each other," he had said, puffing a few times on his clumsily rolled cigarette before snubbing it out. "We've first got to admit to it." Laing had sat in silence for a few minutes; he had a kind of tick of literally turning his eyeballs inwards when he was thinking, and I could see their fitful white gleaming from the shadow-pond of his high-backed chair. "But it's not all dust and ash. The paradox is that by completely renouncing togetherness, we discover real communion.

"Of course," he had added with a sharp laugh, "when you apply that to romance, most people throw in the towel."

For now, I've thrown it in. In the absence of romance, I've been trying to be more conscientious about friendship. I've reconstituted a few old ones, found some new ones. Previously, my friendships tended to be functional, work-related, brittle and so prone to breakage. Now I prefer to spend time together doing things that in no way augment the GNP or the free flow of global information, or even necessarily diminish my quotient of existential loneliness.

I find I want less from others. I expect more from myself, I suppose. I try to think what I can do to support the people I care about, rather than asking them to hoist me on their shoulders so I can do them the favor of reporting the view. It's a painstaking, craftsmanly process, this making of relationship, built from tiny bricks of generosity and restraint.

I try especially to restrain myself from judging, though it's a difficult habit to break. I'm an editor by temperament. I value my fine distinctions. But I know that judgment piles upon judgment, like tiny sea animals forming a coral reef, until one day there is an ossified hump in the sea, the island that John Donne counseled from his sickbed, no man is wise to become. I'm trying to allow people their so-called imperfections, realizing these may be mazeways to their own vital mystery.

I'm not doing this because I'm a nice guy: I'm doing it for my health. I know that the equation I was presented with—Change or Die—is one I still have to try to solve. There is some part of me which, though I might not agree with what it says, will defend to the death its right to say it. I'm left with an imperative to be as truthful as I can manage—however wrenching that might be to relationships, finances, or my own peace of mind—knowing that anything less might be fatal. I have posted next to Leah's poem W. H. Auden's trenchant observation:

> *We would rather be ruined than changed;*
> *We would rather die in our dread*
> *Than climb the cross of the moment*
> *And let our illusions die.*

My experiences of the past years have divided my life into neat halves, like an apple sliced lengthwise through the core. Yesterday I was young, still schoonering on the winds of my twenties. Now I know the woodier, more earthbound resonances of age, of time; the lordship of limits. I am taking on definite shape: I have a newly white forelock of hair, the traditional badge of the man who, on some occasion or other in his life, has nearly been scared to death.

Endnotes

CHAPTER 1—THE VARIETIES OF HEALING EXPERIENCE

1. Juan Ramón Jiménez, *Light and Shadows: Selected Poems of Juan Ramón Jiménez*, trans. Dennis Maloney and Clark Zlotchew (Buffalo, N.Y.: White Pine Press, 1987).

2. George Crile, Jr., "Controversies in Thyroid Surgery," *New York State Journal of Medicine* 80 (November 1980): 1834. Commenting on the common practice of removing the entire thyroid gland for even *non*cancerous benign nodules, Crile writes, "In short, has there not been brewed up a tempest in a teapot? The final question is whether or not the medical profession's widely broadcast scare about cancer of the thyroid has induced the public to expose itself to remedies that are more dangerous than the disease."

3. James Hillman, *Re-Visioning Psychology* (New York: Harper & Row, 1975), p. 80.

4. Ernest Lawrence Rossi, *The Psychobiology of Mind-Body Healing: New Concepts of Therapeutic Hypnosis* (New York: W. W. Norton, 1986).

5. Jeanne Achterberg, *Imagery in Healing: Shamanism and Modern Medicine* (Boston: Shambhala Publications, 1985), p. 174.

6. Rossi, op. cit., p. 187.

7. T. Everson and W. Cole, *Spontaneous Regression of Cancer* (Philadelphia and London: W. B. Saunders, 1966).

8. C. I. V. Franklin, "Spontaneous Regression of Cancer," in *Prolonged Arrest of Cancer*, B. A. Stoll, editor (New York: John Wiley and Sons, 1982), pp. 103–107.

9. Caryle Hirshberg and Brendan O'Regan, *Spontaneous Remission: An Annotated Bibliography* (Sausalito, Calif.: Institute of Noetic Sciences, 1993).

10. *USA Today*, April 1, 1992, p. D1.

11. Oliver Sacks, *Awakenings* (New York: Vintage Books, 1976), p. 265.

12. Rossi, op. cit., p. 108.

13. Achterberg, op, cit., p. 177.

14. Ibid., p. 182.

15. Ibid.

16. E. Benedict and T. Porter, "Native American Medicine Ways," quoted in Achterberg, op. cit., p. 146.

17. Evon Z. Vogt, *Zinacantán: A Maya Community in the Highlands of Chiapas* (Cambridge: Harvard University Press, Belknap Press, 1969), pp. 369–374.

18. C. A. Meier, *Ancient Incubation and Modern Psychotherapy,* trans. Monica Curtis (Evanston, Ill.: Northwestern University Press, 1967), p. 128.

CHAPTER 2—THE HEALING PATH:
MAPS FOR THE JOURNEY

1. A term suggested by the late radical psychiatrist R. D. Laing in *The Politics of Experience* (New York: Ballantine Books, 1967).
2. L. Frank Baum, with introduction and annotation by Michael Patrick Hearn, *The Annotated Wizard of Oz* (New York: Clarkson N. Potter, Inc., 1973), pp. 69–76.
3. Dr. George M. Gould and Dr. Walter L. Pyle, *Anomalies and Curiosities of Medicine* (Philadelphia and London: W. B. Saunders, 1896; reprint, New York: The Julian Press, 1956), pp. 787–88.
4. Ivan Illich, *Medical Nemesis: The Expropriation of Health* (New York: Pantheon Books, 1976), p. 152.
5. John A. Sanford, *Healing and Wholeness* (New York: Paulist Press, 1977), p. 33.
6. D. Patrick Miller, "My Healing Journey Through Chronic Fatigue," *Yoga Journal,* November–December 1992, p. 61.
7. W. H. Polonsky et al., "Psychological Factors, Immunological Function, and Bronchial Asthma," *Psychosomatic Medicine* 47 (1985):77. This study is of particular interest because it utilizes modern research methodology, which some psychoanalytically oriented studies in the 1940s and 1950s that linked disease and personality were faulted for neglecting.
8. Yujiro Ikemi, et al., "Psychosomatic Consideration on Cancer Patients Who Have Made a Narrow Escape from Death," *Dynamic Psychiatry* 8 (1975): p. 86.
9. Joan Halifax, *Shaman: The Wounded Healer* (London: Thames and Hudson, Ltd., 1982), p. 21.
10. Sir John Eccles, quoted in Gotthard Booth, "Psychobiological Aspects of Spontaneous Regressions of Cancer," *Journal of the American Academy of Psychoanalysis* 1 (1973): 306.
11. Ernest Lawrence Rossi, *The Psychobiology of Mind-Body Healing* (New York: W. W. Norton, 1986), p. 72.

CHAPTER 3—THE TANGLED ROOTS OF DISEASE

1. Steven Locke and Douglas Colligan, *The Healer Within: The New Medicine of Mind and Body* (New York: New American Library, 1986), p. 169.
2. John Harrison, M.D., *Love Your Disease: It's Keeping You Healthy* (Santa Monica: Hay House, 1988), p. 100.
3. Maggy Howe, "Youthing: The Inner Alchemy of Breath," *Taxi,* October 1989, p. 127.
4. Marcia Angell, "Disease as a Reflection of the Psyche" (editorial), *New England Journal of Medicine* 312 (June 1985): 1570–1572.

5. B. M. Cormier et al., "Psychological Aspects of Rheumatoid Arthritis," *Canadian Medical Association Journal* 77 (1957): 539–541.

6. L. Temoshok, B.W. Heller, et. al., "The Relationship of Psychosocial Factors to Prognostic Indicators in Cutaneous Malignant Melanoma," *Journal of Psychosomatic Medicine* 29(1985): 139–54.

7. Beth Kirsch, "Stress Control," *Health Journal*, Spring 1989, p. 10.

8. Beatrice Blyth Whiting, *Paiute Sorcery,* abridged in *Culture, Disease, and Healing: Studies in Medical Anthropology,* ed. David Landy (New York: Macmillan, 1977), p. 210.

9. Leonard B. Glick, "Medicine as an Ethnographic Category: the Gimi of the New Guinea Highlands," in Landy, op. cit., pp. 58–70.

10. Forrest Clements, "Primitive Concepts of Disease," University of California Publications in American Archaeology and Ethnology, 32(1932): pp. 185–252.

11. Jeanne Achterberg, "The Shaman: Master Healer in the Imaginary Realm," in *Shamanism,* comp. Shirley Nicholson (Wheaton, Ill.: Theosophical Publishing House, 1987), p. 105.

12. Carl Jung, quoted in Elida Evans, *A Psychological Study of Cancer* (New York: Dodd, Mead, 1926), p. 44.

13. Alice Miller, *Thou Shalt Not Be Aware: Society's Betrayal of the Child* (New York: Meridian Books, 1986), p. 58.

14. Ibid.

15. Jeanne Achterberg, quoted in *Shaman's Path: Healing, Personal Growth and Empowerment,* comp. and ed. Gary Doore (Boston: Shambhala Publications, 1988), p. 121. "We have evidence that stress precedes disease, and that stress inhibits the immune response, but no one has shown conclusively that the inhibited immune response associated with stress actually results in physical disease." On the other hand, she suggests, "An injury to the inviolate core which is the essence of a person's being" may manifest as "despair, immunological damage, cancer, and a host of very serious disorders."

16. Russell A. Lockhart, "Cancer in Myth and Dream," *Spring*, (1977): p. 23n.

17. Roger J. Booth and Kevin R. Ashbridge, "A Fresh Look at the Relationship between the Psyche and Immune System: Teleological Coherence and Harmony of Purpose," *Advances* 9 (Spring, 1993): 2, p. 4.

18. Meredith Sabini and Valerie Hone Maffly, "An Inner View of Illness: The Dreams of Two Cancer Patients," *Journal of Analytical Psychology* 26 (1981): p. 124. (Sabini and Maffly are quoting Claus B. and M. B. Bahnson, footnote 25, below).

19. Susan Sontag, *Illness as Metaphor* (New York: Vintage Books, 1978), p. 50.

20. Ibid., pp. 45–46.

21. Lawrence LeShan, *You Can Fight for Your Life: Emotional Factors in the Treatment of Cancer* (New York: M. Evans, 1977), p. 34.

22. D. M. Kissen, "Personality characteristics in males conduce to lung cancer," *British Journal of Medical Psychology,* 36 (1963): p. 27; and Kissen, D. M., et al., "A further report on personality and psychosocial factors in lung cancer," *Annals of the New York Academy of Science,* 164 (1969): 535–45.

23. S. Greer and Tina Morris, "Psychological Attributes of Women Who Develop Breast Cancer," *Journal of Psychosomatic Research* 19 (1975): pp. 147–53.

24. Steven Locke and Douglas Colligan, *The Healer Within: The New Medicine of Mind and Body* (New York: New American Library, 1986), pp. 167–68.

25. Claus B. Bahnson and M. B. Bahnson, "Ego Defenses in Cancer Patients," *Annals of the New York Academy of Science* 164 (1969): 546.

26. Typical cancer-prone personalities, says psychoanalyst Gotthard Booth, experienced "traumatic frustration in their mother relationship," with the resulting fixation played out all through life as "a desperate need for control of a . . . personal relationship [or] a socioeconomic career." The cancer process begins when, in a sense, insult is added to injury, and the patient experiences "the irreparable loss of control of his idiosyncratic object." (Gotthard Booth, "Psychobiological Aspects of 'Spontaneous' Regressions of Cancer," *Journal of the American Academy of Psychoanalysis*, 1(3)[1973]: pp. 303–17.)

27. Rossi, op. cit., p. 109.

28. It is relevant to mention here a famous study of personality and disease begun in the mid-1940s: Hundreds of members of a Johns Hopkins graduating class were given extensive psychological testing, after which researchers monitored their health over a twenty-year period. One of the most striking findings was that *suicides and cancer victims had nearly identical psychological profiles.* (Caroline Bedell Thomas, "Precursors of Premature Disease and Death: The Predictive Potential of Habits and Family Attitudes," *Annals of Internal Medicine,* 85 [1976]: pp. 653–58.) For an informed and judicious critique of Temoshok's thesis, the reader is referred to a review of her work in *Advances* (9), 4, Fall, 1993, pp. 99–107. Regarding the so-called Type C personality, editor Harris Dienstfrey argues, "Nothing necessarily connects these pieces."

29. Redford Williams, "The Trusting Heart," *Psychology Today,* January–February 1989, p. 36.

30. Ibid.

31. Jeanne Achterberg, *Imagery in Healing: Shamanism and Modern Medicine* (Boston: Shambhala Publications, 1985), p. 130.

32. *Journal of the American Medical Association,* "Medical News and Perspectives" (July 18, 1986), pp. 312–13. Cf. Charles Silberstein, "Psychobiological Considerations in the Development of Acquired Immunodeficiency Syndrome"), *Einstein Quarterly Journal of Biological Medicine,* 3(1985): pp. 136–43.

33. Meredith Sabini, personal communication, October 8, 1985.

34. Claus B. Bahnson and M. B. Bahnson, ibid.

35. John Perry, *The Far Side of Madness* (Englewood Cliffs: Prentice-Hall, 1974), pp. 25–36.

36. Dean Ornish, M.D., personal communication, November 1988.

37. Redford Williams, ibid.

38. Meyer Friedman, M.D., personal communication, April 20, 1993.

39. Redford Williams, op. cit., p. 51.

CHAPTER 4—THE HERALD: THE UNHEARD CALL

1. Joan Halifax, *Shaman: The Wounded Healer* (London: Thames and Hudson, Ltd., 1982), p. 11.

2. Ruth Inge-Heinze, personal communication, May 1988.

3. Ilza Veith, trans., *The Yellow Emperor's Classic of Internal Medicine* (Berkeley: University of California Press, 1972), p. 134.

4. Aristotle, *De Divinatione per Somnum (On Prophesying by Dreams)* quoted in Russell A. Lockhart, "Cancer in Myth and Dream," *Spring* (1977): p. 24n.

5. Ernest Lawrence Rossi, *The Psychobiology of Mind-Body Healing: New Concepts of Therapeutic Hypnosis* (New York: W. W. Norton, 1986), p. 187.

6. Sigmund Freud, *The Interpretation of Dreams* trans. and ed. James Strachey (New York: Avon Books, 1965), p. 67.

7. Edward Thornton, *Diary of a Mystic* (London: George Allen and Unwin, 1967), p. 126.

8. Ibid., p. 132.

9. Robert M. Stein, "Body and Psyche: An Archetypal View of Psychosomatic Phenomena," *Spring* (1976): p. 79.

10. C. A. Meier, "Psychosomatic Medicine from the Jungian Point of View," *Journal of Analytical Psychology* 8 (1963): 103.

11. Joseph Campbell, *The Hero with a Thousand Faces*, Bollingen Series, no. 17 (Princeton: Princeton University Press, 1973), p. 51.

CHAPTER 5—THE SYMPTOM:
THE VOICE OF THE BODYMIND?

1. C. G. Jung, *Collected Works*, quoted in James Hillman, *Re-Visioning Psychology* (New York: Harper & Row, 1975), p. 104.

2. Ted J. Kaptchuk. *The Web That Has No Weaver: Understanding Chinese Medicine* (New York: Congdon & Weed, 1983).

3. Bernadin de Saint-Pierre, carrying forward Aristotle's notions of "natural telelogy."

4. Glenda Hawley, unpublished dissertation, "The Role of Holistic Variables in the Attribution of Cancer Survival" (San Francisco: Saybrook Institution, 1989), p. 53. Referring to C. Garfield (ed.), *Stress and survival: The emotional realities of life-threatening disease* (St. Louis: C. V. Mosby, 1979).

5. A. David Feinstein, "Conflict over childbearing and tumors of the female reproductive system: symbolism in disease," *Somatics,* Fall/Winter 1982, 4(1), pp. 36–41.

6. Leslie D. Weatherhead, *Psychology, Religion and Healing* (New York: Abingdon Press, 1951), p. 385.

7. Michael Murphy, *The Future of the Body* (Los Angeles: Jeremy P. Tarcher, 1992), pp. 491–92.

8. Michael Murphy, op. cit., p. 234.

9. Ibid., p. 488.

10. Ibid., p. 234.

11. Alfred Ribi, *Demons of the Inner World* (Boston: Shambhala Publications, 1990), p. 81.

12. C. G. Jung, *On the Nature of the Psyche*, trans. R. F. C. Hull, Bollingen Series, no. 20, vol. 8 (Princeton: Princeton University Press, 1973), p. 80.

13. Laurence Foss and Kenneth Rothenburg, *The Second Medical Revolution: From Biomedicine to Infomedicine* (Boston: Shambhala Publications, 1987), pp. 289–93. From an "infomedical" point of view, say Foss and Rothenberg, the physical expression of blushing can be seen as a sentence expressing an idea: "[T]o erase the sentence—through an antiblushing drug, for instance—is not to eradicate its meaning: the immaterial proposition survives the physical sentence. (Were the body denied its natural expression, it would likely seek another, apparently unrelated pathway for that expression.)"

14. Ernest Lawrence Rossi, *The Psychobiology of Mind-Body Healing: New Concepts of Therapeutic Hypnosis* (New York: W. W. Norton, 1986), p. 173.

15. R. M. Ford, "The Treatment of Intractable Childhood Asthma by Medium-Term Separation from Home Environment," *Medical Journal of Australia* 1 (1968): 653–656.

16. Ivan Illich, *Medical Nemesis* (New York: Pantheon, 1976), p. 112.

17. Raymond Berté, quoted in Paul C. Roud, *Making Miracles: An Exploration Into the Dynamics of Self-Healing* (New York: Warner Books, 1990), pp. 13–37.

18. Ibid., p. 26.

19. James Hillman, *Healing Fiction* (Barrytown, N.Y.: Station Hill Press, 1983), pp. 99–100.

20. Michel Foucault, *The Birth of the Clinic: An Archaeology of Medical Perception* (New York: Vintage Books, 1975), p. 178.

21. Dr. Charles Weinstock, quoted in Greg Levoy, "Inexplicable Recoveries from Incurable Diseases," *Longevity*, October 1989, p. 41. Dr. Weinstock was formerly director of New York's Psychosomatic Cancer Study Group.

22. Yujiro Ikemi et al., "Psychosomatic Consideration on Cancer Patients Who Have Made a Narrow Escape from Death," *Dynamic Psychiatry* 8 (1975): 77–93.

23. Albert Kreinheder, *Body and Soul: The Other Side of Illness* (Toronto: Inner City Books, 1991), p. 37.

24. Arnold Mindell, *Working with the Dreaming Body* (New York: Routledge & Kegan Paul, 1987), pp. 11–13.

25. Ibid., p. 3.

26. Eric J. Cassell, "Ideas in Conflict: The Rise and Fall (and Rise and Fall) of New Views of Disease," *Daedalus* 115 (1986): 29. An experimental clinic on a Navajo reservation in the 1950s that practiced modern medicine side by side with Navajo healing traditions fell athwart of precisely this problem: "[T]he afflictions of the Navajo (with the important exception of tuberculosis and perhaps *otitis media*) did not fall within the ken of technological medicine. It is not that 1950s medicine did not have solutions to their major diseases, it is that the major causes of morbidity and mortality of the Navajo do not fall within the system of entities that count as 'diseases' in our medicine."

27. Selma Hyman, "Death-in-Life—Life-in-Death," *Spring* (1977): pp. 34–35.

28. Albert Kreinheder, op. cit., p. 16.

29. Joseph Campbell, *The Hero with a Thousand Faces*, Bollingen Series, no. 17 (Princeton: Princeton University Press, 1973), p. 51.

CHAPTER 6—DIAGNOSIS: THE POWER OF NAMING

1. Jane Cowles, *Informed Consent* (New York: Coward-McCann, 1976), p. 22.

2. Ted J. Kaptchuk, *The Web That Has No Weaver: Understanding Chinese Medicine* (New York: Congdon & Weed, 1983), p. 6.

3. Hippocrates, summarized in Howard Clark Kee, *Medicine, Miracle and Magic in New Testament Times* (Cambridge: Cambridge University Press, 1986), pp. 29–30.

4. Ivan Illich, *Medical Nemesis: The Expropriation of Health* (New York: Pantheon Books, 1976), pp. 159–60.

5. Ibid., p. 96.

6. James Hillman. *Re-Visioning Psychology* (New York: Harper & Row, 1975), p. 75.

7. John Richardson, "Picasso's Last Mystery," *Vanity Fair*, May 1988, p. 124.

8. Robert Burton, *The Anatomy of Melancholy*, quoted in C. A. McMahon, "The Role of Imagination in the Disease Process: Pre-Cartesian History," *Psychological Medicine* 6 (1976): 179–184.

9. Drs. John Zurlo and H. Clifford Lane, quoted in Mary Walker, "Surviving AIDS," *East West Journal*, January 1991, p. 39.

10. Daniel Goleman, "Positive Denial: The Case for Not Facing Reality," interview with Dr. Richard S. Lazarus, *Psychology Today*, November 1979, p. 447.

11. Johann Georg Zimmerman, quoted in Michel Foucault, *The Birth of the Clinic: An Archaeology of Medical Perception* (New York: Vintage Books, 1975), p. 14.

12. Eric J. Cassell, "Ideas in Conflict: The Rise and Fall (and Rise and Fall) of New Views of Disease," *Daedalus* 115 (1986): 26.

13. Interview with then–Arkanasas Governor Bill Clinton, "All Things Considered," National Public Radio, broadcast over KGNU, Boulder, Colorado, September 26, 1989.

14. Maurice S. Fox, Ph.D., "On the Diagnosis and Treatment of Breast Cancer," *Journal of the American Medical Association*, February 2, 1979, 241: 5, pp. 489–94.

15. Damon Phinney, "High 10-Year Survival Rate in Patients with Early, Untreated Prostatic Cancer," in *Boulder Daily Camera*, December 20, 1992, p. E3.

16. Sandra Blakeslee, "Routine Removal of Wisdom Teeth Wastes Millions, Report Contends," *The New York Times*, June 26, 1991, pp. A1, B8.

17. Ted J. Kaptchuk, op. cit., p. 4.

18. In Jeanne Achterberg, *Imagery in Healing: Shamanism and Modern Medicine* (Boston: Shambhala Publications, 1985), p. 190.

19. Leonard B. Glick, "Medicine as an Ethnographic Category: The Gimi of the New Guinea Highlands," in *Culture, Disease, and Healing: Studies in Medical Anthropology*, ed. David Landy (New York: Macmillan, 1977), p. 69.

20. Elida Evans, *A Psychological Study of Cancer* (New York: Dodd, Mead, 1926), p. 15.

CHAPTER 7—THE MEETING WITH THE DOCTOR

1. E. Fuller Torrey, M.D., "What Western Psychotherapists Can Learn from Witchdoctors," *American Journal of Orthopsychiatry,* 42 (1972): 69–75.

2. H. Wilmer, "Transference to a Medical Center," quoted in Torrey, op. cit., p. 72.

3. Laurence Foss and Kenneth Rothenberg, *The Second Medical Revolution: From Biomedicine to Infomedicine* (Boston: Shambhala Publications, Inc., 1987), p. 271.

4. David Hellerstein, M.D.F., "The Hope Epidemic," *Mirabella,* October 1989, p. 87.

5. Mark Nichter, M.D., "Holistic Health: An Ethnomedical Perspective," a lecture at the American Holistic Medical Association's annual conference, "Expanding the Spectrum of Medicine," Breckenridge, Colorado, March 17–23, 1991.

6. Brendan O'Regan, "Healing, Remission, and Miracle Cures," Institute of Noetic Sciences Special Report, May 1987, p. 4.

7. S. L. Feder, "Psychological Considerations in the Care of Patients with Cancer," *Annals of the New York Academy of Science* 125 (1966): 1020–1027.

8. Study by psychiatrist Sandra Levy and Yale University psychologist Judith Rodin, reported in *Hippocrates,* November/December 1989, p. 93.

9. Dr. James Gordon, lecture delivered at American Holistic Medical Association's annual conference, Breckenridge, Colorado, March 17–23, 1991.

10. Ivan Illich, *Medical Nemesis: The Expropriation of Health* (New York: Pantheon Books, 1976), p. 30.

11. Ikuko Osumi, *The Shamanic Healer* (Rochester, Vermont: Healing Arts Press, 1988), pp. 54–55.

12. "Abuse of Medical Students Is Found," *The New York Times,* January 26, 1990, p. A12.

13. Dr. Larry Dossey, *Recovering the Soul: A Scientific and Spiritual Search* (New York: Bantam Books, 1989), p. 56.

14. Dr. Larry Dossey, *Healing Words: The Power of Prayer and the Practice of Medicine* (San Francisco: HarperSanFrancisco, 1993), pp. 13–14.

CHAPTER 8—BIG GUNS, MAGIC BULLETS:
THE CITADEL OF MEDICINE

1. See James Hillman, *Re-Visioning Psychology* (New York: Harper & Row, 1975), for a broader discussion of this idea..

2. Oliver Sacks, *Awakenings* (New York: Vintage Books, 1973), p. 264.

3. John C. Bailar and Elaine M. Smith, "Progress against Cancer?" *New England Journal of Medicine* 314:19 (1986), pp. 1225–1232.

4. Martin F. Shapiro, "Chemotherapy: Snake-Oil Remedy?" *Los Angeles Times,* January 9, 1987, II, p. 5.

5. John Cairns, "The Treatment of Diseases and the War against Cancer," *Scientific American,* November 1985, p. 59. Cairns cites a trial of chemotherapy in 600 cases of colon cancer who received standard surgery. Half then also received cytotoxic chemotherapy, but they showed no improvement over the control group who received no additional treatment.

6. U.S. Congress, Office of Technology Assessment, *Assessing the Efficacy and Safety of Medical Technologies,* Report No. OTA-H-75 (Washington, D.C.: U.S. Government Printing Office, September, 1978).

7. Dr. Peter H. Wiernik, quoted in "Patient's Marrow Emerges as Key Cancer Tool," *The New York Times,* March 27, 1990, p. B1.

8. Dr. Steven Heisel, neuropsychiatrist, personal communication, February 1988.

9. Ivan Illich, *Medical Nemesis: The Expropriation of Health* (New York: Pantheon Books, 1976), p. 196.

10. Mark Nichter, M.D., "Holistic Health: An Ethnomedical Perspective," a lecture delivered at the American Holistic Medical Association's annual conference, "Expanding the Spectrum of Medicine," Breckenridge, Colorado, March 17–23, 1991.

11. David Brown, "Surgery for prostate in men has little or no benefit," *Boulder Daily Camera,* May 26, 1993, p. 4A.

12. Lynn Payer, *Medicine and Culture: Varieties of Treatment in the United States, England, West Germany, and France* (New York: Henry Holt, 1988), p. 130.

13. Ibid., pp. 124, 125.

14. James LeMoyne, "Out of the Jungle in El Salvador: Rebels with a New Cause," *The New York Times Magazine,* February 9, 1992, p. 67.

15. Richard Grossinger, *Planet Medicine: From Stone Age Shamanism to Post–Industrial Healing* (New York: Doubleday, 1985), p. 404n.

16. "Doing the Crime, Not the Time," *Time,* September 11, 1989, p. 81.

17. Plato, *Symposium,* quoted in C. A. Meier, *Ancient Incubation and Modern Psychotherapy,* trans. Monica Curtis (Evanston, Ill.: Northwestern University Press, 1967), p. 186.

18. Alfred Ribi, *Demons of the Inner World: Understanding Our Hidden Complexes* (Boston: Shambhala Publications, 1990), p. 69.

19. Dr. Eugene Duboff, quoted in "Getting Back to Their Roots," *Westword,* January 10–16, 1990, p. 76. Dr. Duboff is a Denver psychiatrist and Anafranil proponent.

20. Pamela King, "The Chemistry of Doubt," *Psychology Today,* October 1989.

21. Ronald Kotulak, "Therapy, like drugs, can physically alter the brain," *Chicago Tribune* article in *Boulder Daily Camera,* May 20, 1993, p. C4.

22. Ernest Lawrence Rossi, *The Psychobiology of Mind-Body Healing: New Concepts of Therapeutic Hypnosis* (New York: W. W. Norton, 1986), p. 16.

23. Laurence Foss and Kenneth Rothenberg, *The Second Medical Revolution: From Biomedicine to Infomedicine* (Boston: Shambhala Publications, 1987), p. 70.

24. Ibid.

25. Rose J. Papac, M.D., Chief, Section of Hematology/Oncology, Veterans

Administration Medical Center, West Haven, Connecticut, personal communication, June 7, 1993.

26. Rose J. Papac, M.D., "Spontaneous Regression of Cancer," *Connecticut
Medicine*, 54: 4, April 1990, p. 180.

27. Jeanne Achterberg, *Imagery in Healing* (Boston: Shambhala Publications,
1985), p. 170.

28. Deepak Chopra, *Quantum Healing: Exploring the Frontiers of Mind/Body
Medicine* (New York: Bantam Books, 1989), p. 94.

29. Hillman, op. cit., pp. 102–103.

30. Larry Dossey, *Recovering the Soul: A Scientific and Spiritual Search* (New
York: Bantam Books, 1991), p. 71.

31. Roger Penrose, *The Emperor's New Mind: Concerning Computers, Minds, and
the Laws of Physics* (New York: Penguin Books, 1991), pp. 3–29.

CHAPTER 9—TAKING BACK CONTROL:
FINDING NEW FOOTING

1. Gopi Krishna, *Kundalini: The Evolutionary Energy in Man* (Boston: Shambhala Publications, 1971), pp. 70–72.

2. Victor Turner, *The Ritual Process: Structure and Anti-Structure*, The Lewis
Henry Morgan Lectures, delivered 1966, Ithaca, New York (Ithaca: Cornell
Paperbacks, 1977), p. 95.

3. Hans J. Eysenck, "Health's Character," *Psychology Today*, December 1988,
pp. 27–36.

4. Elida Evans, *A Psychological Study of Cancer* (New York: Dodd, Mead, 1926),
p. 41.

5. Richard Moss, *How Shall I Live: Transforming Surgery or Any Health Crisis
into Greater Aliveness* (Berkeley: Celestial Arts, 1985), p. 50.

CHAPTER 10—THE QUEST FOR MEDICINE:
A WORLD OF ALTERNATIVES

1. Edwin H. Ackerknecht, "Problems of Primitive Medicine," *Bulletin of the
History of Medicine* 11(1942): 46.

2. David M. Eisenberg, M.D., et al. "Unconventional Medicine in the United
States," *New England Journal of Medicine*, January 28, 1993, p. 246.

3. Barrie Cassileth et al., "Contemporary unorthodox treatments in cancer
medicine," *Annals of Internal Medicine* 101(1984): pp. 105–112.

4. Media General and the Associated Press, poll published in November 1985.
Half of respondents said that clinics that treat cancer in ways opposed by
mainstream researchers should be allowed to operate in the U.S.

5. "Why New Age Medicine is Catching On," *Time*, November 4, 1991, p.
68.

6. Loring M. Danforth, "The Role of Dance in the Ritual Therapy of An-
astenaira," *Byzantine and Modern Greek Studies* 5 (1979): 144–48.

7. Lucinda McCray Beier, *Sufferers and Healers: The Experience of Illness in Seventeenth-Century England* (London: Routledge & Kegan Paul, 1987), p. 31.

8. Pliny, *Natural History,* quoted in Howard Clark Kee, *Medicine, Miracle and Magic in New Testament Times* (Cambridge: Cambridge Univesity Press, 1986), p. 21.

9. John F. Avedon, *In Exile from the Land of Snows* (New York: Vintage Books, 1986), p. 138.

10. Dr. Donald Baker, quoted in John F. Avedon, *In Exile from the Land of Snows* (New York: Alfred A. Knopf, 1984), pp. 137.

11. Yeshi Dhonden, "Sleep and the Inner Landscape," *Parabola* 7 (1982): 1, pp. 24–38.

12. Ibid., p. 45.

13. William K. Stevens, "Shamans and Scientists Seek Cures in Plants," *The New York Times,* January 28, 1992, p. B5.

14. Dr. William Bennett, *The Medical Tribune,* October 13, 1988, p. 16, quoted in Andrew Weil, "A New Look at Botanical Medicine," *Whole Earth Review* 64, Fall 1989, pp. 55–56.

15. Weil, op. cit., pp. 54–61.

16. Stevens, op. cit.

17. Sharon Begley and Elizabeth Ann Leonard, "Take Two Roots; Call Me: How Wild Animals Use Nature's Medicine Chest," *Newsweek,* February 3, 1992, pp. 53–54.

18. U.S. Office of Technology Assessment, *Unconventional Cancer Treatments* (Washington, D.C.: U.S. Government Printing Office, 1990), p. 80.

19. "Study Says Unproven Cancer Treatment No Worse Than Standard Care," *Boulder Daily Camera,* April 25, 1991, p. 9A.

20. Natalie Angier, "Where the Unorthodox Gets a Hearing at N.I.H., *The New York Times,* March 16, 1993, p. 85.

21. Barry Bryant, *Cancer and Consciousness* (Boston: Sigo Press, 1990), pp. 165–176.

22. Molly O'Neill, "Eating to Heal: The New Frontiers," *The New York Times,* February 7, 1990, p. B1.

23. Peter Barry Chowka, personal communication, May 5, 1989.

24. Richard Grossman, *The Other Medicines: An Invitation to Understanding and Using Them for Health and Healing* (New York: Doubleday, 1985), pp. 124–25.

CHAPTER 11—THE HELPER: THE WAY OF THE WOUNDED HEALER

1. Joseph Campbell, *The Hero with a Thousand Faces,* Bollingen Series, no. 17 (Princeton: Princeton University Press, 1973), p. 72.

2. Joseph Campbell, op. cit., pp. 70–73.

3. Brooke Medicine Eagle, quoted in *Healers on Healing,* ed. Richard Carlson and Benjamin Shield (Los Angeles: Jeremy P. Tarcher, 1989), p. 61.

4. Dr. Richard Moss, *The Black Butterfly: An Invitation to Radical Aliveness* (Berkeley: Celestial Arts, 1986), p. 54.

5. Ibid., p. 57.

6. Carlson and Shield, op. cit., p. 94.

7. Oliver Sacks, *A Leg to Stand On* (New York: Summit Books, 1984), pp. 142–143.

8. Dr. Bernie Siegel, quoted in Carlson and Shield, op. cit., p. 6.

9. Ibid., p. 140.

10. Washington Matthews, quoted in *Navaho Legends*, Memoirs of the American Folklore Society, vol. 5 (New York: American Folklore Society, 1897), p. 109.

11. Carlson and Shield, op. cit., p. 121.

12. Ibid., p. 71.

13. Frederick G. Levine, "What Is the Truth about Psychic Healing?" *Natural Health*, Jan/Feb 1993, pp. 64+.

14. Jeanne Achterberg, "The Shaman: Master Healer in the Imaginary Realm," in *Shamanism*, comp. Shirley Nicholson (Wheaton, Ill.: Theosophical Publishing House, 1987), p. 105.

15. Barry Bryant, *Cancer and Consciousness* (Boston: Sigo Press, 1990), p. 202.

16. Paraphrased in David Landy, ed., *Culture, Disease, and Healing: Studies in Medical Anthropology* (New York: Macmillian, 1977).

17. Ivan Illich, *Medical Nemesis: The Expropriation of Health* (New York: Pantheon Books, 1976), p. 115.

CHAPTER 12—VISION QUEST: DISCOVERING THE HEALER WITHIN

1. A. Guggenbuhl-Craig, *Power in the Helping Professions,* quoted in Selma Hyman, "Death-in-Life, Life-in-Death," *Spring* (1977): p. 29.

2. C. E. McMahon, "The Role of Imagination in the Disease Process: Pre-Cartesian History," *Psychological Medicine* 6 (1976): 179–84.

3. Jeanne Achterberg, *Imagery in Healing: Shamanism and Modern Medicine* (Boston: Shambhala Publications, 1985), p. 127.

4. Ibid.

5. Ibid., p. 101.

6. C. W. Smith et al., "Imagery and Neutrophil Function Studies: A Preliminary Report," discussed in Achterberg, op. cit., pp. 198–201.

7. Ainslee Meares, "Vivid Visualization and Dim Visual Awareness in the Regression of Cancer in Meditation," *Journal of the American Society of Psychosomatic Dentistry and Medicine* 25 (1978): 3, p. 85.

8. Alice Hopper Epstein, *Mind, Fantasy and Healing: One Woman's Journey from Conflict and Illness to Wholeness and Health* (New York: Delacorte, 1989), p. xxi.

9. Ibid., p. xxiii: "In one study of 141 patients with metastasized kidney cancer, including thirty-three whose affected kidney had been removed, there was none who survived beyond three years."

10. C. G. Jung, *Memories, Dreams, Reflections* (New York: Vintage Books, 1965), p. 183.

11. Harner, Michael, *The Way of the Shaman: A Guide to Power and Healing* (San Francisco: Harper & Row, 1980), p. 99.

12. C. G. Jung, *Dreams,* trans. R F. C. Hull, Bollingen Series, no. 20 (Princeton: Princeton University Press, 1974), p. 98.

13. Ibid., p. 76.

14. Charles Dickens, *The Annotated Christmas Carol: A Christmas Carol,* introduction and notes by Michael Patrick Hearn (New York: Clarkson N. Potter, 1976), p. 87.

15. Dr. Leonard Wisneski "From Biochemistry to Bioenergetics," lecture delivered at American Holistic Medical Association Conference, Breckenridge, Colorado, Spring 1991.

16. P. M. West, "Discussion—comparative case studies," quoted in Augustin M. De la Pena, *The Psychobiology of Cancer: Automatization and Boredom in Health and Disease* (New York: Praeger Press, 1983), p. 74.

CHAPTER 13—INNER WORK: THE RECOVERY OF FEELING

1. James M. Robinson, ed., *The Nag Hammadi Library* (New York: Harper & Row, 1981), p. 118.

2. Alice Miller, *The Drama of the Gifted Child: The Search for the True Self* (New York: Basic Books, 1981), pp. 12–13.

3. Abraham Maslow, *Towards a Psychology of Being,* 2nd ed. (New York: D. Van Nostrand, 1968), p. vii.

4. Dr. Raymond Price, "Shamans and Endorphins: Exogenous and Endogenous Factors in Psychotherapy," (1980) quoted in Rob Schultheiss, *Bone Games* (New York: Random House, 1984), p. 108.

5. Robert Schultheiss, *Bone Games: One Man's Search for the Ultimate Athletic High* (New York: Random House, 1984), pp. 11–12.

6. Marie-Louise von Franz, *On Dreams and Death,* trans. Emmanuel Xipolitas Kennedy and Vernon Brooks (Boston: Shambhala Publications, 1984), p. 150.

7. C. G. Jung, *Mysterium Coniunctionis,* trans. R. F. C. Hull, Bollingen Series 20, Vol. 14 (Princeton: Princeton University Press, 1977), pp. 334–343.

8. Ainslee Meares, "The Quality of Meditation Effective in the Regression of Cancer," *Journal of the American Society of Psychosomatic Dentistry and Medicine* 25 (1978): 4, p. 131.

9. Ian Wickramesekera, "A Conditioned Response Model of the Placebo Effect: Predictions from the Model," quoted in Ernest Lawrence Rossi, *The Psychobiology of Mind-Body Healing: New Concepts of Therapeutic Hypnosis* (New York: W. W. Norton, 1986), p. 31.

10. Garrett Porter and Patricia Norris, *Why me? Harnessing the Healing Power of the Human Spirit* (Walpole, N.H.: Stillpoint Publishing, 1985), p. 159.

11. Ibid.

12. Richard Carlson and Benjamin Shield, eds., *Healers on Healing* (Los Angeles: Jeremy P. Tarcher, 1989), pp. 160–161.

13. C. A. Meier, *Ancient Incubation and Modern Psychotherapy,* trans. Monica Curtis (Evanston, Ill.: Northwestern University Press, 1967), p. 109.

14. Joseph Campbell, *The Hero with a Thousand Faces,* Bollingen Series 17 (Princeton: Princeton University Press, 1973), p. 17.

15. Charles Dickens, *The Annotated Christmas Carol: A Christmas Carol,* intro-

duction and notes by Michael Patrick Hearn (New York: Clarkson N. Potter, 1976), p. 85.

16. Campbell, op. cit., p. 17.

17. Michael Murphy, *The Future of the Body* (Los Angeles: Jeremy P. Tarcher, 1992), pp. 320–21.

18. Ibid., p. 243.

19. Ibid., pp. 242, 244.

20. In Stephen Mitchell, ed. and trans., *The Selected Poetry of Rainer Maria Rilke* (New York: Vintage Books, 1984), p. 259.

21. Meredith Sabini and Valerie Hone Maffly, "An Inner View of Illness: The Dreams of Two Cancer Patients," *Journal of Analytical Psychology* 26 (1981): p. 123.

22. Dickens, op. cit., p. 93.

23. James W. Pennebaker et al., "Disclosure of Traumas and Immune Function: Health Implications for Psychotherapy," *Journal of Consulting Clinical Psychology* 56 (1988): pp. 239–45.

24. Baum, L. Frank, *The Wizard of Oz* (New York: Ballantine Books, 1966), pp. 133–134.

25. Caryle Hirshberg, "Spontaneous Remission: The Spectrum of Self-Repair," introduction to *Spontaneous Remission: An Annotated Bibliography* by Caryle Hirshberg and Brendan O'Regan (Sausalito: Institute of Noetic Sciences, 1993), pp. 19, 22.

26. Richard Katz, *Boiling Energy: Community Healing Among the Kalahari Kung* (Cambridge: Harvard University Press, 1982), pp. 96–97.

27. Ibid., p. 97.

28. D. Patrick Miller, "My Healing Journey Through Chronic Fatigue," *Yoga Journal*, November–December 1992, p. 61.

29. Chogyam Trungpa, *Shambhala: The Sacred Path of the Warrior* (Boulder: Shambhala Publications, 1984), p. 47.

CHAPTER 14—COMING ALIVE: EXPLORING THE HEALING SELVES

1. Joseph Campbell, *The Hero with a Thousand Faces,* Bollingen Series 17 (Princeton: Princeton University Press, 1973), p. 337.

2. Ivan Illich, *Medical Nemesis* (New York: Pantheon Books, 1976), p. 130.

3. Meredith Sabini and Valerie Hone Maffly, "An Inner View of Illness: The Dreams of Two Cancer Patients," *Journal of Analytical Psychology* 26 (April 1981): pp. 126–27.

4. Jeanne Achterberg, Stephanie Matthews, Carl Simonton, "Psychology of the Exceptional Cancer Patient: A Description of Patients Who Outlive Predicted Life Expectancies" (Sausalito: Institute of Noetic Sciences, 1976), pp. 2–3.

5. C. G. Jung, in Marie-Louise von Franz, *On Dreams and Death*, trans. Emmanuel Xipolitas Kennedy and Vernon Brooks (Boston: Shambhala Publications, 1984), p. 44.

6. Albert Kreinheder, *Body and Soul: The Other Side of Illness* (Toronto: Inner City Books, 1991), p. 63.

7. Richard Moss, *The Black Butterfly: An Invitation to Radical Aliveness* (Berkeley: Celestial Arts, 1986), p. 59.

8. Oliver Sacks, *A Leg to Stand On* (New York: Summit Books, 1984), pp. 118–19.

9. Ibid., p. 130.

10. Joan Halifax, quoted in *Healers on Healing*, ed. Richard Carlson and Benjamin Shield (Los Angeles: Jeremy P. Tarcher, 1989), p. 169.

11. John P. Conger, quoted in Carlson and Shield, op. cit., p. 85.

12. C. A. Meier, *Ancient Incubation and Modern Psychotherapy*, trans. by Monica Curtis (Evanston, Ill: Northwestern University Press, 1967), p. 83.

13. Kreinheder, op. cit., pp. 42–44.

14. Kenneth Ring, *The Omega Project: Near-Death Experiences, UFO Encounters, and Mind at Large* (New York: William Morrow, 1992), pp. 145–146.

15. Michael Talbot, *The Holographic Universe* (New York: HarperCollins, 1991), p. 100.

16. Ibid.

17. Alice Hopper Epstein, *Mind, Fantasy and Healing: One Woman's Journey from Conflict and Illness to Wholeness and Health* (New York: Delacorte, 1989), p. 136.

18. C. G. Jung, *Analytical Psychology: Its Theory and Practice* (New York: Vintage Books, 1968), p. 80.

19. Johannes Nicolas Schilder, M.D., "Idiopathic Regression of Cancer," lecture at the First International Conference on Healing Beyond Suffering or Death, Montreal, Canada, June, 1993.

20. Richard Katz, *Boiling Energy: Community Healing Among the Kalihari Kung* (Cambridge: Harvard University Press, 1982), pp. 235, 236.

21. Michael Murphy, *The Future of the Body* (Los Angeles: Jeremy P. Tarcher, 1992), p. 245.

22. Ring, op. cit., p. 143.

23. Quoted in Ernest Lawrence Rossi, *The Psychobiology of Mind-Body Healing: New Concepts of Therapeutic Hypnosis* (New York: W. W. Norton, 1986), p. 41.

24. Ibid.

25. Rossi, op. cit., p. 22.

26. Ibid., p. 67.

CHAPTER 15—THE SOCIAL FABRIC AND THE LOOM OF THE SELF

1. Richard Katz, *Boiling Energy: Community Healing Among the Kalihari Kung* (Cambridge: Harvard University Press, 1982), p. 52.

2. Nancy Scheper-Hughes and Margaret M. Lock, "The Mindful Body," *Medical Anthropology Quarterly* (1987):1, p. 31.

3. Oliver Sacks, *A Leg to Stand On* (New York: Summit Books, 1984), p. 163.

4. Job 13:12–13.

5. Yujiro Ikemi et al., "Psychosomatic Consideration on Cancer Patients Who

Have Made a Narrow Escape from Death," *Dynamic Psychiatry* 8 (1975), pp. 84–86.

6. Charles Weinstock, M.D., "Notes on 'Spontaneous' Regression of Cancer," *Journal of the American Society of Psychosomatic Dentistry and Medicine* 24 (1977): 4, p. 107.

7. Alice Miller, *For Your Own Good: Hidden Cruelty in Child-Rearing and the Roots of Violence,* trans. by Hildegarde and Hunter Hannu (New York: Farrar, Straus & Giroux, 1983), pp. 248–49.

8. Richard Katz, *Boiling Energy: Community Healing Among the Kalahari Kung* (Cambridge: Harvard University Press, 1982), pp. 52–53.

9. Deena Metzger, "Cancer Is the Answer: Illness as Cure," *The Sun* 110: 15.

10. Personal communication, June 1989.

11. Evy McDonald, "A Healing in the Theatre of Life," *Canadian Holistic Healing Association Newsletter* 7 (Winter 1986–87): 4.

12. Evy McDonald, closing address, International Congress on Therapeutic and Psychological Aspects of Amyotrophic Lateral Sclerosis, Varese, Italy, March 27–31, 1985.

13. Sacks, op. cit., pp. 161–62.

14. Meredith B. McGuire, *Ritual Healing in Suburban America* (New Brunswick: Rutgers University Press, 1988), p. 6.

15. Dr. Ruth Hubbard, quoted in Nat Hentoff, "Creating a Master Race," *Village Voice,* June 4, 1991, p. 19.

16. "Poverty Blamed for Blacks' Higher Cancer Rates," *The New York Times,* April 16, 1991, p. A16.

17. Chellis Glendinning, *When Technology Wounds: The Human Consequences of Progress* (New York: William Morris, 1990), pp. 18–20.

18. Dan Fagin, "Growing Evidence Links Breast Cancer, Pesticides," *Boulder Daily Camera,* September 9, 1993, p. c3.

19. Nancy Scheper-Hughes and Margaret M. Lock, "The Mindful Body: A Prolegomenon to Future Work in Medical Anthropology," *Medical Anthropology Quarterly* 1 (1987): 1, p. 9.

20. Metzger, op. cit., p. 17.

CHAPTER 16—THE RETURN: TREASURES FROM THE DARK

1. Oliver Sacks, *A Leg to Stand On* (New York: Summit Books, 1984), p. 160.

2. Joseph Campbell, *The Hero with a Thousand Faces,* Bollingen Series 17 (Princeton: Princeton University Press, 1973), p. 233.

3. Marie-Louise von Franz, *On Dreams and Death,* trans. Emmanuel Xipolitas Kennedy and Vernon Books (Boston: Shambhala Press, 1984), p. xiii.

4. Steven Levine, *Healing into Life and Death* (New York: Anchor Books/Doubleday, 1987), pp. 126–27.

5. I am grateful to Glenda Hawley for introducing me to this highly unusual case. I have drawn in part from her unpublished dissertation "The Role of Holistic Variables in the Attribution of Cancer Survival" (San Francisco: Saybrook Institute, 1989) in preparing this account.

6. Yujiro Ikemi and Akira Ikemi, "An Oriental Point of View in Psychosomatic Medicine," *Psychotherapy and Psychosomatics* 45 (1986): pp. 118–26.

7. Sacks, op. cit., pp. 110–11.

8. Ibid.

9. Ibid., pp. 113–14.

10. Niro Asistent sent me photocopies of her two blood tests. A fuller account can be found in her book, *Why I Survive AIDS* (New York: Simon & Schuster, 1991). For further discussion and four studies, see Farzadegan, H., et al. "Loss of Human Immunodeficiency Virus Type I (HIV-1) Antibodies with Evidence of Viral Infection in Asymptomatic Homosexual Men," *Annals of Internal Medicine* 108 (6): June 1988; pp. 785–790.

11. Alice Epstein, *Mind, Fantasy and Healing* (New York: Delacorte, 1926), p. 171.

12. Arnold Mindell, *Working with the Dreaming Body* (New York: Routledge & Kegan Paul, 1987), p. 81.

13. Mircea Eliade, *Rites and Symbols of Initiation* (New York: Harper & Row, 1975), p. 27.

14. Marilyn Ferguson, *The Aquarian Conspiracy* (Los Angeles: Jeremy P. Tarcher, 1980), p. 165.

EPILOGUE: A SECOND BIRTH

1. André Breton, *Earthlight* (Los Angeles: Sun and Moon Press, 1993), pp. 65–66.

2. Adapted from a translation by Roger Sherman Loomis, *The Grail: From Celtic Myth to Christian Symbol* (New York: Columbia University Press, 1963), pp. 30–45.

BIBLIOGRAPHY

BOOKS

Achterberg, Jeanne. *Imagery in Healing: Shamanism and Modern Medicine.* Boston: Shambhala Publications, 1985.

———. *Woman as Healer: A Panoramic Survey of the Healing Activities of Women from Prehistoric Times to the Present.* Boston: Shambhala Publications, 1990.

Achterberg, J., and G. F. Lawlis. *Imagery and Disease: A Diagnostic Tool.* Champaign, Ill.: Institute for Personality and Ability Testing, 1985.

———. *Bridges of the Bodymind.* Champaign, Ill.: Institute of Personality and Ability Testing, 1980.

Adams, F., trans. *Hippocrates: The Genuine Works of Hippocrates.* 2 vols. Baltimore: Williams & Wilkins, 1939.

Aristotle. *De Anima (On the Soul).* Translated by Hugh Lawson-Tancred. Harmondsworth: Penguin Books, 1986.

Asimov, Isaac. "Doctor, Doctor, Cut My Throat." In *The Tragedy of the Moon.* Doubleday, 1979.

Avedon, John F. *In Exile from the Land of Snows: The First Full Account of the Dalai Lama and the Tibetans since the Chinese Conquest.* New York: Alfred A. Knopf, 1984.

Baum, L. Frank. *The Annotated Wizard of Oz.* Introduction and notes by Michael Patrick Hearn. New York: Clarkson N. Potter, 1973.

Baum, L. Frank. *The Wizard of Oz.* New York: Bobbs-Merrill, 1903. Reprint. New York: Ballantine Books, 1956.

Beier, Lucinda McCray. *Sufferers and Healers: The Experience of Illness in Seventeenth-Century England.* London: Routledge & Kegan Paul, 1987.

Berman, Louis. *The Glands Regulating Personality: A Study of the Glands of Internal Secretion in Relation to the Types of Human Nature.* College Park, Md: McGrath Publishing Company, 1970.

Bettelheim, Bruno. *Symbolic Wounds.* Glencoe, Ill.: Free Press, 1955.

Birnbaum, Raoul. *The Healing Buddha.* Foreword by John Blofeld. Boston: Shambhala Publications, 1989.

Blacking, John, ed. *The Anthropology of the Body.* New York: Academic Press, 1977.

Bly, Robert. Translation and commentary, *Selected Poems of Rainer Maria Rilke.* New York: Harper & Row, 1981.

Borysenko, Joan. *Minding the Body, Mending the Mind.* New York: Bantam Books, 1987.

Boyd, Peggy. *The Silent Wound: On Psychology and Breast Cancer.* New York: Addison-Wesley, 1984.

Bradshaw, John. *Healing the Shame That Binds You.* Deerfield Beach, Fl.: Health Communications, 1988.

Bryant, Barry. *Cancer and Consciousness.* Boston: Sigo Press, 1990.

Cairns, John. *Cancer: Science and Society.* San Francisco: W. H. Freeman, 1978.

Campbell, Joseph. *The Hero with a Thousand Faces.* Bollingen Series, no. 17. Princeton: Princeton University Press, 1973.

Carlson, Richard, and Benjamin Shield, eds. *Healers on Healing.* Los Angeles: Jeremy P. Tarcher, 1989.

Chopra, Dr. Deepak. *Quantum Healing: Exploring the Frontiers of Mind/Body Medicine.* New York: Bantam Books, 1989.

Clifford, Terry. *Tibetan Buddhist Medicine and Psychiatry: The Diamond Healing.* York Beach, Me.: Samuel Weiser, 1984.

Connelly, Dianne M. *Traditional Acupuncture: The Law of the Five Elements.* Columbia, Md.: The Centre for Traditional Acupuncture, 1979.

Cousins, Norman. *Head First: The Biology of Hope.* New York: E. P. Dutton, 1989.

Crile, George, Jr. *Practical Aspects of Thyroid Disease.* Philadelphia: Saunders, 1949.

Damon, S. Foster. Introduction and commentary, *Blake's Job: William Blake's Illustrations of the Book of Job.* New York: E. P. Dutton, 1969.

De la Pena, Augustin M. *The Psychobiology of Cancer: Automatization and Boredom in Health and Disease.* New York: Praeger Press, 1983.

Dhonden, Dr. Yeshi. *Health Through Balance: An Introduction to Tibetan Medicine.* New York: Snow Lion Publications, 1986.

Dickens, Charles. *The Annotated Christmas Carol: A Christmas Carol.* Introduction and notes by Michael Patrick Hearn. New York: Clarkson N. Potter, 1976.

Doore, Gary, ed. and comp. *Shaman's Path: Healing, Personal Growth and Empowerment.* Boston: Shambhala Publications, 1988.

Dossey, Dr. Larry. *Space, Time, and Medicine.* Boulder: Shambhala Publications, 1982.

———. *Meaning and Medicine: A Doctor's Tales of Breakthrough and Healing.* New York: Bantam Books, 1991.

———. *Recovering the Soul: A Scientific and Spiritual Search.* New York: Bantam Books, 1989.

Dourley, John P. *The Illness That We Are: A Jungian Critique of Christianity.* Toronto: Inner City Books, 1984.

Eliade, Mircea. *Rites and Symbols of Initiation: The Mysteries of Birth and Rebirth.* Trans. Willard R. Trask. 1958. Reprint. New York: Harper & Row, 1965.

Epstein, Alice Hopper. *Mind, Fantasy and Healing: One Woman's Journey from Conflict and Illness to Wholeness and Health.* New York: Delacorte, 1989.

Evans, Elida. *A Psychological Study of Cancer.* New York: Dodd, Mead, 1926.

Everson, Tilden C. and Warren H. Cole. *Spontaneous Regression of Cancer.* Philadelphia: W. B. Saunders Company, 1966.

Feher, Michel and Ramona Naddaff and Nadia Tazi, eds. *Fragments for a History of the Human Body.* 3 vols. New York: Zone, 1989.

Ferguson, Marilyn. *The Aquarian Conspiracy: Personal and Social Transformation in the 1980s.* Los Angeles: Jeremy P. Tarcher, 1980.

Foss, Laurence, and Kenneth Rothenberg. *The Second Medical Revolution: From Biomedicine to Infomedicine.* Boston: Shambhala Publications, 1987.

Foucault, Michel. *The Birth of the Clinic: An Archaeology of Medical Perception.* New York: Vintage Books, 1975.

———. *Madness and Civilization: A History of Insanity in the Age of Reason.* New York: Vintage Books, 1973.

Frank, Arthur W. *At the Will of the Body: Reflections on Illness.* New York: Houghton Mifflin, 1991.

von Franz, Marie-Louise. *On Dreams and Death.* Trans. Emmanuel Xipolitas Kennedy and Vernon Brooks. Boston: Shambhala Publications, 1984.

Freud, Sigmund. *The Interpretation of Dreams.* London: Hogarth Press, 1953. Reprint. New York: Avon Books, 1965.

Garland, Joseph E. *Every Man Our Neighbor: A Brief History of the Massachusetts General Hospital, 1811–1961.* Boston: Little, Brown, 1961.

Gerson, Max. *A Cancer Therapy: Results of Fifty Cases and the Cure of Advanced Cancer by Diet Therapy.* Bonita, Calif.: The Gerson Institute, 1958. Reprint, 1990.

Goodman, F. D., J. H. Henney, and E. Pressel. *Trance, Healing and Hallucination: Three Field Studies in Religious Experience.* Malabar, Fla.: Krieger, 1982.

Goodrick-Clarke, Nicholas, trans. *Paracelsus: Essential Readings.* Northampton-shire, U.K.: Aquarian Press, 1990.

Grossinger, Richard. *Planet Medicine: From Stone Age Shamanism to Post-Industrial Healing.* Berkeley: North Atlantic Books, 1987.

Grossman, Richard. *The Other Medicines: An Invitation to Understanding and Using Them for Health and Healing.* New York: Doubleday, 1985.

Halifax, Joan. *Shaman, the Wounded Healer.* New York: Crossroad, 1982.

———. *Shamanic Voices: A Survey of Visionary Narratives.* New York: E. P. Dutton, 1979.

Harner, Michael. *The Way of the Shaman: A Guide to Power and Healing.* San Francisco: Harper & Row, 1980.

Hillman, James. *Healing Fiction.* Barrytown, N.Y.: Station Hill Press, 1983.

———. *Re-Visioning Psychology.* New York: Harper & Row, 1975.

Hirshberg, Caryle and Brendan O'Regan. *Spontaneous Remission: An Annotated Bibliography.* Sausalito: Institute of Noetic Sciences, 1993.

Illich, Ivan. *Medical Nemesis: The Expropriation of Health.* New York: Pantheon, 1976.

James, William. *The Varieties of Religious Experience.* New York: First Vintage Books, 1990. Reprint. New York: Mentor, 1958.

Jung, C. G. *Analytical Psychology: Its Theory and Practice.* New York: Vintage Books, 1968.

———. *Dreams.* Trans. R. F. C. Hull. Bollingen Series, no., 20. Princeton: Princeton University Press, 1974.

———. *Man and His Symbols.* New York: Doubleday, 1983.

———. *Memories, Dreams, Reflections.* Ed. Aniela Jaffé, trans. R. F. C. Hull. New York: Vintage Books, 1965.

———. *Modern Man in Search of a Soul.* San Diego: Harcourt Brace Jovanovich, 1933. Reprint, 1955.

———. *On the Nature of the Psyche.* Trans. R. F. C. Hull. Bollingen Series, no. 20, vol. 8. Princeton: Princeton University Press, 1973.

——. *Psyche and Symbol: A Selection from the Writings of C. G. Jung.* Ed. Violet S. de Laszlo. New York: Doubleday, 1958.

Kalweit, Holger. *Dreamtime and Inner-Space: The World of the Shaman.* Boston: Shambhala Publications, 1988.

Kaptchuk, Ted J. *The Web That Has No Weaver: Understanding Chinese Medicine.* New York: Congdon & Weed, 1983.

Katz, Richard. *Boiling Energy: Community Healing Among the Kalahari Kung.* Cambridge: Harvard University Press, 1982.

Kee, Howard Clark. *Medicine, Miracle and Magic in New Testament Times.* Cambridge: Cambridge University Press, 1986.

Kreinheder, Albert. *Body and Soul: The Other Side of Illness.* Toronto: Inner City Books, 1991.

Krishna, Gopi. *Kundalini: The Evolutionary Energy in Man.* Commentary by James Hillman. Boston: Shambhala Publications, 1971.

Kübler-Ross, Elisabeth. *On Death and Dying.* New York: Macmillan, 1969.

Laing, R. D. *The Divided Self.* London: Tavistock Publications, 1959. Reprint. New York: Penguin Books, 1974.

——. *The Politics of Experience.* New York: Ballantine Books, 1967.

Landy, David, ed. *Culture, Disease and Healing: Studies in Medical Anthropology.* New York: Macmillian, 1977.

LeShan, Lawrence. *You Can Fight for Your Life: Emotional Factors in the Treatment of Cancer.* New York: M. Evans, 1977.

Levine, Stephen. *Healing into Life and Death.* New York: Doubleday, 1987.

Locke, Steven, and Douglas Colligan. *The Healer Within: The New Medicine of Mind and Body.* New York: New American Library, 1986.

Locke, Steven E. *Psychological and Behavioral Treatments for Disorders Associated with the Immune System: An Annotated Bibliography.* New York: Institute for the Advancement of Health, 1986.

Loomis, Roger Sherman. *The Grail: From Celtic Myth to Christian Symbol.* New York: Columbia University Press, 1963.

Majno, G. *The Healing Hand: Man and Wound in the Ancient World.* Cambridge: Harvard University Press, 1975.

Maslow, Abraham. *Towards a Psychology of Being.* 2nd ed. New York: D. Van Nostrand, 1968.

McGuire, Meredith B. *Ritual Healing in Suburban America.* New Brunswick, N.J.: Rutgers University Press, 1988.

Meier, C. A. *Ancient Incubation and Modern Psychotherapy.* Trans. by Monica Curtis. Evanston, Ill.: Northwestern University Press, 1967.

Miller, Alice. *The Drama of the Gifted Child: The Search for the True Self.* New York: Basic Books, 1981. (Originally published as *Prisoners of Childhood.*)

——. *Thou Shalt Not Be Aware: Soceity's Betrayal of the Child.* New York: Meridian Books, 1986.

——. *For Your Own Good: Hidden Cruelty in Child-Rearing and the Roots of Violence.* Trans. Hildegarde and Hunter Hannum. New York: Farrar, Straus & Giroux, 1989.

Mindell, Arnold. *Working with the Dreaming Body.* New York: Routledge & Kegan Paul, 1987.

———. *Dreambody: The Body's Role in Revealing the Self.* Ed. Sisa Steinback-Scott and Becky Goodman. Boston: Sigo Press, 1982.

Mitchell, Stephen, ed. and trans. *The Selected Poetry of Rainer Maria Rilke.* New York: Vintage Books, 1984.

Moss, Richard. *The Black Butterfly: An Invitation to Radical Aliveness.* Berkeley: Celestial Arts, 1986.

Murphy, Michael. *The Future of the Body.* Los Angeles: Jeremy P. Tarcher, 1992.

Nicholson, Shirley, comp. *Shamanism.* Wheaton, Ill.: Theosophical Publishing House, 1987.

Ornstein, Robert, and David Sobel. *The Healing Brain: Breakthrough Medical Discoveries About How the Brain Keeps Us Healthy.* New York: Simon & Schuster, 1987.

Osumi, Ikuko, and Malcolm Ritchie. *The Shamanic Healer: The Healing World of Ikuko Osumi and the Traditional Art of Seiki-Jutsu.* Rochester, Vt.: Healing Arts Press, 1988.

Payer, Lynn. *Medicine and Culture: Varieties of Treatment in the United States, England, West Germany, and France.* New York: Henry Holt, 1988.

Pelgrin, J. *And a Time to Die.* Ed. S. Moon and E. B. Howes. Wheaton, Ill.: Theosophical Publishing House, 1962.

Perry, John Weir. *The Far Side of Madness.* Englewood Cliffs: Prentice-Hall, Inc., 1974.

Ponce, Charles. *Working the Soul: Reflections on Jungian Psychology.* Berkeley: North Atlantic Books, 1988.

Ribi, Alfred. *Demons of the Inner World: Understanding Our Hidden Complexes.* Boston: Shambhala Publications, 1990.

Ricoeur, Paul. *The Symbolism of Evil.* Trans. Emerson Buchanan. Boston: Beacon Press, 1967.

Ring, Kenneth. *The Omega Project: Near-Death Experiences, UFO Encounters, and Mind at Large.* New York: William Morrow, 1992.

Rossi, Ernest Lawrence. *The Psychobiology of Mind-Body Healing: New Concepts of Therapeutic Hypnosis.* New York: W. W. Norton, 1986.

———. *Dreams and the Growth of Personality: Expanding Awareness in Psychotherapy.* New York: Pergamon Press, 1972. Reprint. New York: Brunner/Mazel, 1985.

Rossi, Ernest L., and David B. Cheek. *Mind-Body Therapy: Methods of Ideodynamic Healing in Hypnosis.* New York: W. W. Norton, 1988.

Roud, Dr. Paul C. *Making Miracles: An Exploration into the Dynamics of Self-Healing.* New York: Warner Books, 1990.

Sacks, Oliver W. *A Leg to Stand On.* New York: Summit Books, 1984.

———. *Awakenings.* Garden City, N.Y.: Doubleday, 1974.

Saint John of the Cross. *Dark Night of the Soul.* Trans. New York: Doubleday, 1959.

Sanford, John A. *Healing and Wholeness.* New York: Paulist Press, 1977.

Siegel, Bernie S. *Peace, Love and Healing: Bodymind Communication and the Path to Self-Healing: An Exploration.* New York: Harper & Row, 1989.

———. *Love, Medicine, and Miracles: Lessons Learned About Self-Healing from a Surgeon's Experience with Exceptional Patients.* New York: Harper & Row, 1986.

Simonton, O. Carl, Stephanie Matthews-Simonton, and James L. Creighton. *Getting Well Again.* New York: Bantam Books, 1978.

Sontag, Susan. *Illness as Metaphor.* New York: Vintage Books, 1978.

———. *AIDS and Its Metaphors.* New York: Farrar, Straus & Giroux, 1989.

Sylvester, Edward J. *Target Cancer.* New York: Charles Scribner's Sons, 1968.

Talbot, Michael. *The Holographic Universe.* New York: HarperCollins, 1991.

The Holy Bible. New York: Meridian Books, The World Publishing Company, 1964.

Thornton, Edward. *Diary of a Mystic.* London: George Allen & Unwin, 1967.

Trungpa, Chogyam. *Shambhala: The Sacred Path of the Warrior.* Boulder: Shambhala Publications, 1984.

Turner, Victor. *The Ritual Process: Structure and Anti-Structure.* The Lewis Henry Morgan Lectures, 1966. Ithaca, N.Y.: Cornell University Press, 1969.

U.S. Office of Technology Assessment. *Unconventional Cancer Treatments.* Washington, D.C.: U.S. Government Printing Office, 1990.

Veith, Ilza, trans. *The Yellow Emperor's Classic of Internal Medicine.* Berkeley: University of California Press, 1972.

Vogl, Adalbert Albert. *Therese Neumann: Mystic and Stigmatist, 1898–1962.* Rockford, Ill.: Tan Books, 1987.

Weatherhead, L. D. *Psychology, Religion, and Healing.* New York: Abingdon-Cokesbury Press, 1951.

Whitman, Walt. *Leaves of Grass.* Ed. Harold W. Blodgett and Sculley Bradley. New York: W. W. Norton, 1968.

Zweig, Connie and Jeremiah Abrams, eds. *Meeting the Shadow: The Hidden Power of the Dark Side of Human Nature.* Los Angeles, Jeremy P. Tarcher, 1991.

JOURNAL ARTICLES

Achterberg, J. "A Canonical Analysis of Blood Chemistry Variables Related to Psychological Measures of Cancer Patients." *Multivariate Experimental Clinical Research* 4 (1979): 1–10.

Achterberg, J., O. C. Simonton, and S. Simonton. "Psychology of the Exceptional Cancer Patient: A Description of Patients Who Outlive Predicted Life Expectancies." *Psychotherapy: Theory, Research, and Practice* 14 (1977): 416–422.

Ackerknecht, E. "Psychopathology, Primitive-Medicine, and Primitive Culture." *Bulletin of the History of Medicine* 14 (1943): 30–67.

Adler, Rolf H. "Letters to the Editor." *New England Journal of Medicine* 313 (1985): 1358–1359.

Angell, Marcia. "Letters to the Editor." *New England Journal of Medicine* 313 (1985): 1359.

———. "Disease as a Reflection of the Psyche." *New England Journal of Medicine* 312 (June 1985): 1570–1572.

Bahnson, Claus B., and M. B. Bahnson. "Ego Defenses in Cancer Patients." *Annals of the New York Academy of Science* 164 (1969): 546.

———. "Role of Ego Defences: Denial and Repression in Etiology of Malignant Neoplasms." *Annals of the New York Academy of Science* 125 (1966): 3.

Bailar, John C. and Elaine M. Smith. "Progress Against Cancer." *New England Journal of Medicine* 314 (1986): 1225–1232.

Bastien, Joseph. "Quollahuaya-Andean Body Concepts." *American Anthropologist* 87 (1985): 595–611.

Bennett, Graham. "Psychic and Cellular Aspects of Isolation and Identity Impairment in Cancer: A Dialectic of Alienation." *Annals of the New York Academy of Science* 164 (1969): 352.

Booth, G. "General and Organic Specific Object Relationships in Cancer." *Annals of the New York Academy of Science* 164 (1969): 568.

Booth, Gotthard. "Psychobiological Aspects of Spontaneous Regressions of Cancer." *Journal of the American Academy of Psychoanalysis* 1 (1973): pp. 103 +.

———. "The Irrational Complications of the Cancer Problem." *American Journal of Psychoanalysis* 25 (1965): 1.

Braud, William. "Exploring the Interface Between Parapsychology and Psychoneuroimmunology." *Parapsychology Review* 17 (1986): 4.

Brown, G. M. "Psychiatric and Neurologic Aspects of Endocrine Disease." *Hospital Practice:* 10 (1975): 71–79.

Cairns, J. "The Treatment of Diseases and the War Against Cancer." *Scientific American,* May 1985, pp. 51–59.

Cassell, Eric. "Ideas in Conflict: The Rise and Fall [and Rise and Fall] of New Views of Disease." *Daedalus* 115 (1986): 19–42.

Cassileth, Barrie R. "Letters to the Editor." *New England Journal of Medicine* 313 (1956).

Cassileth, Barrie R., et al. "Psychosocial Correlates of Survival in Advanced Malignant Disease?" *New England Journal of Medicine* 312 (1985): 15.

Clower, C. G., A. J. Young, and D. Kepas. "Psychotic States Resulting from Disorders of Thyroid Function." *Johns Hopkins Medical Journal* 124 (1969): 305–10.

Crile, George, Jr. "Controversies in Thyroid Surgery." *New York State Journal of Medicine* 80 (1980): 12, pp. 1832–35.

———. "A Conservative Approach to Treatment of Thyroid Cancer." *Postgraduate Medicine* 57 (1975): 7, pp. 111–15.

Fordham, Michael. "Jungian Views of the Mind-Body Relationship." *Spring* (1974): 176.

Gibson, J. C. "Emotions and the Thyroid Gland: A Critical Reappraisal." *Journal of Psychosomatic Research* 6 (1962): pp. 93–116.

Goleman, Daniel. "Strong Emotional Response to Disease May Bolster Patient's Immune System." *New York Times,* October 22, 1985, p. 29.

———. "Matter of Mind: Interview with Soloman Snyder." *Psychology Today,* June 1980, pp. 66–76.

Hahn, Robert, and Arthur Kleinman. "Belief as Pathogen, Belief as Medicine." *Medical Anthropology Quarterly* 14 (1983): 16–19.

Hall, H. R. "Hypnosis and the Immune System: A Review with Implications for Cancer and the Psychology of Healing." *Journal of Clinical Hypnosis* 2 (1982): 92–103.

Ikemi, Yujiro, et al. "Psychosomatic Consideration on Cancer Patients Who Have Made a Narrow Escape from Death." *Dynamic Psychiatry* 8 (1975): 77–93.

Inglefinger, F. J. "Medicine: Meritorious or Meretricious?" *Science.* 200 May 26, 1978.

Kavetsky, R. E., N. M. Turkewich, and K. P. Balitsky. "On the Psychophysiological Mechanism of the Organism's Resistence to Tumor Growth." *Annals of the New York Academy of Sciences* 125 (1966): 933.

Kent, Jaylene, et al. "Unexpected Recoveries: Spontaneous Remission and Immune Functioning." *Advances* (journal of the Institute for the Advancement of Health) 6 (1990): pp. 66–73.

Kleinman, A. "Some Issues for a Comparative Study of Medical Healing." *International Journal of Social Psychiatry* 19 (1973): 159.

Klopfer, B. "Psychological Variables in Human Cancer." *Journal of Projective Techniques* 21 (1957): 331–340.

Kowal, S. J. "Emotions as a Cause of Cancer: Eighteenth and Nineteenth Century Contributions." *Psychoanalytical Review* 42 (1955): 217–227.

Laudenslager, M. L., et al. "Inescapable Shock Suppresses Lymphocyte Proliferation, but Escapable Shock Doesn't." *Science* 221 (1983): 568–570.

Le Shan, Dr. Lawrence. "An Emotional Life-History Pattern Associated with Neoplastic Disease." *Annals of the New York Academy of Science* 125 (1966): pp. 780–93.

———. "A Basic Psychological Orientation Apparently Associated with Malignant Disease." *The Psychiatric Quarterly* 35 (1961): 314.

Libow L. S., and J. Durell. "Clinical Studies on the Relationship Between Psychosis and the Regulation of Thyroid Gland Activity." *Psychosomatic Medicine* 27 (1965): pp. 377–82.

Lockhart, Russell. "Cancer in Myth and Dream." *Spring* (1977): pp. 1–26.

McDonald, Evy, "A Healing in the Theatre of Life," *Canadian Holistic Healing Association Newsletter,* 7:4, Winter 1986–87.

McMahon, C. E. "The Role of Imagination in the Disease Process: Pre-Cartesian History." *Psychological Medicine* 6 (1976): 179–184.

McWhinney, Ian R. "Medical Knowledge and the Rise of Technology." *Journal of Medicine and Philosophy* 3 (1978): pp. 293–304.

Meerloo, J. "The Initial Neurologic and Psychiatric Picture Syndrome of Pulmonary Growth." *Journal of the American Medical Association* 146 (1951): pp. 558–59.

———. "Psychological Implications of Malignant Growths." *British Journal of Medical Psychology* 27 (1954): 210.

Meier, C. A. "Psychosomatic Medicine from the Jungian Point of View." *Journal of Analytical Psychology* 8 (1963): 103.

Metzger, Deena. "Cancer Is the Answer: Illness as Cure." *The Sun,* no. 110: pp. 15–18.

O'Regan, Brendan. "Healing, Remission, and Miracle Cures." *Whole Earth Review,* Winter 1989, pp. 126–35.

Risenberg, Donald E. "Can Mind Affect Body Defenses Against Disease?" and "Nascent Speciality Offers Host of Tantalizing Clues." *Journal of the American Medical Association.* 256 (1986): 313–17.

Sabini, Meredith. "Imagery in Dreams of Illness." *Quadrant* 14 (1981): 85.

Sabini, M., and V. Hone Maffly. "An Inner View of Illness: Dreams of Two Cancer Patients." *Journal of Analytical Psychology* 26 (1981): 123.

Scheper-Hughes, Nancy, and Margaret Lock. "The Mindful Body: A Prolegomenon to Future Work in Medical Anthropology." *Medical Anthropology Quarterly* New Series 1(1987): 1, pp. 6–41.

Schleifer, S. J., et al. "Suppression of Lymphocyte Stimulation Following Bereavement." *Journal of the American Association* 250 (1983): 374–377.

Shapiro, Dr. Martin F. "Chemotherapy: Snake Oil Remedy?" *Los Angeles Times,* January 9, 1987, section II, p. 5.

Smith, C. K., et al. "Psychiatric Disturbance in Endocrinologic Disease." *Psychosomatic Medicine* 34 (1972): 69–86.

Stein, Robert M. "Body and Psyche: An Archetypal View of Psychosomatic Phenomena." *Spring* (1976): 66.

———. "Introducing Not-Self." *Journal of Analytical Psychology* 12 (1967): 2, pp. 97–113.

Thomas, Caroline Bedell. "Precursors of Premature Disease and Death: The Predictive Potential of Habits and Family Attitudes." *Annals of Internal Medicine* 85 (1976): pp. 653–58.

Wallace, A. F. C. "Dreams and Wishes of the Soul: A Type of Psychoanalytic Theory Among the Seventeenth Century Iroquois." *American Anthropologist* 60 (1958): 234–248.

Wanebo, Harold J., Wilson Andrews, and Donald L. Kaiser. "Thyroid Cancer: Some Basic Considerations." *Cancer Journal for Clinicians* 142 (1981): 474–479.

Weinstock, Charles. "Notes on 'Spontaneous' Regression of Cancer." *Journal of the American Society of Psychosomatic Dentistry and Medicine* 24 (1977) 4: p. 106.

———. "Recent Progress in Cancer Psychobiology and Psychiatry." *Journal of the American Society of Psychosomatic Dentistry and Medicine* 24 (1977): 1, pp. 4–14.

West, P. M., E. M. Blumberg, and F. W. Ellis. "An Observed Correlation Between Psychological Factors and Growth Rate of Cancer in Man." *Cancer Research* 12 (1955): 306–307.

INDEX

Hubbard, Ruth, 352
Huichol Indians, 152
Humility, Helpers and, 250
Hyman, Selma, 133
Hypnosis, 326
Hysterectomies, 182–83

emotional inventory in, 301
fantasy self in, 91
Helpers in, 65, 241
identity loss in, 64
life crisis in, 63
roots of predicament in, 65
turning point in, 368
wounded child in, 89

I

Ikemi, Yujiro, 73, 129, 341–42, 366
Illich, Ivan, 72, 126, 141, 171, 181, 206, 260, 310, 352
Illness as Metaphor (Sontag), 48, 86
Imagery in Healing: Shamanism and Modern Medicine (Achterberg), 192
Images. *See* Visualization
Immune system, role of, 83–84
Immunoglobulin A, 55
Indian sweat lodge, 31–32
Individuation, Helpers and, 250
In Exile from the Land of Snows (Avedon), 223
Inge-Heinze, Ruth, 102, 171, 250, 260
Inglefinger, Franz J., 163
Institute for Noetic Sciences, 51
Insurance companies, alternative medicine and, 237
Involution, 293
Involvement, Helpers and, 250
Isolation, 336
It's a Wonderful Life (Capra)
changes in social relations in, 330
confrontation with death in, 66

J

Jacobs, Joseph, 237
Jahenny, Marie-Julie, 123
James, William, 54
Janeway, Charles A., 168
Ji-on, 210–11, 265–67, 303
Job, 60–61, 62, 64, 65, 66, 284, 331, 334–35
Journal of the American Medical Association (JAMA), 150, 183
Journal of Women's Health, 182
Jung, Carl, 29–30
blushing and, 124
diagnosis and, 158
encounter with the psyche and, 64
guides and visualizations and, 281, 282–83
healing and, 313
horse symbol and, 156
physical reactions to emotions and, 324, 326
rediscovery of self and healing and, 60
sacrificum intellectus and, 108
symptoms and, 128
time perception and, 292
transformation and, 373

FOR THE BEST IN PAPERBACKS, LOOK FOR THE

In every corner of the world, on every subject under the sun, Penguin represents quality and variety—the very best in publishing today.

For complete information about books available from Penguin—including Pelicans, Puffins, Peregrines, and Penguin Classics—and how to order them, write to us at the appropriate address below. Please note that for copyright reasons the selection of books varies from country to country.

In the United Kingdom: For a complete list of books available from Penguin in the U.K., please write to *Dept E.P., Penguin Books Ltd, Harmondsworth, Middlesex, UB7 0DA.*

In the United States: For a complete list of books available from Penguin in the U.S., please write to *Consumer Sales, Penguin USA, P.O. Box 999— Dept. 17109, Bergenfield, New Jersey 07621-0120.* VISA and MasterCard holders call 1-800-253-6476 to order all Penguin titles.

In Canada: For a complete list of books available from Penguin in Canada, please write to *Penguin Books Canada Ltd, 10 Alcorn Avenue, Suite 300, Toronto, Ontario, Canada M4V 3B2.*

In Australia: For a complete list of books available from Penguin in Australia, please write to the *Marketing Department, Penguin Books Ltd, P.O. Box 257, Ringwood, Victoria 3134.*

In New Zealand: For a complete list of books available from Penguin in New Zealand, please write to the *Marketing Department, Penguin Books (NZ) Ltd, Private Bag, Takapuna, Auckland 9.*

In India: For a complete list of books available from Penguin, please write to *Penguin Overseas Ltd, 706 Eros Apartments, 56 Nehru Place, New Delhi, 110019.*

In Holland: For a complete list of books available from Penguin in Holland, please write to *Penguin Books Nederland B.V., Postbus 195, NL-1380AD Weesp, Netherlands.*

In Germany: For a complete list of books available from Penguin, please write to *Penguin Books Ltd, Friedrichstrasse 10-12, D-6000 Frankfurt Main 1, Federal Republic of Germany.*

In Spain: For a complete list of books available from Penguin in Spain, please write to *Longman, Penguin España, Calle San Nicolas 15, E-28013 Madrid, Spain.*

In Japan: For a complete list of books available from Penguin in Japan, please write to *Longman Penguin Japan Co Ltd, Yamaguchi Building, 2-12-9 Kanda Jimbocho, Chiyoda-Ku, Tokyo 101, Japan.*